SHOCK
Comprehensive nursing management

ANNE GRIFFIN PERRY, R.N., M.S.N.

Assistant Professor, St. Louis University School of Nursing,
St. Louis, Missouri

PATRICIA ANN POTTER, R.N., M.S.N.

Assistant Director of Nursing Service, Barnes Hospital,
St. Louis, Missouri; formerly Assistant Professor,
St. Louis University School of Nursing,
St. Louis, Missouri

LINDA NIEDRINGHAUS, R.N., M.S.N.

Instructor, St. Louis University School of Nursing,
St. Louis, Missouri

ANGELA SMITH-COLLINS, R.N., M.S.N.

Clinical Nurse Specialist, Critical Care, North Mississippi
Medical Center, Tupelo, Mississippi; formerly Instructor,
St. Louis University School of Nursing,
St. Louis, Missouri

JUDITH L. MYERS, R.N., M.S.N.

Assistant Professor, St. Louis University School of Nursing,
St. Louis, Missouri

SHOCK

Comprehensive nursing management

Editors

ANNE GRIFFIN PERRY, R.N., M.S.N.

PATRICIA ANN POTTER, R.N., M.S.N.

Co-authors

LINDA NIEDRINGHAUS, R.N., M.S.N.

ANGELA SMITH-COLLINS, R.N., M.S.N.

JUDITH L. MYERS, R.N., M.S.N.

Illustrated

The C. V. Mosby Company

x

ST. LOUIS • TORONTO • LONDON   1983

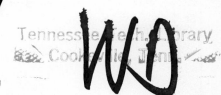

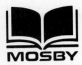

MOSBY

A TRADITION OF PUBLISHING EXCELLENCE

Editor: Pamela Swearingen
Assistant editor: Bess Arends
Editing supervisor: Lin Dempsey Hallgren
Manuscript editor: Diane Ackermann
Book design: Kay M. Kramer
Cover design: Diane Beasley
Production: Judy England, Sue Soehngen

The C.V. Mosby Company
11830 Westline Industrial Drive, St. Louis, Missouri 63141

Library of Congress Cataloging in Publication Data

Main entry under title:

Shock, comprehensive nursing management.

    Includes index.
    1. Shock. 2. Shock—Nursing. I. Perry,
Anne Griffin. II. Potter, Patricia Ann.
III. Niedringhaus, Linda. IV. Smith-Collins, Angela.
V. Myers, Judith L. [DNLM: 1. Shock—
Nursing. QZ 140 S676]
RB150.S5S485   617′.21   82-3424
ISBN 0-8016-3827-5   AACR2

GW/VH/VH 9 8 7 6 5 4 3 2 1   01/D/035

Introduction

The definition of shock has changed over the years concomitant with an improved understanding of its pathophysiology. Beland* described shock as a disproportion between the volume of blood and the capacity of the vascular chamber. The nature of shock is seen on the basis of this earlier conceptualization as a circulatory imbalance in which the ability to maintain blood flow is impaired by either a deficiency in blood volume or an expanded capacity of the vascular system. Conceptualizing shock as a circulatory imbalance gave clinicians a whole-organ perspective. This allowed for the recognition that multiple body systems become involved as a result of inadequate organ perfusion resulting from decreased venous return and cardiac output. However, the whole-organ concept did not direct therapy toward the real culprit. The pathophysiology of shock can now be dissected to a cellular level, giving physicians and nurses the information needed to initiate early preventive therapy.

Currently shock is defined as a deficiency of tissue perfusion associated with the inadequate delivery of oxygen and nutrients to the cells.† A cellular conceptualization of the alterations created by shock provides improved insight into the origin of clinical manifestations, the etiology of complications, and the rationale for comprehensive therapy. This insight has implications for the nurse.

Management of the patient in shock is of course no simple task. A comprehensive understanding of the pathological interrelationships that exist is a basic requirement for the clinician. The nurse must not be guided only by the physician's eyes. This is to say that he or she should not become complacent in relying on the focus of medical therapy as the only direction for assessment or intervention. It is the nurse who will spend the most time caring directly for the acutely ill shock patient. It is imperative that the nurse be prepared with a sound theoretical background to make the independent decisions necessary for management of critically ill individuals.

The purpose of this text is to provide the nurse with the most current information from medical and nursing research to explain the entity of shock. An emphasis on physiology as well as pathophysiology equips the nurse with the essential background of knowledge to make quick and insightful observations, decisions, and interventions. Likewise, the emphasis on pathophysiology aids in clarifying the rationale for various treat-

*Beland, I.: Clinical Nursing: pathophysiological and psychosocial approaches, New York, 1965, Macmillan Publishing Co., Inc.

†O'Donnell, T.F., Jr., and Belkin, S.C.: The pathophysiology, monitoring, and treatment of shock, Orthopedic Clinics of North America **9:**589, 1978; Groer, M.E., and Shekelton, M.: Basic pathophysiology: a conceptual approach, St. Louis, 1979, The C.V. Mosby Co.; Guyton, A.C.: Textbook of medical physiology, ed. 5, Philadelphia, 1976, W.B. Saunders Co.

ment modalities. Throughout the text the relationship of the function of one body system to that of another is stressed. Content representing the biological, physiological, and social sciences is integrated. A holistic approach is utilized to stress the need for the nurse to remain aware of how the patient is affected psychologically as well as physically by serious illness.

In planning the textbook's contextual format, it was decided an attempt would be made to provide readers with a simple referential approach to shock. Being able to conceptualize the nature of major pathological alterations on the basis of a knowledge of normal physiological mechanisms would enable the clinician to gain a fuller understanding of shock syndromes. For this reason the chapters on physiological mechanisms have been thoroughly developed.

The initial portion of the text introduces the reader to a physiologically centered conceptual framework. Four physiological concepts are developed: the heart, the blood vessels, the blood volume, and the lung. Syndromes of shock create pathological alterations that influence the homeostasis of each of these physiological entities. With an inadequacy in tissue perfusion there exist alterations in blood volume distribution. Changes occur in the regulatory status of the vessels themselves that alter vessel integrity and fluid balance. The heart, if able, must compensate as a result of the disturbance in venous return. Of the many organ systems involved, the lung is a crucial one, for there must be an adequate provision of oxygen to reverse the progression of shock. When the pathological nature of a specific shock syndrome directly affects the heart, vessels, blood volume, or lung, the ability of the whole organism to adapt to the insult is seriously impaired.

Chapters on the heart, cardiovascular control mechanisms, and microcirculation provide an in-depth understanding of normal circulatory regulation. The reader is able to recognize the adaptive responses that occur when circulatory equilibrium is threatened. The chapter on microcirculation explores the physiology of fluid balance and exchange. It provides a reference for understanding the mechanisms of cellular pathology described later in the chapter on the classification of shock. The oxygenation chapter explores in depth the requirements for adequate delivery of oxygen at the cellular level.

Each chapter on physiology provides readers with an exploration of anatomical structures as well as a detailed look at physiological function. Terminology familiar to the critical care nurse is carefully explained and applied to relevant physiological processes. The reader gains a comprehensive knowledge of the compensatory and interdependent mechanisms existing within the heart, blood vessels, and lung to maintain perfusion and oxygen delivery to cells. Understanding regulatory responses that maintain circulation and oxygenation will aid the nurse in the early recognition of signs of shock. In completing the physiological review, the reader will be prepared to understand all of the ramifications of the pathogenic process known as shock.

The reader is introduced to the varieties and nature of shock in the next section. The introduction to the classification system for shock reveals to the reader that shock is not a single disease entity but rather a complex syndrome. The clinical status of a given patient can change dramatically during the course of shock. The different causes of shock as well as the different levels of severity create a challenge for the practitioner seeking the most appropriate means of therapy. The current classification systems are presented in a concise manner to provide the reader a means of learning terminology and concepts.

A chapter on hemodynamic monitoring follows the review of the classification systems of shock. Sophisticated machinery is now utilized to record subtle changes in a patient's hemodynamic status. The use of hemodynamic monitoring is consistent with the management of all shock types. The nurse must be responsible for the efficient functioning of this monitoring equipment as well as the analyzing and reporting of significant data findings. The chapter on hemodynamic monitoring explores the use of the Swan-Ganz catheter in carefully recording the ongoing condition of the shock patient. A thorough look at the function and purpose of Swan-Ganz monitoring is presented.

The text next presents an in-depth look at four different types of shock. The clinical pictures of hypovolemic, cardiogenic, septic, and anaphylactic shock are described in detail. Each clinical picture begins with a look at its specific pathological nature. The most recent medical research directed toward understanding the nature of the various shock entities is utilized. A summary of clinical signs and symptoms accompanied by a physiological rationale for each is also given. This informs the nurse of the types of assessment measurements required as well as the significance of the findings gathered. Current diagnostic methods and criteria for their use are also explored.

Within the management section of each clinical picture, both medical and nursing therapies are carefully presented. A goal-oriented approach is utilized to organize the content of the management section. The authors have taken care to explain the most current forms of therapy and the proposed therapeutic rationale for each. In cases in which the form of therapy is controversial, each treatment modality is explored for its benefits and disadvantages. In situations in which similar types of nursing therapy are utilized for all types of shock, one chapter is used to explore that therapy in depth. Within all of the clinical pictures the nursing implications that evolve from therapeutic measures are highlighted. The reader is prepared with a complete picture of the nurse's responsibilities concerning each type of shock. Current pharmacological therapy is integrated throughout all of the chapters.

To assist the reader in assimilating theory with practice, patient vignettes are presented at the end of each clinical picture. A hypothetical patient-care situation is presented, and the reader is asked to reflect on the previously discussed theory. A series of four to six questions requires the reader to make decisions similar to those confronted in the clinical setting. A final explanation of the answers affords a useful summarization of theoretical viewpoints.

The final section of the text deals with common complications resulting from shock. Adult respiratory distress syndrome, disseminated intravascular coagulation, and renal failure, although common complications of shock, are disease entities in their own right. The amount of recent literature dealing with each is voluminous. However, there have been few attempts to thoroughly explore these complications as they relate to shock from a nursing focus. Each complication is given the same comprehensive presentation as the clinical pictures of shock. Prevention as well as management of the complications is considered.

A question a reader might ask is, Will this textbook serve to improve nursing care? The theme of the text is to do just that. As the nurse faces the challenge of caring for a shock patient many questions arise:

What conditions favor the development of shock?

Can these conditions be prevented by nursing measures?

What clinical signs and symptoms can the nurse expect to see?

What is the significance of these signs and symptoms?

What assessment measurements are critical for the nurse to make?

What subtle findings help to discriminate the nature of different forms of shock?

What interventions become a priority during the acute onset of shock?

What is the specific scientific rationale for these interventions?

What measures are utilized to monitor the patient's progress?

How can the nurse specifically maintain and support existing functions to prevent complications?

What is the therapeutic rationale for controversial treatment modalities?

How can the nurse maintain the patient's identity and sense of worth during a time of critical illness?

This text attempts to provide answers to all of these questions. With the rapid expansion of knowledge and technology, it is imperative that the nurses be prepared to continually expand their learning. The field of critical care has grown by leaps and bounds during the last decade.

The authors have attempted to prepare a concise, cohesive, and comprehensive look at shock. Texts often provide a cookbook approach to a particular nursing care problem without giving thought to the ''cook's'' background or knowledge. This text has been developed with the goal of providing the nurse the most complete and accurate information available. Each chapter has been prepared with the whole text in mind.

Patricia Ann Potter

Acknowledgments

The uniqueness of this book lies in the collaborative effort of all the co-authors. A true team effort was utilized in developing the style, format, and content. Each author's goal is to provide content for the sophisticated learning needs of the professional nurse.

In addition we wish to offer our sincere appreciation to:

Helen Wells for excellent manuscript preparation. Despite multiple revisions and requests she remained helpful, organized, and consistently tolerant.

Jeanne Robertson, an outstanding medical illustrator whose work was consistently excellent and creative.

Nancy Mullins, Assistant Editor, and **Pamela Swearingen,** Editor, Nursing Division, at The C.V. Mosby Company for their support and advice during the manuscript preparation.

Bess Arends, Assistant Editor, Nursing Division, at The C.V. Mosby Company who provided much support in the final manuscript preparation.

Diane Ackermann, Manuscript Editor, and **Lin Hallgren,** Supervising Editor, at The C.V. Mosby Company for their editorial expertise.

St. Louis University School of Nursing for the academic environment that served to stimulate this book's creation.

Our respective **families, friends,** and **colleagues** for their support while this book consumed time and energy.

We also appreciate the review and suggestions on portions of this manuscript by **Elaine Hurley, Elaine Larson, Linda Lazure,** and **Judith Masiak.**

Anne Griffin Perry
Patricia Ann Potter
Linda Niedringhaus
Angela Smith-Collins
Judith L. Myers

Contents

PART ONE

PHYSIOLOGICAL CONTROLS

1 Cardiovascular control systems

LINDA NIEDRINGHAUS

The function of the cardiovascular system is to supply oxygen and nutrients to all tissues of the body according to their metabolic requirements. Normally, each tissue and organ receives the exact blood flow required for adequate nutrition. To meet these variations in circulatory requirements, the cardiovascular system responds through a multitude of regulatory mechanisms. These mechanisms respond to stress by increasing the blood supply to active tissues. When the challenge is severe, blood flow to the vital organs such as the heart and brain is maintained at the expense of the circulation to the rest of the body. An understanding of the manner in which this system responds to stress is of importance to the nurse since signs and symptoms of shock are caused by an impairment of these responses.

COMPONENTS OF THE CARDIOVASCULAR SYSTEM

The cardiovascular system is a closed transport system composed of a heart serving as a pump, blood serving as the carrier, and vessels serving as conduits for the blood. All three of these components must be functioning to provide all of the body tissues with adequate oxygen and nutrients.

The heart

The heart is a pulsatile four-chambered pump composed of two atria and two ventricles. The atria function as entryways to the two ventricles and also serve to pump blood into the ventricles during the latter part of diastole. The ventricles generate the main force that propels blood through the lungs and peripheral circulatory system. The functional activities of the heart are related to three of the physiological properties of heart muscle: rhythmicity, conductivity, and contractility. Each of these properties is developed to different degrees in various areas of the heart. *Rhythmicity* is well developed in the pacemaker region of the heart, which is responsible for initiating impulses conducted to the rest of the heart. The property of *conductivity* is especially developed in the region of the Purkinje network, which is responsible for the rapid conduction of impulses from the pacemaker cells to the ventricles. *Contractility* is developed in the walls of the atria and to a greater extent in the muscular walls of the ventricles. The cardiac muscle, valves, conduction system, blood supply, and neural mechanisms must be intact for the heart to function normally. All of these components work together to ensure that the rate, force, and volume of blood pumped into the circulation will be adequate to supply all body tissues when the person is at rest or when metabolic demands are increased by illness, exercise, or stress. (See Chapter 2 for a complete discussion of the heart as a pump.)

The blood

Blood serves as the carrier of the cardiovascular transport system. The normal circulating blood volume of a man weighing 70 kg is approximately 8% of the body weight, or 5600 ml. About 55% of this volume is plasma. Whole blood contains plasma proteins, red blood cells, white blood cells, and platelets, which are suspended in the plasma. Although small amounts of oxygen and carbon dioxide are dissolved in the plasma, most of it is bound to hemoglobin in the red blood cells. Nutrients are dissolved in the plasma, and hormones are bound to plasma proteins for transport from their endocrine glands to sites of action (target tissues). Nitrogenous and other wastes are also transported by the blood to the kidney for excretion. Blood volume must be adequate to ensure that the cardiovascular transport system functions normally.

The vessels

The system of vascular conduits, the third component of the cardiovascular transport system, is composed of arteries, arterioles, capillaries, venules, and veins. Each of these structures has a particular function, which correlates directly with its individual vessel size and wall structure (Table 1-1).

The aorta and large arteries serve as temporary storage facilities, storing some pressure in their elastic walls during systole and releasing or returning pressure to the cardiovascular system during diastole. These elastic properties prevent large fluctuations in pressure and provide for even distribution of blood flow to the peripheral tissues. The aorta is the largest vessel in the body with a lumen diameter of 2.5 cm and a wall thickness of 2 mm. The arteries have a lumen diameter of about 0.4 cm and a wall thickness of 1 mm. A large diameter and wall thickness are necessary for these vessels to tolerate the full force of the pumping action of the left ventricle.

The arterioles serve as resistance vessels. The lumen diameter of the arterioles is about 30 μm with a wall thickness of 20 μm. These relatively thick, muscular vessels

Table 1-1. Characteristics of various types of blood vessels

	Lumen diameter	Wall thickness	Function
Aorta	2.5 cm	2 mm	Pressure storage
Artery	0.4 cm	1 mm	Pressure storage
Arteriole	30 μm	20 μm	Resistance
Capillary	6 μm	1 μm	Exchange
Venule	20 μm	2 μm	Volume storage
Vein	0.5 cm	0.5 mm	Volume storage

are richly innervated by sympathetic and parasympathetic nerves that allow them to constrict or dilate, thereby controlling systemic blood pressure and allowing for capillary runoff, which lowers arterial pressure. Thus arterioles are the major site of resistance to blood flow. Small changes in their caliber cause large changes in the total peripheral resistance and blood pressure.

The arterioles divide into smaller, muscle-walled vessels called metarterioles. These divide further into capillaries that are the exchange vessels. Porelike openings in the walls of the capillaries allow for the exchange of oxygen and nutrients from capillaries to body cells and the exchange of carbon dioxide and wastes from cells to capillaries. The rate of blood flow from an arteriole into a capillary bed is influenced by metarterioles and precapillary sphincters. These alter capillary circulation in response to the increased oxygen needs of the body cells served by a particular capillary bed.

The walls of the venules are only slightly thicker than those of the capillaries. These vessels are the capacitance vessels that function as reservoirs for volume storage. Veins, which are slightly larger, also serve the same function. The walls of venules and veins are thin and easily distended allowing them to store large volumes of blood with minimal changes in pressure. More than one half of the body's blood supply is normally contained in these capacitance vessels. These vessels are innervated by sympathetic nerves, which can respond to stimulation by constriction, thus providing a way of mobilizing this blood reserve when the system is stressed.

FUNCTIONS OF THE CARDIOVASCULAR SYSTEM
Transport of oxygen, nutrients, hormones, and waste products

The primary function of the cardiovascular system is to serve the capillary bed or microcirculation as a transport system to meet individual tissue needs. Blood delivers oxygen, glucose, amino acids, fatty acids, hormones, and electrolytes to cells while removing carbon dioxide, urea, lactic acid, and other waste products.

Transport and distribution of heat

The cardiovascular system helps to regulate body temperature by transporting warmed blood from active tissues, such as exercising muscle, to the skin where some of the heat is radiated to the environment. Blood flow to active tissues is regulated by the cardiovascular center in the medulla in response to the temperature-regulating center in the hypothalamus. The cardiovascular center receives nervous impulses from the hypothalamus and, in turn, regulates blood flow in the peripheral tissues by causing alternate vasodilation and constriction of blood vessels in the skin to dissipate the heat.

Maintenance of fluid and electrolyte balance

The cardiovascular system serves as a storage and transport system for body water and electrolytes. These two substances are delivered to body cells by the interstitial fluid that is formed by continuous filtration, diffusion, and reabsorption from the blood. In addition to providing the cells with adequate water and electrolytes, the cardiovascular system pumps 1700 L of blood to the kidneys each day. Here the quantity of water and electrolytes in the body can be adjusted and maintained. The blood itself serves as an important buffering mechanism to maintain an optimum pH of 7.35 to 7.45. Hemoglobin and plasma proteins play key roles in this buffering mechanism.

REGULATORY MECHANISMS

The human body has multiple cardiovascular regulatory mechanisms that increase the blood supply to active tissues by increasing the cardiac output. Cardiac output is regulated by variations in heart rate, stroke volume, and venous return. The remainder of this chapter will focus on control mechanisms that influence heart rate, stroke volume, and venous return.

Mechanisms controlling heart rate

Under normal resting conditions the heart beats about 70 times each minute. This rate of contraction is controlled by the heart's own intrinsic control mechanism regulated by the sinoatrial node (SA node), atrioventricular node (AV node), and Purkinje system (Chapter 2).

During periods of emotional excitement or muscular exercise, the heart can contract up to 200 times each minute. Normally the heart rate is regulated by the insertion of the sympathetic and parasympathetic branches of the autonomic nervous system; sympathetic stimulation increases the heart rate, whereas parasympathetic stimulation has an inhibiting effect on the heart rate via the vagus nerve.

Cardiovascular reflexes. There are four major reflexes mediated by the autonomic nervous system. These four reflexes, the baroreceptor reflex, the chemoreceptor reflex, the Bainbridge reflex, and the respiratory reflex, regulate the heart rate.

The *baroreceptor reflex* is perhaps the most important reflex controlling heart rate and blood pressure. The baroreceptors are stretch or pressure receptors located in the carotid sinus and aortic arch. These receptors are stimulated by the distention or stretching of the walls of the aorta or carotid artery. When these receptors are stretched by an increase in blood pressure or blood volume, they increase their firing rate of nervous impulses over their afferent fibers to the inhibitor portion of the cardiovascular center in the medulla. From the cardiovascular center in the medulla, efferent impulses are transmitted over autonomic nerves to the heart and to the peripheral blood vessels, thereby causing a decrease in heart rate and peripheral vascular resistance (Fig. 1-1).

The range of the baroreceptor response can be illustrated by two examples, hypertensive crisis and hypovolemic shock. In hypertensive crisis, the baroreceptor response to an increase in carotid sinus and aortic pressure is to decrease the sympathetic nervous discharge to the heart and peripheral blood vessels. At the same time, parasympathetic nervous discharges over the vagal nerves to the SA node are increased. This combination of reactions slows the heart rate and causes vasodilation; thus blood pressure falls.

During hypovolemic shock, the low mean arterial blood pressure causes fewer

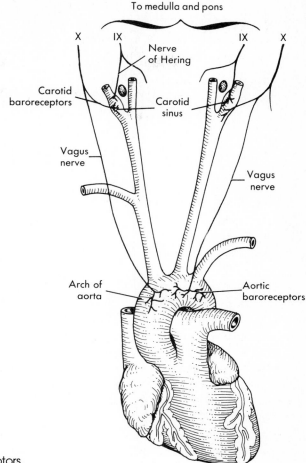

Fig. 1-1. Location of baroreceptors.

afferent impulses to be conducted to the cardiovascular center in the medulla. Following the drop in the rate of transmission of impulses from the baroreceptors, sympathetic stimulation to the SA node and the peripheral vessels increases. Heart rate, as well as peripheral vascular resistance, is increased. Both of these reactions serve to increase the blood pressure and cardiac output for the patient suffering from hypovolemic shock. Initially these compensatory mechanisms can save a patient's life until medical and nursing care are available.

The *chemoreceptor reflex* produces changes in heart and respiratory rates in response to changes in partial pressure of oxygen (Pao_2), partial pressure of carbon dioxide ($Paco_2$), and changes in serum hydrogen ion concentration (pH).

Cardiac response to chemoreceptor stimulation can be divided into primary and secondary reflex mechanisms. At first, the primary reflex causes bradycardia in re-

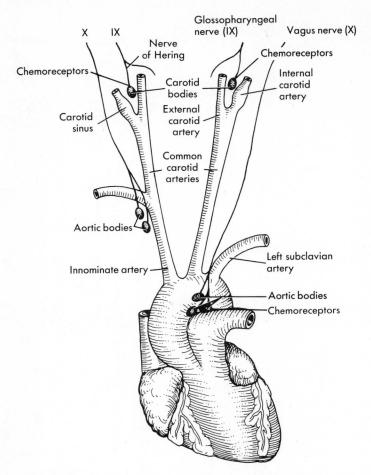

Fig. 1-2. Location of peripheral chemoreceptors.

sponse to a decrease in partial pressure of oxygen, an increase in partial pressure of carbon dioxide, and a decrease in pH. Next, the secondary reflex causes an increase in respiratory activity that will usually increase the heart rate. These primary and secondary reflexes exert opposing effects on the heart rate in response to the same stimuli, thus minimizing the net result of chemoreceptor activity on heart rate.

This response is mediated by peripheral and central chemoreceptors (Fig. 1-2). The peripheral chemoreceptors are clusters of sensory nerve cells located in the carotid and aortic bodies. The aortic bodies are located close to the aortic arch. The carotid bodies are located at the bifurcation of the common carotid artery. These afferent fibers converge on the vasomotor center in the medulla. Although the main effect of the chemoreceptor reflex is on respiration, increased activity in these chemical receptors is respon-

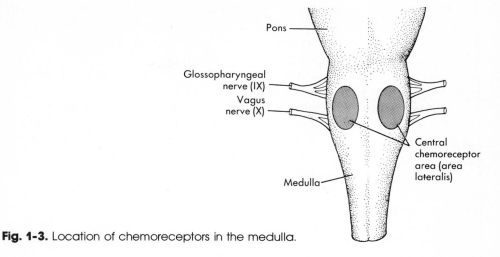

Fig. 1-3. Location of chemoreceptors in the medulla.

sible for the hypertension produced by hypoxia (Heistad and Abboud, 1980). Under normal physiological conditions, chemoreceptor influence is exerted primarily on peripheral resistance rather than on cardiac function.

Peripheral chemoreceptors are constantly sampling the arterial blood for changes in Pa_{O_2}, Pa_{CO_2}, and pH. In contrast, central chemoreceptors (Fig. 1-3) located in the medulla monitor the composition of the cerebral spinal fluid and the extracellular fluid of the brain. The central chemoreceptors are primarily sensitive to changes in Pa_{CO_2} and pH. Chemoreceptors, by nature of their location, receive a very large blood supply.

The *Bainbridge reflex* provides for an increase in heart rate in response to an increase in venous return. The receptors for the Bainbridge reflex are located in the atria, large veins, and pulmonary artery. When these stretch receptors are stimulated by an increased blood volume, afferent nervous impulses are transmitted at an increased rate to the cardiovascular center in the medulla. The cardiovascular center responds by increasing the efferent sympathetic discharge that increases the heart rate and cardiac output. This reflex provides a mechanism for the heart to pump all of the blood that is returned to it. The Bainbridge reflex is very important during strenuous exercise when the amount of venous return is increased by the pumping action of skeletal muscles.

The *respiratory reflex,* also known as sinus arrhythmia, is a normal physiological phenomenon. It refers to the normal fluctuations in the heart rate that occur with the phases of respiration. This effect of respiration on the heart rate may be absent during quiet breathing but is readily seen when the depth of breathing is increased. During inspiration the heart rate accelerates and during expiration it decelerates. The vagus nerve mediates this reflex. During inspiration the intrathoracic pressure decreases, causing a greater venous return to the right side of the heart. This increased venous return stimulates the stretch receptors in the lungs, which fire impulses to the cardiovascular center in the medulla at an increased rate. The tonic vagal discharges that keep the heart rate stable are inhibited, causing the heart rate to rise. This momentary increase in heart rate is enough to increase the cardiac output so that it compensates for the momentary increase in venous return. In contrast, heart rate is slowed during expiration, when increased intrathoracic pressure inhibits venous return.

Effect of ions on heart rate. The SA node, or pacemaker, of the heart is a collection of nerve cells that serves as the intrinsic regulator of the heart rate. Changes in extracellular fluid concentrations of electrolytes (ions) will alter the heart rate because the electrical activity of the heart depends on the balanced distribution of these ions across the cell membrane. Three cations, potassium, sodium, and calcium, have marked effects on the rate of contraction of cardiac muscle. Therefore changes in the normal concentration of these positively charged ions in the extracellular fluids will have marked effects on cardiac function.

Hypokalemia, a decreased plasma concentration of potassium ions, is a serious condition but is not as rapidly fatal as hyperkalemia. Potassium levels below 3 mEq/L can cause increased sensitivity to digitalis and can cause ECG changes. The ECG abnormalities could include flat or inverted T waves, prominent U waves, and depressed S-T segments.

Hyperkalemia, an increased plasma concentration of potassium, is a potentially lethal condition because of its effects on the heart. Cardiac symptoms can be observed when the serum potassium level exceeds 8 mEq/L. These symptoms include bradycardia, hypotension, ventricular fibrillation, and cardiac arrest, and are caused by the depressant action of excessive potassium ions on the pacemaker's firing potential. ECG monitoring will show tall, peaked T waves, depressed ST segments, decreased amplitude of R waves, prolonged PR interval, and widening of the QRS complex.

Clinically, a fall in plasma sodium concentration *(hyponatremia)* may be associated with low-voltage ECG complexes that signify a depressed heart. Excessive plasma sodium *(hypernatremia)* has a depressant action on cardiac function by competing with and replacing calcium ions in the contractile process of the cardiac muscle cells. When sodium ions are increased in the plasma, fewer calcium ions are available to participate in contraction. Death from cardiac fibrillation can result. It must be emphasized that extremes in sodium ion concentration almost never occur clinically. Low sodium concentration can result from water intoxication.

Calcium ion concentration changes can alter cardiac function because of the importance of calcium in cardiac contraction. *Hypocalcemia,* a decrease in calcium ion concentration, will cause death by tetany of the respiratory muscles before it will affect the heart (Guyton, 1976). When hypocalcemia is present, the ECG may be normal or may demonstrate a prolonged QT interval.

Hypercalcemia, an increased plasma concentration of calcium, increases the force of contractility of the heart muscle by its direct participation in the contractile process. Infusion of large amounts of calcium in laboratory animals has caused cardiac standstill

---

Summary of factors affecting heart rate

Increase heart rate

Sympathetic stimulation
Inspiration
Decreased baroreceptor activity
Bainbridge reflex
Excitement
Exercise
Fever
Hypoxia

Decrease heart rate

Vagal stimulation
Expiration
Increased baroreceptor activity
Increased intracranial pressure
Hyperkalemia

---

during systole. The plasma calcium level in humans is rarely high enough to affect the heart. When calcium ion concentration begins to rise, calcium is deposited in the bones and other body tissues as insoluble calcium salts before a toxic level can be reached.

Effect of temperature on heart rate. Fever causes an increase in heart rate. When the temperature of the pacemaker cells is increased, the permeability of the cell membrane to various ions is increased. This increase in permeability accelerates the depolarization of the pacemaker cells and thus increases the heart rate. Contractile strength of the heart muscle also increases temporarily. Prolonged elevation of body temperature causes exhaustion and weakness. Heart rate changes of 50 beats/minute have been demonstrated to occur with 1° C change in right atrial temperature (Guyton and Cowley, 1976).

Mechanisms controlling stroke volume

Cardiac output is determined by heart rate multiplied by stroke volume. By definition, stroke volume is the difference between the end-diastolic volume and the end-systolic volume of the heart. End-diastolic volume is the volume of blood in the heart just before contraction occurs. This volume measures approximately 130 ml of blood in the adult male. The end-systolic volume is the volume of blood remaining in the heart at the end of systole. This volume measures approximately 60 ml. If we subtract the end-systolic volume (60 ml) from the end-diastolic volume (130 ml), we find that the average stroke volume for an adult male is 70 ml. This means that 70 ml of blood is ejected from the left ventricle with each heart beat.

Determinants of stroke volume. The stroke volume can be altered by changes in the following three factors:

1. Preload, or left ventricular filling pressure, which reflects the left ventricular filling volume. This volume can be measured by the Swan-Ganz catheter.
2. Afterload, which reflects the peripheral resistance against which the left ventricle must pump. The afterload is equivalent to the systemic blood pressure and represents the resistance to ventricular ejection.
3. Contractile state of the heart, or the ability of the heart to alter its pumping force and speed.

All of these factors, preload, afterload, and contractility, are regulated by intrinsic and extrinsic control mechanisms that provide each tissue and organ with the exact blood flow required for adequate nutrition and function (O'Donnell and Belkin, 1978).

The heart automatically pumps all the volume of blood returned to the right atrium by the venous circulation. The intrinsic regulation of stroke volume is subdivided into heterometric and homeometric autoregulation. The extrinsic regulation of stroke volume is subdivided into nervous and chemical control.

Intrinsic mechanisms. Regulation of blood output caused by changes in myocardial fiber length is called heterometric regulation. The intrinsic ability of the heart to adapt to changing volumes of blood by changing the fiber length of myocardial cells is described by the Frank-Starling law of the heart. This law states that the more the left ventricle is filled during diastole (preload), the greater the volume of blood that is pumped into the aorta. This ability of stretched muscle to contract with increased force is characteristic of all striated muscle. This increased force of contraction is caused by an optimal degree of interdigitation of actin and myosin filaments (Guyton, 1976).

Within physiological limits, the heart pumps all the blood that enters it without allowing excessive backup of blood into the veins. The heart can pump a large or a small amount of blood. It automatically adapts to the blood volume as long as the total quantity of blood does not rise above physiological limits.

Homeometric regulation is defined as the intrinsic adjustment of stroke volume that is independent of changes in myocardial fiber length. The pumping efficiency of the heart and the cardiac output can be increased by an increase in heart rate (treppe). In treppe, an increase in the frequency of cardiac stimulation increases the contractility of the cardiac muscle by increasing its tension development. This mechanism is called homeometric regulation because the increased contractile strength returns myocardial muscle fibers to their original length causing cardiac output to increase without changing fiber length (Guyton, 1976).

Extrinsic mechanisms

Nervous control. The major extrinsic control of stroke volume is exerted by the autonomic nervous system. Sympathetic and parasympathetic stimulation can alter the stroke volume by changing the heart rate (chronotropic effect). The autonomic nervous

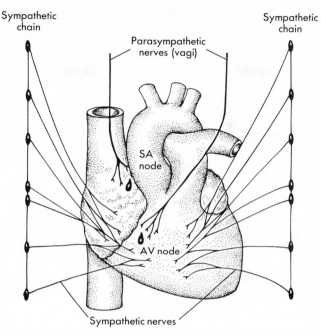

Fig. 1-4. Sympathetic and parasympathetic nerves supplying the heart.

system also alters the stroke volume by changing the strength of cardiac contraction (inotropic effect). These changes in contractility parallel changes in heart rate. When sympathetic stimulation decreases, parasympathetic tone predominates, resulting in a decreased heart rate, contractility, and stroke volume. When sympathetic stimulation increases, heart rate, contractility, and stroke volume increase (Fig. 1-4).

The two atria are well supplied with sympathetic and parasympathetic nerve fibers. The ventricles are supplied mainly by sympathetic fibers. Under normal conditions, the sympathetic nerve fibers to the heart discharge at a slow rate that maintains a strength of ventricular contraction about 20% above what its strength would be with no sympathetic stimulation (Guyton, 1976). Therefore the nervous system can decrease the strength of ventricular contraction by slowing or stopping sympathetic impulses to the heart. Maximal sympathetic stimulation can increase the strength of ventricular contraction to 100% above normal. Maximal parasympathetic stimulation decreases ventricular contraction strength by only 30%. Therefore the effect of parasympathetic stimulation on the heart is small when compared to the effect of sympathetic stimulation.

The nerve fibers that mediate sympathetic control of the heart are adrenergic fibers. These fibers contain the chemical transmitter norepinephrine (noradrenalin). Norepinephrine is also secreted by the adrenal medulla. Adrenergic nerve endings supply the heart with norepinephrine whenever they are stimulated by the cardiovascular center located in the medulla, resulting in an overall increase in heart activity. The heart rate increases (chronotropic effect) and the force of cardiac contraction increases (inotropic effect).

This mechanism is activated in the following manner. Norepinephrine increases the permeability of the heart to sodium and calcium ions. In the SA node, an increase of sodium ions decreases the resting membrane potential so that the firing of the pacemaker cells is accelerated. In the AV node, increased sodium permeability makes it easier for each fiber to excite the succeeding fiber, causing decreased conduction time from the atria to the ventricles. The increased permeability to calcium ions accounts for the increased contractility. Calcium ions excite the contractile process of the myocardial muscle fibers.

Acetylcholine is the transmitter released at the nerve endings of the parasympathetic fibers. When acetylcholine is released at these vagal endings, increased permeability of the SA node to potassium ions causes a decrease in the rate of firing of the SA node. This vagal stimulation also decreases the excitability within the AV junctional fibers between the atrial musculature and the AV node, causing slowing of impulse transmission to the ventricles. This decrease in impulse transmission slows the heart rate, thereby decreasing its stroke volume and cardiac output.

Changes in cardiac output can also be elicited when the central nervous system becomes hypoxic and ischemic. When cerebral blood flow is interrupted, massive sympathetic stimulation from the medulla increases ventricular contractility. This response is referred to as the cerebral ischemic response. It is a final effort by the nervous system to restore the cardiac output to normal. This pressor response is an attempt by the sympathetic nervous system to restore adequate circulation to vital tissues such as the heart and brain during periods of profound hypotension (Heistad and Abboud, 1980).

Any damage to the myocardium, valves, or conduction system of the heart will affect the stroke volume. The more serious the damage, the less the cardiac output will be. Specific causes of a decreased stroke volume include myocardial infarction, valvular heart disease, intense vagal stimulation, inhibition of sympathetic stimulation, congenital heart disease, myocarditis, cardiac anoxia, and myocardial damage caused by chest trauma.

Chemical control. The second form of extrinsic control of stroke volume is concerned with such chemicals as hormones and blood gases. The catecholamines (epinephrine and norepinephrine) are the most important circulating hormones that have an effect on stroke volume. When the amounts of these two hormones are increased, both heart rate and stroke volume are increased. The heart becomes more effective as a pump and provides better perfusion to vital organs and muscles. Several other hormones affect the stroke volume of the heart. The thyroid hormones (triiodothyronine [T_3] and thyroxine [T_4]) potentiate the actions of the catecholamines. T_3 and T_4 sensitize the beta receptors in the heart to norepinephrine, thereby increasing heart rate and stroke volume (Berk et al., 1976). Glucagon, the antihypoglycemic hormone produced by the alpha cells of the pancreas, has an inotropic effect on the heart by stimulating and energizing the

---

Effect of various activities or conditions on stroke volume

Increase stroke volume

Anxiety
Cerebral ischemic response
Eating
Epinephrine
Excitement
Exercise
Glucagon
High environmental temperature
Thyroid hormone

Decrease stroke volume

Acidosis
Decreased blood volume
Hypercapnia
Hypoxia
Myocardial infarction
Rapid arrhythmias

---

contractile mechanism of the heart muscle. Berk et al. (1976) cite the use of glucagon in intensive care units to increase cardiac output of patients suffering mild to moderate left ventricular failure.

The chemoreceptors in the medulla and carotid and aortic bodies constantly measure the blood gases (Pa_{CO_2} and Pa_{O_2}) as well as the hydrogen ion concentration (pH). An increased carbon dioxide tension in the blood stimulates the vasomotor center to increase the heart rate and peripheral vascular constriction. Anoxia, or a decreased oxygen tension, appears to have a direct effect on the SA node itself. When oxygen tension is lowered, the heart rate increases in an effort to increase the cardiac output to supply ischemic cells.

Mechanisms controlling venous return

Venous return regulates cardiac filling during diastole and has a subsequent effect on cardiac output. The rate of diastolic filling determines what the end-diastolic volume will be and hence what the stroke volume will be for each beat of the heart. The rate of venous return to the heart is related to two factors, venous pressure and blood volume.

Venous pressure. Blood returns to the heart because a pressure gradient exists. When the heart pumps blood, arterial pressure ranges from 120 mm Hg during systole to 70 mm Hg during diastole. This pressure falls as the blood moves throughout the arterioles, capillaries, and venules. The pressure in the venules is 12 to 18 mm Hg and falls steadily in the larger veins to about 5.5 mm Hg in the great veins outside the thorax. The pressure at the entrance to the right atrium (central venous pressure) averages 4.6 mm Hg (Ganong, 1977).

This drop in pressure as blood circulates through the body back to the heart is caused by the capacitance of the veins and arteries. Capacitance describes the ability of the vessels to distend to accept larger volumes of blood. The venous system is a high-capacitance system that can accept a large volume of blood with minimal pressure change. Capacitance by the venous system is possible because of the characteristics of the vessel walls, which are elastic and richly innervated by the sympathetic nervous system. Through capacitance and sympathetic innervation, venous pressure is altered to regulate venous return to the heart. Venous constriction caused by sympathetic stimulation will reduce capacitance and increase venous pressure, thus improving venous return to the heart. Venous dilation will achieve the opposite effect. Capacitance will increase; venous pressure and venous return will decrease.

Blood volume. When blood volume is reduced, as occurs in shock caused by hemorrhage, venous pressure will fall and venous return to the heart will become inadequate. Compensatory responses include an increase in venous tone that decreases capacitance of the vascular system. This will result in an increase in venous pressure and venous return.

The opposite effect occurs in cardiogenic shock caused by failure of the left ventricle to deliver an adequate cardiac output. Complex hormonal and renal mechanisms (aldosterone and angiotensin) will conserve salt and water and expand the circulating blood volume in an attempt to raise venous pressure and venous return. As cardiogenic shock progresses, the venous pressure becomes too high and the system can no longer compensate. At this point, the increased venous pressure no longer improves the cardiac output but actually causes symptoms of congestive heart failure (Green, 1977).

Gravity. In the standing position, the venous pressure in the areas of the body above the heart is decreased by the force of gravity while the gravitational force opposing the return of blood to the heart from the legs is increased. This increases the amount of blood in the distensible veins, promoting translocation of fluid into the interstitial tissues and thus reducing venous pressure and venous return. One factor that counteracts this effect of gravity is the presence of one-way valves in the large veins to prevent the backflow of blood.

Skeletal muscle pump. Muscle contraction aids venous return. When muscles contract, the veins located between the muscle bundles are compressed and blood in the veins is squeezed toward the heart. Pulsations of nearby arteries may also compress the veins. During quiet standing, venous pressure at the ankle may be as high as 85 to 90 mm Hg. Rhythmic contractions of the leg muscles while standing can lower the venous pressure in the legs to less than 30 mm Hg by propelling blood toward the heart. The pooling of blood in the lower extremities is a common cause of fainting, as experienced by young recruits forced to stand at attention for long periods of time. Rhythmic con-

---

Effect of various factors on venous return

Increase venous return

Increased blood volume
Vasoconstriction
Inspiration
Skeletal muscle contraction
Ventricular systole
Early diastole

Decrease venous return

Decreased blood volume
Vasodilation
Expiration
Incompetent venous valves
Gravity (feet in dependent position)

---

tractions of the calves and thighs will activate the muscle pump to increase venous return and cardiac output, thereby preventing fainting.

Thoracic pump. During inspiration the intrapleural pressure falls from approximately -2.5 to -6 mm Hg. This negative pressure is transferred to the larger veins and atria so that central venous pressure falls from 6 mm Hg during expiration to 2 mm Hg during inspiration. This drop in venous pressure aids venous return by providing a more negative pressure within the thoracic cavity. During inspiration the diaphragm descends and intra-abdominal pressure rises, squeezing blood toward the heart. Backflow into the leg veins is prevented by the venous valves.

Heartbeat. During ventricular systole there is a rapid inflow of venous blood into the atria caused by the downward movement of the ventricle. During ventricular diastole there is a rapid increase in venous return from the vena cava to the right atrium resulting in increased atrial pressure. Therefore venous return is accelerated during systole and diastole. At a rapid heart rate, most of the blood enters the heart during systole because of the sucking action of the ventricle on the atria and great veins. This compensates for the shortened diastolic filling time at rapid heart rates (Ganong, 1977).

EVALUATION OF CARDIAC FUNCTION
Cardiac output

The effectiveness of the cardiovascular system can be determined by measuring the cardiac output. The cardiac output is the product of the heart rate and the stroke volume. The amount of blood pumped out of either the right or the left ventricle with each heart beat is the stroke volume. The normal stroke volume for a resting male in the supine position is 70 ml/beat. This figure can be substituted in the following formula to obtain the cardiac output when the heart rate is 70 beats/min:

$$Cardiac\ output\ (CO) = Stroke\ volume\ (SV) \times Heart\ rate\ (HR)$$
$$CO = 70\ ml \times 70$$
$$CO = 4900\ ml$$
$$CO = 4.9\ L/min$$

Normal cardiac output is 4.5 to 5.5 L/min for the adult at rest. The cardiac index correlates cardiac output and body surface area. Use of the cardiac index (the cardiac output per minute per square meter of body surface) will compensate for the size difference of patients. The normal cardiac index is 2.8 to 3.2 L/min/m² (Berk et al., 1976).

Variations in the cardiac output and cardiac index can be produced by changes in heart rate or stroke volume. In times of need, such as during strenuous exercise, the heart can increase its output up to 25 L/min by increasing both its rate and stroke volume.

Traditionally, cardiac output has been measured by indirect methods such as circulation time, dye dilution, and a method based on the measurement of oxygen consumption and the arteriovenous oxygen difference. The current method of measurement used at the bedside of critically ill patients is the thermodilution technique using the flow-directed, triple-lumen Swan-Ganz catheter (Del Guercio and Cohn, 1976; Shinn, Woods, and Huseby, 1979). Each of these methods will be described.

Circulation time. The circulation time measurement technique often results in an inaccurate estimate of cardiac function and is no longer used when more reliable methods are available (Little, 1977). This test measures the time a substance takes to move from its injection point to a measuring point. A common substance used is dehydrocholate. It is injected into the cephalic vein in the arm and is recognized as a bitter taste in the tongue 8 to 17 seconds later. Ether can be injected in the arm and will be circulated to the lungs within 4 to 8 seconds. Its arrival in the lungs will be evident by the characteristic ether smell on the patient's breath. This test provides a rough estimate of the effectiveness of the cardiac output and is not a quantitative test of cardiac output.

Dye dilution. The dye dilution technique for measuring cardiac output is based on the Fick principle, which states that the volume of a moving stream can be determined by knowing the amount of a substance that enters or leaves that stream and the difference in concentration resulting from entering or leaving. In this case a known amount of a nontoxic dye that attaches to the plasma proteins is rapidly injected into the right ventricle by way of a catheter. Its dilution and time of initial appearance on the arterial side of the circulation is monitored. By measuring these events carefully, the cardiac output can be calculated. Results are dependent on the patient's plasma protein concentration.

If 5 mg of dye is injected and the duration of the first circulation time is 24 seconds with an average dye concentration of 2.5 mg/L, the following formula can be used to calculate the cardiac output:

$$CO = \frac{\text{Amount of dye injected}}{\text{Mean concentration of dye} \times \text{Duration of first circulation}}$$

$$CO = \frac{5 \text{ mg}}{2.5 \text{ mg/L} \times 24/60 \text{ sec}}$$

$$CO = 5 \text{ L/min}$$

The dye dilution method of measuring cardiac output is also known as the indicator dilution method and was first suggested by G.N. Stewart in 1898 (Little, 1977). Recirculation of some of the dye through the heart begins before the first circulation has been washed completely from the aorta. For this reason, the dye dilution technique is not a quantitative but rather a relative estimate of cardiac output. In spite of this difficulty, this method of measuring cardiac output has proved useful in clinical situations.

Direct Fick method. The Fick method also utilizes the Fick principle to determine cardiac output. The amount of oxygen consumed by the body in a minute is measured. This value is divided by the difference between the oxygen concentration in the arteries (Ao_2) and in the veins (Vo_2). This is known as the arteriovenous oxygen difference (Jensen, 1976).

Oxygen consumption by the lungs is measured by a respirometer. Arterial oxygen concentration can be measured by a blood sample from any convenient artery. A sample of venous blood is obtained by means of a cardiac catheter inserted into the right atrium. Calculation of cardiac output using the direct Fick method and the following values is demonstrated:

$$\text{Oxygen consumption} = 250 \text{ ml/min}$$
$$Ao_2 = 200 \text{ ml/L blood}$$
$$Vo_2 = 160 \text{ ml/L blood}$$

$$CO = \frac{O_2 \text{ consumption (ml } O_2/\text{min)}}{Ao_2 - Vo_2 \text{ (ml } O_2/\text{L blood)}}$$

$$CO = \frac{250 \text{ ml/min}}{200 \text{ ml/L} - 160 \text{ ml/L}}$$

$$CO = \frac{250 \text{ ml/min}}{40 \text{ ml/L}}$$

$$CO = 6.25 \text{ L/min}$$

In general, the level of arteriovenous oxygen difference ($Ao_2 - Vo_2$) is inversely proportional to the cardiac output. That means as the arteriovenous oxygen difference rises, the cardiac output will fall correspondingly. For example, the fall in cardiac output observed in the patient with left ventricular failure will cause an increase in the arteriovenous difference.

Thermodilution. The triple-lumen Swan-Ganz catheter can be used to determine cardiac output by the thermodilution technique. This technique is gaining popularity in intensive care units because of its simplicity, safety, and reliability (Costrini and Thomson, 1977). A small thermistor that measures the temperature of the blood is located close to the tip of the catheter so that it lies in the main pulmonary artery or one of its major branches. In addition to the main lumen used to record pulmonary artery pressure, there is another lumen that opens 28 or 30 cm from the tip. This second lumen opens high in the right atrium or in the right atrial-superior vena cava junction. Cold dextrose solution is injected into the right atrium through this lumen. This injection of cold dextrose changes the temperature of the blood as it flows through the right ventricle into the pulmonary artery. The thermistor in the pulmonary artery records this change. The degree of cooling of the blood is inversely proportional to the volume of blood flowing by the thermistor; the cooler the blood, the less is the volume of flow. In other words, if the blood downstream from the point of dextrose injection is still relatively cool, the cardiac output will be less.

The response of the cardiovascular system to strenuous exercise demonstrates the heart's ability to provide increased amounts of oxygen to body tissues when it is challenged. The resting cardiac output is 5 L/minute. During maximal exercise such as running or cycling, the well-trained athlete can increase his cardiac output to as much as 25 L/minute. This increase is accomplished by increasing both stroke volume and heart rate. At the same time, the pumping of skeletal muscle is causing an increase in the volume of blood returning to the right side of the heart. This increased venous return increases left ventricular filling pressure and volume, thus ensuring an increased cardiac output.

Whenever the cardiovascular control systems are damaged by injury, drugs, surgery, or anesthesia, the heart loses its ability to supply adequate amounts of oxygen to body tissues. Decreased sympathetic nerve activity to the heart and vessels, hypoxia, hypercapnia, and acidosis all lead to a decreased venous return and cardiac output. Damage to the myocardium itself that occurs following an infarction also will cause a decrease in the cardiac output. The damaged myocardium can no longer pump all of the blood returned to the left ventricle. No matter what the cause, interruptions of the normal cardiovascular control systems lead to hypoperfusion of body tissues, ischemia, hypoxia, and cellular death.

REFERENCES

Berk, J.L., et al.: Handbook of critical care, Boston, 1976, Little, Brown & Co.

Costrini, N.V., and Thomson, W.M., editors: Manual of medical therapeutics, ed. 22, Boston, 1977, Little, Brown & Co.

Del Guercio, L.R.M., and Cohn, J.D.: Monitoring: methods and significance, Surgical Clinics of North America **56:**977-994, 1976.

Foster, W.T.: Principles of acute coronary care, New York, 1976, Appleton-Century-Crofts.

Ganong, W.F.: Review of medical physiology, ed. 8, Los Altos, Calif., 1977, Lange Medical Publications.

Green, J.F.: Mechanical concepts in cardiovascular and pulmonary physiology, Philadelphia, 1977, Lea & Febiger.

Guyton, A.C.: Textbook of medical physiology, ed. 5, Philadelphia, 1976, W.B. Saunders Co.

Guyton, A.C., and Cowley, A.W., Jr.: Cardiovascular physiology II. In Guyton, A.C., editor: International review of physiology, vol. 9, Baltimore, 1976, University Park Press.

Hechtman, H.B.: Adequate circulatory responses or cardiovascular failure, Surgical Clinics of North America **56:**929-943, 1976.

Heistad, D.D., and Abboud, F.M.: Circulatory adjustments to hypoxia, Circulation **61:**463-470, 1980.

Hurst, J.W.: The heart, ed. 4, New York, 1978, McGraw-Hill Book Co.

Jensen, D.: The principles of physiology, New York, 1976, Appleton-Century-Crofts.

Little, R.C.: Physiology of the heart and circulation, Chicago, 1977, Year Book Medical Publishers, Inc.

O'Donnell, T.F., Jr., and Belkin, S.C.: The pathophysiology, monitoring, and treatment of shock, Orthopedic Clinics of North America **9:**589-609, 1978.

Sears, M.F., and Heise, C.: Troubleshooting the Swan-Ganz catheter, Heart & Lung **9:**303-305, 1980.

Shah, D.M., et al.: Cardiac output and pulmonary wedge pressure, Archives of Surgery **112:**1161-1164, 1977.

Shinn, J.A., Woods, S.L., and Huseby, J.S.: Effect of intermittent positive pressure ventilation upon pulmonary artery and pulmonary capillary wedge pressure in acutely ill patients, Heart & Lung **8:** 322-327, 1979.

Strand, F.L.: Physiology, New York, 1978, Macmillan Publishing Co., Inc.

2 Myocardial pump

ANGELA SMITH-COLLINS

The myocardial pump (heart) is monitored and controlled by a complex inter-action of neurological, electrochemical, and mechanical events. These events maintain a pressure gradient within the vasculature that ensures adequate perfusion of body tissues (Duggan, 1980). Any dysfunction in the heart requires compensation by other systems of the body for life to continue. Conversely, any significant alteration in any system of the body will affect the heart. Shock may be pathologically linked to myocardial dysfunction, or a functional myocardium may be the principal mediator affecting the patient's survival.

Therapeutic interventions for the patient with shock can appear confusing for the practitioner who does not have a working knowledge of cardiac functioning. Therefore the nurse must have a thorough understanding of the heart's specialized features and cyclic events as a basis for patient care. An understanding of the relationship between the heart and the other systems of the body will enable the nurse to care for these patients more effectively.

FUNCTIONAL ANATOMY OF THE HEART

The heart's major function is to maintain cardiac output in response to the body's oxygen demands. Many specialized structures exist to fulfill this function. The anatomy and physiology of the heart are inextricably linked. Knowledge of both is necessary to provide the nurse a sound basis for assessing the patient's condition. Cardiac physical assessment and the accurate interpretation of ECGs and x-ray films become easier for the nurse who understands the physiological basis for the information.

The human heart is located in the thoracic cavity, usually to the left of the mid-sternal area. It fits snugly between the lungs and the diaphragm, protected by the sternum and rib cage. The tip of the left ventricle is called the apex and rests on the diaphragm. The base of the heart is the location for the origin of the great vessels. This is somewhat confusing to many on their first contact with cardiac anatomy. Usually *apex* simply means top and *base* means bottom. In the heart, however, this is not the case.

The exterior surface of the ventricles is referred to in three sections (Fig. 2-1), which serve as landmarks for assessing cardiac dysfunction. They are the anterior surface, diaphragmatic surface, and posterior surface. The anterior surface is directly under the sternum, the diaphragmatic surface is that portion of the heart closest to the diaphragm, and the posterior surface is closest to the spine.

22

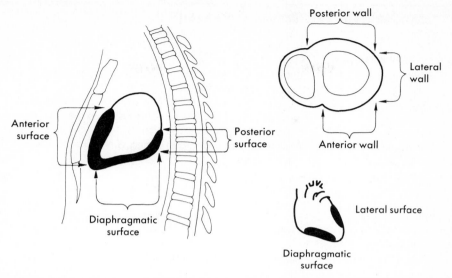

Fig. 2-1. Surfaces of the heart. (From Conover, M.H.: Understanding electrocardiography: physiological and interpretive concepts, ed. 3, St. Louis, 1981, The C.V. Mosby Co.)

Pericardium

The shiny outer covering surrounding the heart and the first centimeter of the great vessels is the pericardium (pericardial sac). It is made up of two thin layers of fibrous tissue, with a lubricating fluid in between. The inner layer, the visceral pericardium, is in direct contact with the heart. The outer layer, the parietal pericardium, touches the lungs and diaphragm. The 10 ml of fluid between the visceral and parietal layers serves to reduce the friction caused by the pumping action of the heart. In addition to lubrication, the pericardial sac performs another function. In the healthy myocardium this tough fibrous tissue resists stretching, thus helping to prevent the heart from becoming overdistended with blood (Holt, 1970).

Chambers

Although it is a single organ, the heart is structured as two pumps separated by a solid wall of muscle called the septum. Each pump, in turn, is separated into two chambers. These chambers, the atrium and ventricle, are separated by an atrioventricular valve.

The right atrium receives blood from the superior and inferior venae cavae. The right side of the heart serves to deliver deoxygenated blood from the venous system into the pulmonary system. This blood then fills the right ventricle and is ejected into the pulmonary artery for gaseous exchange with the lungs. The right side of the heart normally pumps against a low resistance of 18 to 24 mm Hg during ventricular systole.

Gross structure and function of the heart

Structure	Function
Vena cava	Serves as a reservoir for venous blood and a passageway to the right atrium.
Right atrium	Provides 20% of right ventricular stroke volume by atrial contraction ("kick") and acts as passageway for passive filling of right ventricle.
Atrioventricular valves Tricuspid valve Mitral valve	Prevent backflow of blood during ventricular contraction (systole).
Right ventricle	Pumps deoxygenated venous blood to pulmonary circulation.
Semilunar valves Pulmonic valve Aortic valve	Prevent backflow of blood during ventricular relaxation (diastole).
Pulmonary artery	Carries deoxygenated venous blood to lungs from right ventricle.
Pulmonary vein	Carries oxygenated arterial blood to left atrium.
Left atrium	Provides 20% of left ventricular stroke volume by atrial contraction ("kick") and acts as passageway for passive filling of left ventricle.
Left ventricle	Pumps oxygenated arterial blood to systemic circulation.
Aorta	Carries oxygenated arterial blood to systemic circulation.
Septum	Provides a barrier between cardiac chambers, so venous and arterial blood do not mix.

The left side of the heart delivers oxygenated blood from the pulmonary system into the arteries of the body. The left atrium receives blood from the pulmonary vein. This blood then fills the left ventricle and is ejected through the aorta to the systemic circulation. The left side of the heart has more than twice the muscle mass of the right side since it pumps against an arterial pressure of approximately 120 mm Hg (Brecher and Galletti, 1963). Although the left side works against higher resistance, the cardiac output ejected by both ventricles is the same. Normally the amount of blood ejected by each ventricle (stroke volume) is approximately 70 ml/contraction.

Cardiac valves

The cardiac valves keep blood traveling in the proper direction through the chambers and great vessels of the heart (Fig. 2-2). There are two types of valves: atrioventricular (mitral and tricuspid), and semilunar (pulmonary and aortic).

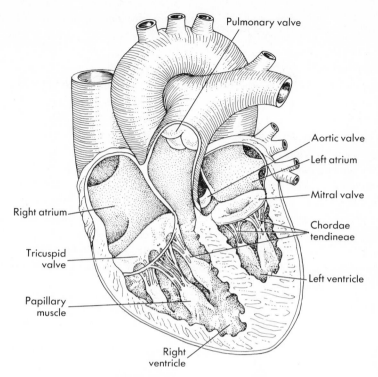

Fig. 2-2. Interior of the heart.

The atrioventricular valves separate the atria and the ventricles of the heart. The mitral and tricuspid valves permit free flow of blood during diastole and prevent back-flow of blood during systole. The tricuspid valve is located between the right atrium and ventricle. It derives its name from the fact that it has three leaflets. The mitral valve is located between the left atrium and ventricle and has two leaflets. Both of the atrioventricular valves are controlled by their attaching structures: the chordae tendineae and the papillary muscles. The chordae tendineae are fibrous bands originating from the pupillary muscle and attached to the valve border. The chordae tendineae provide the support that prevents blood from flowing back into the atrium as ventricular pressure increases. The papillary muscles pull the leaflets together and downward to close the valves at the beginning of systole (Silverman and Schlant, 1978).

The semilunar valves separate the ventricles from the great arteries of the heart. They prevent blood from flowing back into the ventricles during diastole. The pulmonary valve is located between the right ventricle and the pulmonary artery. The aortic valve is located between the left ventricle and the aorta. The semilunar valves have three leaflets, made of fibrous tissue that is anchored in the walls of the pulmonary artery and aorta. These valves open as a result of the increased blood pressure generated during systole. As the pressure decreases, the valves close, preventing blood from flowing back into the ventricles during diastole.

Coronary circulation

The heart itself must be nourished by an ample supply of blood to assure its function. This supply is provided by the coronary arteries (Fig. 2-3), the first two branches off the aorta. These two branches are known as the left and right coronary arteries. The left coronary artery divides into two arteries, the circumflex artery and the left anterior descending coronary artery.

Both the left and right sides of the myocardium normally receive oxygenated blood for metabolic needs. However, the time during which each ventricle is oxygenated differs. This is caused by the greater pressure generated by the left ventricle at the time of systole. The right side of the heart receives a constant flow of oxygenated blood from the coronary circulation because the pressure generated by the right ventricular contraction is always less than the pressure in the aorta, thus allowing the right coronary artery to be perfused. The left side of the heart, on the other hand, exerts a pressure dur-

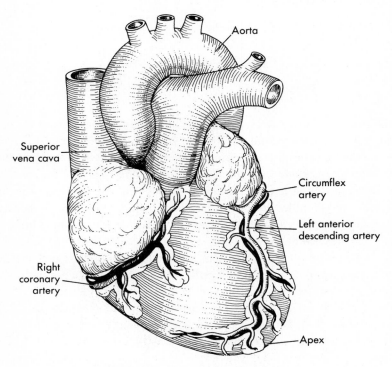

Fig. 2-3. Location of coronary arteries.

ing systole that is equal to or greater than the pressure in the aorta. Perfusion to the left side of the heart is halted during systole. Therefore the left side of the heart receives oxygenated blood only during diastole.

The coronary arteries receive about 5% of the cardiac output. This can be increased up to 25% on exertion. When there is an increase in oxygen requirements, coronary blood flow must increase or metabolic damage to the myocardium will occur.

Four variables affect myocardial oxygen consumption: muscular tension, external work, heart rate, and the contractile state of the cardiac muscle. *Muscular tension* refers to the tension that is produced when myocardial cells shorten, increasing the pressure within the ventricles. Muscular tension is greater during systole than during diastole. The *external work* of the heart is the activity needed to move the stroke volume from the ventricle to the aorta (Fuller, 1980). External work is a product of the pressure that builds as a result of muscle shortening. The third variable, *heart rate,* is significantly affected by changing oxygen requirements of the body. The final variable, *contractile state* of the myocardium, refers to the fact that the ventricles can change the force of their contraction without changing the volume of blood pumped on each contraction. An increase in any one of these four variables results in increased myocardial oxygen consumption. When coronary circulation is compromised, the interaction between these factors becomes very important.

Normal conduction pathway

The heart has a self-contained electrical system (Harris, 1979). This system serves to produce and conduct electrical impulses to all the myocardial cells. This pathway carries the electrical impulses that stimulate the myocardial cells to contract (Fig. 2-4).

The conduction system begins at the sinoatrial node (SA node), which is located

---

Coronary artery blood flow distribution

Artery	Area supplied
Right coronary artery	Right atrium (SA node)
	Right ventricle
	Posterior wall of the left ventricle
Left coronary artery	
Circumflex artery	Lateral and posterior wall of the left ventricle
Left anterior descending	Anterior wall of left ventricle
artery	Two thirds of intraventricular septum
	(These are the most common sites of myocardial infarctions)

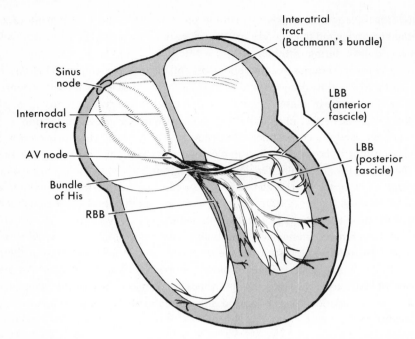

Fig. 2-4. Conductive system of the heart. (From Conover, M.H.: Understanding electro-cardiography: physiological and interpretive concepts, ed. 3, St. Louis, 1981, The C.V. Mosby Co.)

in the upper posterior portion of the right atrium. This node is also called the heart's pace-maker. Under normal circumstances the SA node sets the heart rate. The sinoatrial node is influenced primarily by neural transmitters (e.g., acetylcholine and norepinephrine). The SA node is innervated by a branch of the parasympathetic nervous system (vagus nerve) that has the capacity to slow the rate of SA node firing through the release of acetylcholine. The SA node is also sensitive to the sympathetic neurotransmitter norepi-nephrine. Increased hormone levels in the blood increase the rate of SA node firing.

Three tracts of specialized conduction fibers branch out from the SA node: the anterior, middle, and posterior internodal tracts. The anterior tract has a branch that becomes Bachmann's bundle. Bachmann's bundle travels through the atrial septum to the left atrium. It has no further contact with the other internodal tracts. The three primary internodal tracts converge at the atrioventricular node (AV node). This node is located, as the name implies, near the junction of the atria and ventricles. Its exact location is on the posterior surface of the right atrium directly above the tricuspid valve (Weeks, 1981). A bundle of conductive tissue (bundle of His) emerges from the AV node and follows a path down the septum (Skorga and Nunnery, 1981). This bundle divides into the right and left bundle branch. The right side follows the septal wall and then terminates as many small conductive fibers, the Purkinje fibers, which are embedded throughout the ventricular wall. The left bundle branch has three subdivisions: the posterior fascicle, septal fascicle, and anterior fascicle. These structures conduct electrical impulses over the larger muscle mass of the left ventricle in a time period similar to the right ventricle. These fascicle branches also terminate in Purkinje fibers in the ventricular walls (James, 1963).

CELLULAR ULTRASTRUCTURE AND FUNCTION

Cardiac muscle must generate the pressure and force needed to move the blood through the circulatory system. The atria and ventricles are comprised of bundles of myocardial cells that are aligned in the same direction (Warner, Russel, and Span, 1972). However, adjacent bundles of muscles may take a different course through the heart. Therefore when the heart is examined microscopically, muscle bundles appearing to swirl around the length of different heart chambers are seen.

The myocardial cells are unique. For example, each cell is small, 30 to 60 μm in length and 10 to 15 μm in diameter (Braunwald, Ross, and Sonnenblick, 1967), and contains significantly more mitochondria than other cells. These mitochondria provide adenosine triphosphate (ATP), which supplies the energy necessary for the muscle to contract.

Each myocardial cell contains multiple contractile units called sarcomeres. Sarcomeres are lined up in the cell in parallel rows along the long axis of the cell (Warner, Russell, and Spann, 1972). They have different bands of light and dark reflecting elements, which provide microscopic landmarks for studying all contractions. It is significant that these bands are made up of the contractile elements actin and myosin, which lengthen and shorten by forming biochemical cross-bridges. The formation of these cross-bridges is dependent on the ionic transfer of potassium and sodium and the release of calcium. Calcium is stored and released by the T-tubules, which are located within the myocardium. The length change of countless actin and myosin filaments is mediated by electrochemical changes. The formation of these cross-bridges causes the muscle cell shortening that generates the pressure that pumps blood out of the heart.

A final important anatomical characteristic of cardiac muscle is the presence of intercalated discs. The function of these discs is to reduce the electrical resistance that facilitates the transmission of the electrical impulse from one myocardial cell to another. Because the ions flow easily along the axes of the myocardial fibers, the action potential is propagated from one cell to the next past the intercalated discs (Guyton, 1981). As a result the myocardium is a functional syncytium. Thus when one cell in the atria or ventricles becomes excited, the action potential spreads throughout the chamber. The atria act as one syncytium and the ventricles as another.

PROPERTIES OF CARDIAC MUSCLE

The specialized conductive and contractile cells in the heart possess physiological properties that are clinically relevant. Cardiac tissue has the following properties: conductivity, automaticity, rhythmicity, excitability, and contractility.

Conductivity refers to the movement of an impulse from one cardiac cell to another. The conductive property of the heart is anatomically based; the intercalated discs and the conduction system contribute to the rapid spreading of impulses.

Automaticity is the ability of the cardiac muscle to spontaneously originate electrical impulses. In the conduction system there are electrolyte fluctuations that allow an impulse to occur at regular intervals. In other words, the impulse starts within the cardiac cell without an external stimulus. However, automaticity can be influenced by the parasympathetic and sympathetic nervous systems.

Rhythmicity is a property of cardiac muscle that allows impulses to be evenly spaced. The rhythm of the heart is externally influenced by the vagus nerve and sympathetic nerve fibers. These fibers affect the rate of impulse firing of the SA node.

Excitability is the response of the cardiac muscle to an electrical impulse. The spread of this excitation is a result of the unique electrolyte balance and the sodium pump within the myocardium. The section on electrophysiology details the spread of the electrical impulse and the subsequent mechanical events.

Contractility is the manner in which cardiac muscles shorten in response to a stimulus. Starling's law of the heart describes the normal physiological contractile response to ventricular blood volume. This law states that the amount of myocardial fiber stretched by blood filling the heart will determine the amount of muscle shortening. This

---

Drugs affecting cardiac contractility

Positive inotropic agents
Cardiac glycosides
  Digitalis preparations (most commonly used drug)
Adrenergics
  Dobutamine
  Dopamine hydrochloride
  Epinephrine
  Norepinephrine
  Isoproterenol

Negative inotropic agents
Anti-arrhythmics (decrease force of contraction)
  Propranolol
  Quinidine
  Lidocaine
  Disopyramide*

*Disopyramide is the most negatively inotropic agent.

muscle shortening increases the contractile force of the ventricle. In short, the more blood that fills the ventricle during diastole (end-diastolic volume), the greater will be the force of the muscular contraction. However, there is an optimal filling point, and once physiological limits are reached, increasing end-diastolic volume will not increase contractility or subsequent stroke volume.

Contractility may also be altered by the presence of biochemical agents. These agents are called either positive or negative inotropic agents. Positive inotropic agents (e.g., norepinephrine and digitalis) increase cardiac contractility. Negative agents (quinidine and propranolol) decrease cardiac contractility (Graboys, 1979).

ELECTROPHYSIOLOGY

Transmission of the impulse that stimulates heart muscle contraction is by way of a series of electrochemical events. These events must precede muscle contraction. The basis for these events is the semipermeable cardiac cell membrane that maintains an electrical disequilibrium between the inside and the outside of the cell and requires energy. Prominent electrolytes involved in the electrochemical events of the heart are cations (positively charged ions): sodium, potassium, and calcium.

Resting membrane potential

The resting cardiac cell has a -90 mV charge. This electrical charge is created by the concentration of cations and anions on either side of the cell wall. In the resting cardiac cell the potassium is about 140 mEq/L. Outside the cell wall the potassium level is about 3.5 to 5.0 mEq/L (Tilkian, Converse, and Tilkian, 1979). The semipermeable

---

Terminology of electrophysiology

ions Positively or negatively charged atoms or groups of atoms.
anion Negative ion.
cation Positive ion.
polarization A situation in which there are more negative ions inside a cell than outside.
depolarization The process by which a cardiac cell loses its negative charge.
repolarization The process by which a cardiac cell regains its negative charge.
action potential A period of electrical depolarization and repolarization.
threshold A point of depolarization that must be reached before an impulse can be transmitted.
millivolts (mV) A measure of electrical charge; 1 mV equals 0.001 volt.
milliequivalent (mEq) A measure of the concentration of ions. It is related to electrical charge. "One equivalent" means one molecular weight of ions; 1 mEq equals 0.001 equivalent.

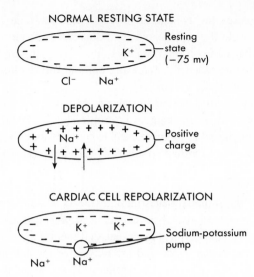

NORMAL RESTING STATE

Resting state (−75 mv)

K⁺

Cl⁻   Na⁺

DEPOLARIZATION

Positive charge

Na⁺

CARDIAC CELL REPOLARIZATION

K⁺   K⁺

Sodium-potassium pump

Na⁺   Na⁺

Fig. 2-5. Cellular electrophysiology. (From Pathophysiology: Clinical Concepts of Disease Processes by S. Price and L. Wilson. © 1978 McGraw-Hill Book Company. Used with permission of McGraw-Hill Book Company.)

cell membrane prevents potassium from diffusing down its concentration gradient and out of the cell. Sodium concentration outside the cell wall is about 140 mEq/L. Intracellularly the concentration is 10 mEq/L (Tilkian, Converse, and Tilkian, 1979). The tendency of sodium to flow down its concentration gradient is also counteracted by the semipermeable membrane. Therefore a polarity exists between the two sides of the cell membrane. The outer side has a positive electrical charge and the inner side has a negative electrical charge (Fig. 2-5). With this ionic difference, electrical current can flow from one cell to another (Conover, 1980).

Action potential

As long as the cellular walls of the myocardium are undisturbed the resting membrane potential remains at −90 mV. A stimulus of the cell membrane will increase the permeability of the cell membrane to sodium and potassium. This stimulus is called the action potential and occurs in two separate stages: depolarization and repolarization.

During depolarization the cardiac cell membrane becomes more permeable to cations. Sodium and potassium move down their concentration gradients. The actual number of ions that enter or leave the cell is very small and is entirely separate from the action potential or depolarization of the cell membrane. Almost immediately after depolarization the cellular membrane again becomes impermeable to sodium and potassium. This is the phase of rapid repolarization when the cell membrane potential ap-

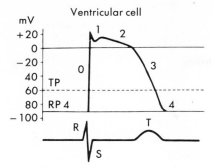

Fig. 2-6. Action potential. *TP*, threshold potential; *RP*, resting potential. (From Conover, M.H.: Understanding electrocardiography: physiological and interpretive concepts, ed. 3, St. Louis, 1981, The C.V. Mosby Co.)

proaches the resting state, -90 mV (Fig. 2-6). During final repolarization the small number of potassium ions that were extruded are pumped into the cell, and the excess sodium is removed via the sodium-potassium ATP-dependent pump.

All or none principle

Each cardiac cell transmits the flow of current from one cell to another. This characteristic is called the "all or none principle" of cardiac muscle. The basis for this characteristic is the cardiac cell wall anatomy that reduces impedence to electrical flow. The concept of the functional syncytium is demonstrated by the all or none principle.

Normally action potentials originate in the SA node from pacemaker cells. The resting membrane potential of these cells is less negative than other cardiac cells, which is attributed to a slow, constant, inward leak of calcium. This leak prevents the attainment of a normal resting potential, and the cells' resting potential gradually increases to -40 mV. This causes an action potential to fire and be conducted throughout the heart.

Conduction of action potentials

The normal conduction pathway provides a timed sequence of delivery action potentials to the cardiac cells. The SA node originates the impulse and sends it down the internodal tracts and Bachmann's bundle, and the many cells of the atria begin depolarizing. The action potential is delayed at the AV node for a fraction of a second, thereby allowing the atria to contract before the ventricles (Cranefield, 1975). After the delay, the action potential then resumes its speed through the ventricular conduction pathways (the bundle of His and Purkinje fibers). Then the depolarization events occur throughout the ventricles.

Electrocardiogram

Normally in the clinical setting the measurement of individual action potentials is not done. The electrocardiogram, a timed map of how the action potentials spread through the heart, is used instead. The electrocardiogram (ECG) is a useful assessment tool that provides data about the electrochemical activities, heart rate, and integrity of the conduction pathway.

Before a map can be followed, reference points are needed. The main reference points of the electrocardiogram are the P, Q, R, S, and T waves. Each of these has a particular significance. The P wave represents atrial depolarization. The QRS configuration represents ventricular depolarization. The T wave represents the repolarization of the ventricle. The relationship between the ECG points and the heart's conduction system is illustrated in Fig. 2-7.

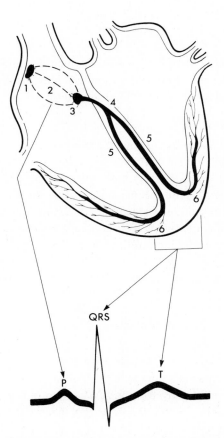

Fig. 2-7. ECG waves as they relate to the depolarization and repolarization of the conduction system. (From Harris, C.C.: A primer of cardiac arrhythmias, St. Louis, 1979, The C.V. Mosby Co.)

Excitation-contraction coupling

Depolarization is not muscle contraction, but rather is the electrical stimulus for the mechanical event of muscle contraction. The process by which depolarization causes the muscle to shorten is called excitation-contraction coupling, which is the basis of the heart's pumping activity.

This process is not fully understood. The current theory is that there are channels in the cardiac cell membrane that become electrically excited. Excitation causes the tubules to release calcium intracellularly during phase one and two of the action potential. Calcium then reacts with the chemicals troponin and tropomyosin (Weeks, 1981). In the presence of calcium, troponin and tropomyosin form chemical cross-bridges between the actin and myosin filaments (Katz, 1970). The creation of these interconnecting cross-bridges shortens the length of the cardiac cell by drawing the actin and myosin filaments physically closer together. After shortening occurs, repolarization removes calcium, which breaks the cross-bridges. The amount of calcium is thought to influence the force of contraction (Langer, 1973). A calcium deficit will depress cardiac function. It is rare for the calcium level to be elevated enough to affect the heart, since calcium precipitates in bone or other tissues. Intravenous calcium may be given as a therapeutic measure because of its positive inotropic effect on the myocardium (Metheny and Snively, 1979).

THE CARDIAC CYCLE

The cardiac cycle is the sum total of all the events occurring from one heartbeat to the next (Guyton, 1981). The term *cardiac cycle* refers primarily to the relationship between electrical and mechanical events. Heart sounds that accompany these processes serve as reference points of the cycle. Each of these events is interrelated and time sequenced. Understanding the cardiac cycle gives the nurse an integrated view of the heart's dynamic activities.

The cardiac cycle is best understood by visualizing the different events (Fig. 2-8). Note that the figure is broadly divided into two parts: ventricular diastole and systole. The length of diastole and systole varies depending upon the heart rate. At a normal heart rate of 72 beats/min, diastole is longer than systole. The cardiac cycle simply interrelates the cardiac physiology with the time sequence of systole and diastole.

Diastole

Diastole is the period of ventricular relaxation and filling. During diastole the metabolic needs of both ventricles are met. In the early portion of diastole, following the T wave, the cross-bridges of actin and myosin disengage and the myocardial cells lengthen. The ventricular chambers relax and aortic and pulmonic valves close, making the second heart sound (S_2). When ventricular relaxation occurs to the point that atrial pressures are greater than ventricular pressures, the atrioventricular valves open. Blood then flows passively, rapidly filling the ventricles. During this time of rapid filling, an abnormal heart sound (S_3) may be heard. This is a pathological sound in adults over the age of 30 years (Malasanos, 1981).

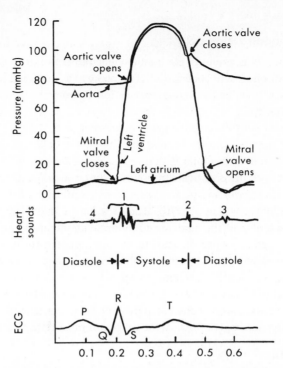

Fig. 2-8. Diagram of the cardiac cycle, showing electrocardiac events, heart sounds, and pressure curves. (From Cardiology for Nurses by N. Wenger, J.W. Hurst, and M.G. McIntyre. © 1980 McGraw-Hill Book Company. Used with permission of McGraw-Hill Book Company.)

The cardiac cycle

cardiac cycle Sum total of electrical, mechanical, volume, and pressure events occurring from ventricular systole to ventricular systole.

diastole Period of ventricular relaxation.

systole Period of ventricular contraction.

stroke volume Difference between end-diastolic and end-systolic volume of the heart.

end-diastolic volume Amount of blood in ventricles after atrioventricular valves close (preload).

end-systolic volume Amount of blood in ventricles after semilunar valves close.

isovolumetric contraction All four valves are closed, and volume in ventricles remains constant. Pressure is increasing in readiness for ejection of stroke volume.

isovolumetric relaxation All four valves are closed, and volume in ventricles remains constant. Ventricular pressures are decreased after ejection of stroke volume.

cardiac output Product of heart rate times stroke volume: $CO = SV \times HR$.

In late diastole, the SA node depolarizes and initiates a wave of atrial depolarization and contraction. This contraction, called the atrial kick, adds an additional 20% to the volume of the ventricles. The blood volume now in the ventricles, the end-diastolic volume, determines the degree of work the ventricles can perform, according to Starling's law of the heart. The ventricular pressure now exceeds the atrial pressure and both atrioventricular valves close. Systole is about to begin.

Systole

Systole is the period of ventricular contraction. It is initiated when the depolarizing impulse that was slightly delayed by the AV node enters the bundle of His. This impulse travels through the bundle of His and its branches, terminating in the Purkinje fibers. As the cells depolarize, calcium causes the actin and myosin cross-bridges to form, and ventricular contraction ensues. At first, the pressures generated by contraction are not high enough to open the aortic and pulmonic valves. This early phase of systole is called isovolumic contraction since all four valves are closed.

As systole progresses, the pressure increases until it becomes greater than the pressure in the great vessels on both the right and left side. The pulmonic and aortic valves open, and blood is ejected outward into the pulmonary and systemic circulation. This period of ejection coincides with the absolute refractory period. The amount of blood ejected into the aorta and pulmonary artery is called the stroke volume, which is equal to approximately 70 ml. As ejection of the left ventricular contents is complete, the pressure in the ventricle falls, and the aortic and pulmonic valves close. When aortic or pulmonary artery pressures exceed the left or right ventricular pressures, respectively, diastole occurs.

ALTERATIONS IN THE MYOCARDIUM

Shock causes a number of alterations in the body's functioning that affect the heart. In order for the patient with shock to survive, either the heart must compensate alone, or therapeutic measures to maximize cardiac functioning must be initiated. Alterations of the heart that may occur during shock include ionic imbalances, excessive oxygen consumption, and impaired stroke volume. These are particularly significant because they are the target of medical and nursing intervention for the shock patient.

Electrolyte imbalances

Serum potassium levels are often elevated in shock. *Hyperkalemia* can result from impaired renal function, metabolic acidosis, and excessive blood transfusion. High levels of potassium increase the positive charge on the outside of the cardiac cell. This increased positive charge depresses the formation of action potentials and results in bradycardia. If the potassium level remains excessive, asystole will ensue.

Hypokalemia can occur in the shock patient as a result of excessive use of potassium-wasting diuretics, excessive diarrhea, vomiting, or prolonged nasogastric suctioning. A lower extracellular concentration of potassium leads to increased discharge of action potentials by the cardiac cells, resulting in cardiac irritability and arrhythmias. Premature beats are particularly common with hypokalemia. A weak irregular pulse is a common assessment finding (Fletcher, 1980).

Hypercalcemia in the shock patient may be caused by acidosis, hyperparathyroidism, or metabolic disease. In contrast to hyperkalemia, hypercalcemia causes excitation of the cardiac muscle. This excitation can result in an elevated heart rate. If the imbalance is pronounced, spastic contraction of the heart may occur.

In the shock patient *hypocalcemia* can result from chronic renal failure, malabsorption, or hypoparathyroidism. Hypocalcemia causes weakened muscular contractions. This is related to the role of calcium in forming the actin and myosin cross-bridges that shorten the muscle. The pulse of a person with hypocalcemia would be diminished in strength.

Ionic imbalances disturb the critical timing of the electrical and mechanical events of the cardiac cycle. The nurse should be aware of how these imbalances affect the heart. The electrocardiogram can be of value in identifying electrolyte imbalances (Table 2-1). Serum electrolyte values should be monitored frequently in the shock patient.

Excessive oxygen consumption

In a patient with shock, the heart is stimulated by the sympathetic nervous system to contract with increased force and at a higher rate. These actions increase cardiac output and are adaptive mechanisms in shock. However, the activation of the sympathetic nervous system also causes increased oxygen consumption by the myocardium that can compromise the functioning of the heart.

Inadequate oxygen delivery to the heart muscle can be the causative factor of cardiogenic shock or can accompany other types of shock. If the heart is unable to provide enough oxygenated blood to meet its own demands, a vicious cycle will result. When the cardiac muscle becomes ischemic, electrical irritability develops and cardiac arrhythmias occur. These arrhythmias impair the proper timing of the filling and pressure events of the cardiac cycle. Arrhythmias further compromise the delivery of adequate oxygen to the cardiac muscle, decreasing the force of muscle contraction (Dracup, Breu, and Tillish, 1981). When the sympathetic nervous system elevates the heart rate excessively, diastole will be shortened, which results in decreased end-diastolic volume and diminished stroke volume.

Stroke volume in shock

The amount of blood that the ventricles eject with each contraction (stroke volume) is determined by three factors: preload, afterload, and contractility. Any or all of these factors can be altered in shock. Preload is the volume of blood that stretches the ventricular muscles at the end of diastole (Dracup, Breu, and Tillish, 1981). This volume results from the amount of blood returning to the heart from the venous system and the amount of blood that remains in the ventricle after systole. The event of preload exemplifies Starling's law of the heart. As end-diastolic volume (preload) increases, so does

Table 2-1. Electrolyte imbalances

Electrolyte	ECG findings	Check points
Potassium (normal range: 3.5-5 mEq/L)		
Hyperkalemia	Heart rate may decrease P wave widens if potassium level is over 7.5 QRS complex widens T wave is tall and peaked	1. Make sure the IV fluids contain no potassium. 2. Check the BUN and creatinine levels for data about renal function. 3. Check medications for potassium content. 4. Restrict potassium foods if level is critical.
Hypokalemia	Heart rate may increase P wave has no change QRS complex has no change ST segment is sagging T wave shows flattening and inversion	1. Check for excessive loss of body fluids; vomiting, diarrhea. 2. Assess for use of potassium-wasting diuretics. 3. If digitalis is being given, assess for toxic effects.
Calcium (normal range: ionized, 2.1-2.6 mEq/L; total, 4.5-5.3 mEq/L)		
Hypercalcemia	Heart rate may increase ST segment shortens T wave rounds Ectopic arrhythmias	1. Check for history of bone metastatic disease. 2. Monitor pH of blood.
Hypocalcemia	Heart rate may decrease QT interval is prolonged	1. Check the BUN and creatinine levels for data about renal function. 2. Check for history of parathyroid disease.

the stretch of the cardiac muscles. This increased stretch improves ventricular functioning by allowing more actin and myosin cross-bridges to form.

In shock, preload may need to be reduced or increased depending on the pumping ability of the heart. Pulmonary artery and pulmonary artery wedge pressures provide the basis for decisions about treatments that manipulate preload. Elevated preload values suggest congestion and inadequate emptying of the ventricles. This condition is most commonly seen in cardiogenic shock. Pharmacological therapies, such as diuretics and vasodilators, can reduce preload. These drugs reduce the preload by either increasing urine production (decreasing intravascular volume) or increasing venous capacitance.

Decreasing preload in the failing heart can actually improve cardiac functioning. This improvement is attributed to the resultant decrease in oxygen consumption of the over-distended ventricles.

When assessment reveals lowered preload values, decreased venous return is usually noted. Decreased venous return is particularly associated with hypovolemic, septic, and anaphylactic shock. However, it can occur in any type of shock. Preload can be elevated by increased infusion of intravenous fluids and plasma-expander colloids.

Afterload is related to the pressure the ventricle must overcome to eject blood. Afterload is controlled by the valves separating the ventricles from the great vessels and the resistance of the vascular system. These structures impede blood ejection. An indirect measure of afterload is the blood pressure.

Afterload is largely controlled by the sympathetic constriction of the arterial system. The higher the pressure in the arterial system, the more work it takes to pump the blood from the ventricle. The myocardium must generate pressure by increasing ventricular muscular tension to overcome afterload. By doing this the heart must generate increased tension that impairs muscle shortening, thus requiring more force to eject the blood.

In shock, interventions may be directed toward changing afterload. If afterload is increased, vasodilators, such as nitroprusside, are given to decrease resistance and thus decrease the heart's workload. Stroke volume can then be ejected with less oxygen expenditure by the myocardium. When afterload is decreased during shock, the arteries offer no resistance to cardiac contraction, and thus perfusion is compromised. Perfusion pressures are essential for nutrient exchange in the capillaries. Afterload can be increased by utilizing sympathomimetic agents that cause arterial vasoconstriction, such as dopamine hydrochloride.

In summary, contractility is the interaction between ionic balance, sympathetic nervous system activity, and oxygen supply. If the contractility of the heart is increased, more stroke volume is ejected. If contractility is decreased, stroke volume is decreased. Contractility can be either increased or decreased in shock. This is primarily caused by the interaction of the aforementioned factors. Positive inotropic agents that maximize contractility are given if necessary but may increase the amount of oxygen needed by the ventricle.

The pumping ability of the heart can be the critical determinant of survival for the patient in shock. Therefore the nurse needs a working knowledge of the heart's specialized features and cyclic events. Nursing interventions are directed toward facilitating normal cardiac functioning and maximizing the heart's adaptive capacity.

REFERENCES

Berne, R.M., and Levy, M.N.: Cardiovascular physiology, ed. 4, St. Louis, 1981, The C.V. Mosby Co.

Braunwald, E., Ross, J., and Sonnenblick, E.: Mechanisms of contraction of the normal and failing heart. Part I, New England Journal of Medicine **277:**794-800, 1967.

Brecher, G., and Galletti, P.: Functional anatomy of cardiac pumping. In Hamilton, W.F., editor: Handbook of physiology, vol. 2, Baltimore, 1963, The Williams & Wilkins Co.

Conover, M.B.: Understanding electrocardiography: physiological and interpretive concepts, ed. 3, St. Louis, 1980, The C.V. Mosby Co.

Cranefield, P.F.: The conduction of the cardiac impulse, New York, 1975, Futura Publishing Co., Inc.

Dracup, K.A., Breu, C.S., and Tillish, J.A.: The physiological basis for combined nitroprusside-dopamine therapy in post-myocardial infarction heart failure, Heart & Lung **10:**114-120, 1981.

Duggan, S.A.: Cardiovascular anatomy, physiology and assessment. In Halfman, M.A., editor: Proceedings of the seventh annual 1980 National Teaching Institute, Irvine, Calif., 1980, American Association of Critical Care Nurses.

Fisch, C.: Relation of electrolyte disturbances to cardiac arrhythmias, Circulation **47:**408-418, 1973.

Fletcher, G.F.: Less common causes of heart disease. In Wenger, N.K., Hurst, J.W., and McIntyre, M., editors: Cardiology for nurses, New York, 1980, McGraw-Hill Book Co.

Fuller, E.O.: The effect of antianginal drugs on myocardial oxygen consumption, American Journal of Nursing **80:**250-254, 1980.

Graboys, T.B.: Clinical pharmacology of antiarrhythmic agents, Heart and Lung **8:**706-710, 1979.

Grossman, W., and Lambert, L.P.: Diastolic properties of the left ventricle, Annals of Internal Medicine **84:**316-325, 1976.

Guyton, A.C.: Textbook of medical physiology, Philadelphia, 1981, W.B. Saunders Co.

Harris, C.C.: A primer of cardiac arrhythmias: a self-instructional program, St. Louis, 1979, The C.V. Mosby Co.

Holt, J.P.: The normal pericardium, American Journal of Cardiology **26:**455-463, 1970.

James, T.N.: The connecting pathways between the sinus node and AV node and between the right and left atriums in the human heart, American Heart Journal **66:**498-508, 1963.

Johnson, E.A., and Lieborman, M.: Heart: excitation and contraction, Annual Review of Physiology **33:** 479-528, 1971.

Katz, A.M.: Contractile proteins of the heart, Physiology Review **50:**63-158, 1970.

Langer, G.A.: Heart: excitation-contraction coupling, Annual Review of Physiology **35:**55-80, 1973.

Malasanos, L., et al.: Health assessment, ed. 2, St. Louis, 1981, The C.V. Mosby Co.

Mason, D.T., Spann, J.F., and Zelis, R.: Quantification of the contractile state of the intact human heart, The American Journal of Cardiology **26:**248-257, 1970.

Metheny, N., and Snively, W.: Nurses' handbook of fluid balance, ed. 3, Philadelphia, 1979, J.B. Lippincott Co.

Silverman, M.E., and Schlant, R.C.: Anatomy of the normal heart and blood vessels. In Hurst, J.W., et al., editors: The heart, ed. 4, New York, 1978, McGraw-Hill Book Co.

Skorga, P., and Nunnery, C.: How to spot and care for patient with Lown-Ganong-Levine syndrome, Nursing '81 **11:**37-42, 1981.

Surawicz, B.: Relationship between electrocardiogram and electrolytes, American Heart Journal **73:** 814-820, 1967.

Tilkian, S.M., Conover, M.B., and Tilkian, A.G.: Clinical implications of laboratory tests, St. Louis, 1979, The C.V. Mosby Co.

Warner, H.F., Russell, M.W., and Spann, J.F.: Heart muscle: clinical applications of basic physiology and cellular anatomy, Heart & Lung **1:**494-507, 1972.

Weber, K.T.: Introduction: physiologic and clinical correlates, The American Journal of Cardiology **44:** 719-720, 1979.

Weeks, L.C.: Cardiovascular physiology. In Kinney, M., et al., editors: AACN's clinical reference for critical care nursing, New York, 1981, McGraw-Hill Book Co.

3 Microcirculation

PATRICIA POTTER

Despite all the intricacies of the systemic circulation that have been described, in terms of cell life, the microcirculation is the most vital division of the circulatory system. The term *microcirculation* is not used simply in the context of a structural definition to describe the microscopic vessels comprising it, but rather it describes a group of blood vessels within the tissues that, as an independent organic unit, regulates blood supply to the tissues. The exchange of nutrients to and the removal of wastes from cells is only part of the function served by the microcirculation. It is designed with the capacity to adjust blood flow in relation to the changing metabolic needs of tissues. Fluid movement across the enormous surface area of the microcirculation is required for the maintenance of osmotic equilibrium in the tissue environment, the facilitation of large molecular movement such as protein through the interstitium, and the regulation of total blood volume (Intaglietta and Zweifach, 1974). Cellular life could not be maintained without the efficient functioning of the microcirculation.

The form and function of the circulatory system are interdependent, and anatomy clearly reflects the physiology of the part (Sobin and Tremer, 1977). The structural organization of the microcirculation is comprised of vessels with unique functionally determined properties. A superficial examination of the microcirculation of different organs shows striking differences related to the functional role of each organ. Yet each vascular unit works in concert with the others to achieve a delicate balance between blood flow and tissue demand. Stabilizing the internal environment of tissue beds requires a precise regulation of the microcirculation. The characteristic ebb and flow of blood moving through the microvasculature is a hallmark of physiological adaptation. When a threat exists to this constancy of blood flow, as in the case of shock, the autonomic nervous system, by modulating vascular tone, assists in the regulation of the microcirculation by controlling the amount of flow delivered to a particular body tissue. Humoral, chemical, and metabolic influences also act to control the microcirculation. The microcirculation is sensitive to the changing metabolic demands of the body's tissues. Any threat to the physiological equilibrium of cellular metabolism will initiate an adaptive response from the microcirculation to improve cellular perfusion.

The role the microcirculation plays in fluid exchange and balance is likewise complex. The microcirculation functions as a biological barrier between the physiological compartments of blood, tissue, and lymph to promote an exchange of substances and to maintain vessel wall integrity (Hauck, 1971). Capillary fluid exchange is regulated by precise interacting mechanisms. Theories to explain the nature of these mechanisms are currently the subject of much research. During the initial stages of any form of shock, the microcirculation becomes a major site of involvement. The delicate nature of microcirculatory physiology should alert the nurse to the widespread influence shock may have. A look into the dynamics of microcirculatory function and regulation provides the nurse with a foundation for understanding shock pathology. Understanding the effects of shock at the cellular level equips the nurse with knowledge necessary for quick assessment and intervention. Likewise it prepares the nurse to anticipate the effects various medical therapies have on the patient's physiological status.

COMPONENTS OF MICROCIRCULATION

A simple definition of what comprises the microcirculation might be: that portion of the vascular bed lying between the arterioles and venules. Chapter 1 notes that beyond the larger arteries blood pressure drops rapidly and the velocity of blood flow is reduced. Vascular pulsations diminish and blood flow changes into a more steady flow as it approaches the capillary bed. There are no distinct boundaries existing between the small vessels comprising the microcirculation. It is important to know that the arrangement and distribution of the microcirculation differs from tissue to tissue, depending on tissue architecture and function. However, the pattern almost uniformly appears to be a variation of that described by Zweifach (1961), who developed the premise that all circulatory beds share certain common structural features (Fig. 3-1). The arrangement of the microcirculation permits large changes in the total amount of blood flow through tissue, as well as the course of that flow.

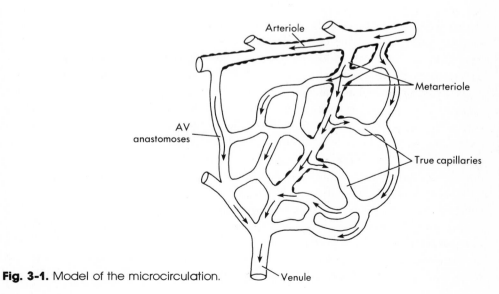

Fig. 3-1. Model of the microcirculation.

Arterioles

Structurally the most prominent landmark of the microcirculatory bed is its arteriolar parent trunk, which gives rise to all other microcirculatory components. The arterioles are small arteries containing up to three layers of smooth muscle. As the arterioles enter the terminal vascular bed, they are already of capillary dimensions but are easily recognized by the high velocity of the blood flow and by their scalloped appearance that is created by the presence of vascular smooth muscle (Zweifach, 1977). These small arterial vessels are also comprised of elastin and collagen fibers that provide the vessels with the property to change diameter size and thereby alter blood flow. These vessels serve not only to direct blood flow to the capillary beds but also to control the pressure of blood delivered to those beds. The capacity of the arterioles to adjust blood flow is a function of vasomotor influences. The arterioles are the first to respond to the hemodynamic assault of shock.

Metarterioles

Blood does not flow directly from arterioles to venules by way of the capillaries. The main path is through thoroughfare channels called the metarterioles (precapillary arterioles). The metarterioles are side branches that leave the arterioles at right angles. Smooth muscle cells coat the metarterioles proximally as they leave the arterioles. This layer of smooth muscle cells is discontinuous along the course of the vessel (Mountcastle, 1980). The smooth muscle cells disappear distally as the vessels approach the true capillaries. The presence of smooth muscle cells provides the metarterioles with active diameter control and serves to regulate the entrance of blood into the capillary network.

Precapillary sphincters

At the point where the true capillaries branch off from the metarterioles often there can be found one or two smooth muscle cells. These muscular junctions called the precapillary sphincters are the only muscular part of a true capillary. The sphincter is a significant structural component responsible for the selective distribution of blood within the capillaries. In effect, contraction of a precapillary sphincter removes the true capillaries from active circulation. This vasoconstrictor activation can close off arterioles, resulting in a decreased perfusion of groups of capillaries fed by the arterioles and a decreased capillary exchange surface area (Rosell and Belfrage, 1975). The action of the precapillary sphincter is functionally significant when the metabolic needs of tissue change. In the case of shock, when perfusion of vital organs is threatened, shunting redirects blood to the tissue bed that is in greater need of blood flow. Although the sphincters can be found in many tissues, there are others (e.g., skeletal muscles) wherein the control for blood distribution to the capillaries depends on the larger arterioles. For this reason researchers differ as to the main structure credited with controlling blood flow distribution (Duling, 1978; Zweifach, 1974). Zweifach (1974) suggested that the branching network of the microcirculation represents the regulatory mechanism for capillary blood flow. He has credited the pressure drop and resistance in the branching system as a function of the parent arterioles and branching vessels. Crone (1975) suggested that the control mechanism actually resided in the entire metarteriole. Despite the disagreement over the exact location of the control site, it is evident there is a mechanism located in the vicinity of the minute arterioles that carefully regulates blood flow distribution.

Capillaries

Branching from the metarterioles there is a network of capillaries. In organs with a high metabolic rate the number of branching capillaries is greater (Wolff, 1977). This branching increases the surface area for greater fluid and nutrient exchange and for the lowering of blood flow velocity to prolong transport time through the capillaries.

Blood entering the true capillaries is surrounded by thin-walled endothelial tubes that are void of smooth muscle and adventitial layers. True capillaries contain no true contractile properties. Regarding circulatory regulation, the capillaries do not respond to vasoactive chemicals, electrical or mechanical stimulation, or pressure across their walls. The endothelial cells are permeable to lipid-soluble materials, such as gases and steroids that diffuse readily across the capillary wall. This is caused by the lipid content found within the cell walls. In contrast, the blood capillary wall acts as a selective filter for water-soluble materials such as water, sugars, and various ions. Water-soluble materials evidently pass through the capillaries by different routes or mechanisms. The range of selectivity seen in capillaries varies considerably in different tissues. Capillaries with seemingly identical structural features have different permeabilities. This consideration leads to a discussion of the pore theory of capillary exchange.

The pore theory, supported by the early work of Pappenheimer (1951) and Soloman (1968), suggested that water-filled channels (pores) could be found within the capillary endothelium. These pores were believed to functionally serve to allow water-soluble materials to cross over the endothelial barrier. The vascular endothelium is highly permeable to water and water-soluble molecules as well as water-soluble macromolecules (e.g., proteins). The fact that a small amount of protein continuously permeates capillaries and venules into the interstitium suggests the presence of some type of larger pore. Intaglietta and Zweifach (1974) have suggested that large pores are present mostly in the venous portion of the capillary network, which explains the high permeability of the venules.

An additional proposed mechanism for fluid transport across capillary walls is micropinocytosis. This active transport mechanism carries elements across the capillary membrane barrier in vesicles formed from invaginations of the cell membrane (Fig. 3-2, A). The vesicles function in two ways: (1) as mass carriers of fluid and solutes across the endothelium and (2) as creators of transendothelial channels by fusion with the vessel lumen (Palade, Simionescu, and Simionescu, 1979). The existence of numerous endothelial cell vesicles suggest these structures serve as transport pathways for large molecules and small water-soluble materials. Their function as small or large pores depends on the porosity of their diaphragms and the size of local strictures along their pathway (Palade, Simionescu, and Simionescu, 1979). Functionally the vesicles act to increase the surface area of the vascular endothelium. The distance across the endo-

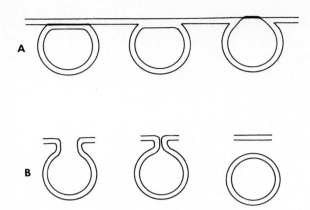

Fig. 3-2. A, Diagram of stages assumed to be involved in the process of membrane fusion-fision. **B,** Diagram presenting assumed steps in the process of detachment of vesicles. (From Palade, G.E., M. Simionescu, & N. Simionescu. Structural Aspects of the Permeability of the Microvascular Endothelium. *Acta Physiologica Scandinavica.* 1979, Suppl. 463, 11-32. Uppsala, Sweden: Almquist and Wiksell.)

thelium (pathway for diffusion) is reduced by the diameter of one or two vesicles. Fig. 3-2, *B,* reveals the stages involved in the membrane fusion-fission process of vesicle formation.

Bendayan, Sandborn, and Rasio (1976) proposed the existence of an intracellular tubular system that allows bulk transport across cells and increases by many times the cell surface area. This system resembles that of the vesicular system in theory, whereby both provide a pathway for intracellular and transcellular transport and provide an increased cell surface area. The classical concept of a uniform permeability of the capillary bed in terms of similar pore structure throughout tissues has been discounted. Not only do permeabilities differ, but the vehicles for transcellular exchange also vary considerably.

Mountcastle (1980) and Wolff (1977) have described three different kinds of capillary walls: continuous, fenestrated, and discontinuous (Table 3-1). The continuous capillary wall is a continuous membrane of endothelial cells containing intercellular channels that connect the capillary with the surrounding interstitial space. These intercellular channels resemble micropinocytic vesicles. The continuous capillaries are the most common type of capillary seen in the tissues and can be found in skeletal and smooth muscle, heart, fat, and connective tissue.

Fenestrated capillaries are found in highly permeable tissues and contain intracellular fenestrations. These small openings or porelike structures can be temporarily closed by very thin membranous diaphragms. The fenestrae are not static structures in that they can proliferate, particularly in inflamed tissue (Wolff, 1977). The permeability of the fenestrated capillaries is high to fluids and certain solutes.

Table 3-1. Location and morphology of three types of capillary walls

Capillary wall type	Location	Structure
Continuous	Connective tissue Fatty tissue Heart Skeletal muscle Smooth muscle	Continuous membrane of intercellular channels Capacity for enlarged surface area
Fenestrated	Choroid plexus Endocrine glands Intestinal villi Muscle fascia Renal glomeruli	Capable of proliferation High permeability
Discontinuous	Bone marrow Liver Spleen	Interrupted by large intracellular gaps Allowing exchange of blood components

The discontinuous capillaries are commonly found in the lining of sinusoids and sinuses of hematopoietic tissue. Their walls are interrupted at intervals by large intracellular gaps that allow for the free exchange of formed blood elements (e.g., red blood cells). As in the case of the other types of capillary endothelium, the discontinuous capillaries are not static. Their shape and structure can change in response to an interplay between cellular, extracellular, local, and humoral factors. The morphology of capillary walls explains the basis for the exchange and transfer of most fluids and substances.

Arteriovenous anastomoses

Another component of the microcirculation is the arteriovenous anastomoses, located on the outskirts of the capillary bed connecting arterioles directly to venules. These vessels, endowed with a smooth muscle coat and rich nerve innervation, serve as thoroughfare channels by shunting blood away from the major portion of the capillary circulation. The arteriovenous anastomoses allow blood to be directed to those tissues that are metabolically the most active and thus in greater demand for nutrition.

Venules

The final structural component in the microcirculatory system is the venules. The venous side of the terminal vascular bed has no clear distinct boundaries between venous capillaries, collecting venules, muscular venules, and small collecting veins. Intaglietta and Zweifach (1974) have clarified that the venous circulation begins where the flow pattern in the microcirculation changes from divergent, or branching, to convergent. The various types of venules may also be distinguished by their diameters. The venous capillaries empty into somewhat larger collecting venules. Lined with endothelium, the collecting venules are surrounded only by an outer sheath of collagen. No smooth muscle can be found within these venular walls. Although the venules are capable of little change in diameter size, their position is strategic in terms of postcapillary resistance, a factor significant in fluid exchange.

Like the capillaries, the venules have a large surface area, small volume capacity, and thin walls, features compatible with fluid exchange. The venules have a relatively high permeability for large molecules and a high sensitivity to vasoactive agents (e.g., histamine). This makes the venules highly susceptible to metabolic alterations present in shock. Hauck (1971) reported that the filtration rate on the venular side of the microcirculation may be two to three times that on the arterial side. This evidence has prompted conclusions that a significant amount of fluid exchange by filtration occurs on the venous side of the capillary network. It challenges the widely accepted view of microcirculatory fluid exchange described by Starling (1896).

The collecting venules flow into larger veins called the muscular venules. Smooth muscle cells can be found between the endothelium and the connective tissue of these larger vessels. Receptors for the catecholamines epinephrine and norepinephrine are found in these smooth muscle cells, giving the venules contractile properties. As a result the muscular veins play a significant role in postcapillary resistance.

CHARACTERISTICS OF BLOOD FLOW THROUGH MICROCIRCULATION

Blood flow through the capillaries is a function of pressure, the capillary itself, and the viscous resistance of blood. Characteristically blood flow through a freely open system such as a capillary bed depends on differences in total fluid energy. It is not simply the pressure difference from the arterial to the venous end, but the total fluid energy that originates from energy being absorbed by the arterial tree as blood is pumped from the myocardium. This movement of energy is a factor in creating the driving force needed to maintain tissue perfusion. Blood delivered to the microcirculation arrives as a result of this pressure differential. However, flow through the microcirculation itself does not resemble a constant even flow.

Vasomotion

At the level of a single capillary, blood flow is erratic. Red blood cells must pass through capillaries in single file. The term *vasomotion* describes the character of blood flow through the microcirculation. Baez (1977) defines vasomotion as the continuous fluctuation in the velocity and distribution of cellular elements both in the same vessel and in different vessels. The capillaries have no active contractile elements. The periodic fluctuations of flow seen in the microcirculation are caused by the partial narrowing and dilatation of terminal arterioles, metarterioles, and precapillary sphincters. Minor changes in the diameter of terminal arterioles or precapillary sphincters can cut off capillary perfusion temporarily and lead to an intermittency of blood flow. With an increase in vasomotion (increased vasomotor activity), blood flow decreases. In a basal metabolic state only a fraction of available microvessels are perfused. Vasomotion is influenced by local metabolism and myogenic and neurogenic influences. It primarily depends on the metabolic activity of tissue. With an increased metabolism, vasomotion decreases, allowing blood flow to increase and resulting in improved cellular perfusion. Vasomotion is not to be equated with autoregulation, wherein a constant perfusion of tissues is maintained under a varying range of blood pressure. However, it does assist in meeting the need for the redistribution of local blood flow to tissues. Zweifach (1977) noted that vasomotion does have a direct effect on a number of basic microcirculatory functions including volume of blood delivered, intercapillary spacing, distribution of blood within the capillaries, hydrostatic pressure within the capillaries, and therefore fluid exchange. Vasomotion can be suppressed by factors such as anesthesia, sympathetic blocking agents, or rising temperature and can be enhanced by stress, as in the case of hemorrhage (Baez, 1977). Thus in hemorrhagic shock vasomotion will increase, reducing blood flow to vital tissues.

Viscosity

The viscosity of blood is an important determinant of blood flow. Viscosity is an internal friction between adjacent fluid layers.

$$\text{Viscosity} = \frac{\text{Stress}}{\text{Shear rate}} = \frac{\text{Force/unit area}}{\text{Change in velocity}}$$

It rises when velocity of blood flow is slowed between layers (shear rate) or when the force applied is increased. Viscosity is influenced by the external factor of temperature. As the temperature falls, the viscosity of blood increases, a response seen during shock. With the increase in viscosity, blood flow through a vessel will be slowed. This becomes significant when the metabolic demands of tissues require an increased flow of blood.

In the microcirculation blood flows as a single row of red blood cells. Red blood cells in general are larger than capillaries and their deformation is necessary for passage through the capillaries. It was once assumed that low shear rates were the rule in the microcirculation, thus proving the existence of high viscosity (Rosenblum, 1977). However, such is not the case, for within the microcirculation shear rates are above the level needed for a high viscosity. Normal capillary flow is not characterized by the presence of viscous blood elements. The major exception to this is during increased vasomotion. During increased vasomotion, when intermittency of blood flow is heightened, viscosity will increase. In shock this resultant increase in viscosity makes the formation of thromboemboli more likely.

REGULATION OF MICROCIRCULATORY FLOW

Within the capillaries, blood flow is only passively influenced by physical factors such as vessel size, branching, and pressure differences. These physical factors of blood flow are not the mechanisms that provide regulation of the microcirculation. An organism does not remain in a basal metabolic state of activity. There are increased demands placed on the organism by metabolic changes and external conditions that require an adjustment of local perfusion of body tissues. Mechanisms must exist to locally regulate blood flow.

Sympathetic nervous system modulation

To assist the nurse to better understand the intricacies of autoregulation, a review of nervous control is necessary. It is impossible to generalize the nature of nervous control for all vascular beds. The mechanism of nervous control has characteristic features uniquely related to tissue function. For purposes of simplifying this explanation, the adrenergic control over integumentary tissue will serve as a useful model for discussion. The adrenergic sympathetic vasoconstriction system is the most extensive one affecting blood flow in most major organs. Furthermore this system is the efferent link to executing reflex readjustments of the blood circulation when changes in blood flow demands occur. Thus the autonomic nervous system does have an influence on the autoregulation of microcirculatory flow.

The microcirculation of the skin is supplied with alpha receptors that respond to the chemical mediators epinephrine and norepinephrine. With the release of catecholamine, adrenergic nerve fibers innervate the smooth muscle cells of the microcirculatory vessels, causing vasoconstriction. This primarily occurs on the arterial side, where the entrance of blood into the capillary network is regulated. Venous innervation is more sparse. The density and function of neural innervation vary greatly in different types of vessels. As the diameters of vessels decrease in size, the number of bundles of adrenergic terminals decrease, small arterioles usually having only two bundles (Rosell and Belfrage, 1975).

The postganglionic terminal nerve endings are a considerable distance from the vascular smooth muscle cells. The distance that a chemical transmitter must diffuse is great and can be significant when local changes occur within tissues, as in the case of edema. The general pattern of neural innervation is the same for small and large arteries. Sympathetic contraction of vascular smooth muscle results in a certain degree of tension on the vascular wall. This vascular tone is largely determined by the frequency of incoming nerve impulses. In a normal resting state adrenergic discharge contributing to the basal tone of vessels is slow. Control over the frequency of sympathetic innervation can raise or lower the resistance of vessels feeding the capillaries. Increased frequency of sympathetic innervation will raise vascular resistance, and a decreased frequency of innervation will lower resistance. The modulation of sympathetic innervation is a central mechanism for controlling local tissue perfusion.

Hemodynamic effects

The hemodynamic effects of vasomotor activity are twofold: changes in compliance of the vessel wall and changes in diameter of the blood vessel lumen. Compliance is the change in volume for a given change in pressure. A vessel that is highly compliant will increase in volume, or distend easily under a slight pressure change. As

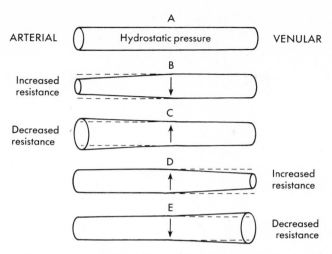

Fig. 3-3. Representation of the effects changes in precapillary and postcapillary resistance have upon intravascular hydrostatic pressure. **A,** Vessel with constant resistance on both arterial and venular ends. **B,** Arterial vasoconstriction. **C,** Arterial vasodilation. **D,** Venular vasoconstriction. **E,** Venular vasodilation. ↑, Increased pressure; ↓ decreased pressure.

vascular tone increases with vasoconstriction, the walls of involved vessels are tense and become less compliant. The combined effect of changes in vessel diameter and compliance induces an increase in the ratio of precapillary to postcapillary resistance. Vasoconstriction of arterioles increases precapillary resistance significantly. The differential effect of raising and lowering resistance is functionally important. The ratio of precapillary to postcapillary resistance influences transvascular fluid exchange and intravascular fluid volume (Fig. 3-3). When postcapillary resistance remains constant, an increased precapillary resistance reduces the volume of blood entering the capillaries. This lowers the capillary hydrostatic pressure (derived from the driving force of the heart), reducing one of the forces required for the movement of fluid out of the capillaries and into the tissues. A decreased precapillary resistance, combined with a constant postcapillary resistance, increases blood flow delivered to the capillary bed, thereby increasing hydrostatic pressure. As a result the increased hydrostatic pressure facilitates fluid movement out of the capillaries. On the postcapillary end similar changes in blood volume and pressures occur. When the precapillary resistance is held constant, an increase in postcapillary resistance traps blood within the microcirculatory bed, increasing hydrostatic pressure. Vasodilation lowers postcapillary resistance, allowing blood to leave the capillary network and lowering capillary hydrostatic pressure.

During the initial stage of shock vasoconstriction of all microcirculatory beds containing alpha receptors (skin, liver, lung, gut, and kidney) ensues. Arteriolar and venular vasoconstriction prevents fluid from entering or leaving the microcirculatory bed

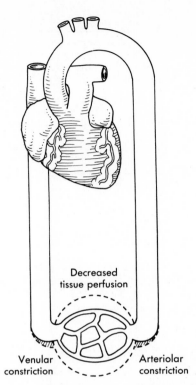

Decreased
tissue perfusion

Venular
constriction

Arteriolar
constriction

Fig. 3-4. Response of the microcirculation to the stress of shock. Initial phase of ischemic anoxia. Arteriolar and venular constriction conserve fluid volume but lower tissue perfusion.

(Fig. 3-4). There is a resultant decrease in intravascular hydrostatic pressure, whereas the colloid osmotic pressure remains unchanged. The net influx of fluid into the vascular system, known as an autotransfusion response, serves to retain circulatory volume. However, decreased tissue perfusion is a harmful side effect. The brain contains no alpha or beta receptors for sympathetic innervation. As a result the cerebral microcirculation receives the largest proportion of the shock patient's already reduced cardiac output. Because of the human organism's normal adaptive response to shock, the introduction of pharmacological agents to further promote vasoconstriction is unnecessary. Continued administration of these medications may accelerate progression from ischemic to stagnant shock.

If shock is allowed to persist for whatever cause, stagnant anoxia develops. Venular constriction persists, but arterioles begin to dilate as a result of anoxia and acidosis (Fig. 3-5). Seemingly the venules are able to resist changes in oxygen tension and pH longer than the arterioles. Blood is able to enter the microcirculation, but it cannot escape. Stagnation and pooling of blood increase hydrostatic forces, which push fluid out of the

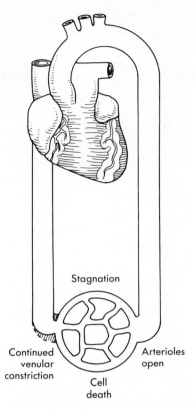

Stagnation

Continued
venular
constriction

Arterioles
open

Cell
death

Fig. 3-5. Stagnant anoxia develops if the course of shock is unabated. There is a continued venular constriction with a reduced or absent arteriolar constriction. Blood within the microcirculation cannot escape but instead is forced into surrounding tissues. Anoxia and cell death ensue.

vascular system. Edema develops within all involved microcirculatory beds, and the vasculatures membrane decays to allow seepage of red blood cells. In humans the organ found to be most sensitive to shock is the lung. Interruption of microcirculatory flow to lung tissue is believed to be the common precursor to adult respiratory distress syndrome (Chapter 12). During the stagnant phase of shock the potential for the aggregation of cellular blood components may lead to disseminated intravascular coagulation (Chapter 13).

This description of shock demonstrates that the integrity of sympathetic vasoconstrictor tone is essential to local blood flow regulation. In contrast, sympathetic cholinergic vasodilator nerves do not play such an important role. In fact, the existence of this type of nerve fiber in humans has been controversial. The precapillary portion of the microcirculatory bed, influential in regulating the number of open capillaries, is not innervated by the cholinergic vasodilator nerves. True vasodilator fibers, causing the relaxation of vascular smooth muscle, are few in number and limited in distribution. Vasodilator fibers are primarily distributed to vessels supplying skeletal muscles. Activation of these vasodilator nerves is part of the vascular adjustment associated with exercise and the defense reaction. In these situations vasodilation causes a pronounced increase in blood flow to the skeletal muscles. Simultaneously, through an integrated cardiovascular response, vasoconstriction is increased to other vascular beds, shunting blood flow to muscle fibers. Heart rate and cardiac contractility increase as adjuncts to the response.

The vascular response seen during exercise and the defense reaction is the only known role played by vasodilator fibers. Analysis shows that true vasodilator nerve fibers are not significant vasomotor influences on local blood flow.

Given an understanding of the structure of the microcirculation, the physical properties of blood flow, and nervous system innervation, the complex question of microcirculatory regulation can better be explained. The question to be raised is: Since blood flow in the microcirculation is influenced by a myriad of factors, what mechanism serves as its primary control? Local regulatory phenomena are designed to sustain the metabolic needs of tissues and to maintain tissue perfusion. These phenomena are challenged by physiological alterations such as exercise, inflammation, and shock. When changes in systemic blood pressure result in corresponding alterations in blood flow, body organs compensate through local readjustments to restore blood flow to normal. This process is known as autoregulation. Autoregulation involves the arteriolar constriction or relaxation of the terminal arterioles and metarterioles, which ensures a constant organ perfusion under conditions of varying blood pressure (Crone, 1975). Impulses from the autonomic nervous system are not the primary stimulant for control, but the modulation of vasomotor tone is the instrument of autoregulation. Through this mechanism blood flow is regulated by adjustments in the number of open capillaries, the exchange surface area, and capillary pressure.

Normally during the resting state blood flows through a small number of capillary channels. The volume of blood that perfuses each organ is highly dependent on that organ's function. The skeletal muscles afford an example of how blood flow within a single organ can vary greatly. In the skeletal muscles the potential total capillary volume during exercise is 1.5 L (Mountcastle, 1980). When the muscles are inactive, 1% of the capillaries are patent, amounting to a blood volume of only 150 ml. Exercise can therefore make a tenfold difference in the amount of blood perfused to the muscles. The increase in the number of active capillaries is essential in decreasing the diffusion distance of oxygen molecules and improving the delivery of oxygen to active muscle fibers. Autoregulation plays a significant role in this physiological adjustment.

Chemical, humoral, and metabolic influences

Vasomotor tone is altered by neural, hormonal, chemical, and metabolic influences. The interaction of these control systems regulates peripheral blood perfusion as well as the exchange processes between blood and tissue (Dahlberg, 1979). Autoregulation is thought to be mainly dependent on the liberation of blood-borne chemical and humoral mediators in the area of small vessels or in vascular smooth muscle endothelial cell complexes (Altura, 1978). These mediators and their specific influence on the auto-regulation of the microcirculation will be further explored.

Autoregulation controls the degree of intermittency of blood flow, a character-istic within the microcirculation and a manifestation of vasomotion. August Krogh in 1922 proposed that tissue oxygen pressure was the mediator affecting intermittency of blood flow. His theory was basically simple. The number of open or closed capillaries was dependent on oxygen content in the tissues. The relationship was an inverse one in that a decreased oxygen content would result in an increased number of open capillaries and vice versa. With a decrease in oxygen content, vasomotion decreases, allowing the ar-terioles and precapillary sphincters to open and allow for blood flow. In terms of meta-bolic function Krogh's theory was quite functional. Any increase in tissue metabolism calling for an increase in oxygen delivery would diminish the intermittency of flow com-monly seen at rest. Blood perfusion would therefore improve in tissues where the oxygen content was low. An opening of capillary beds then makes available a greater surface area for gas and nutrient exchange.

Krogh's hypothesis had gone unchallenged for many years. The Po_2 of tissue (partial pressure of oxygen) or the Po_2 of some fraction of the tissue continues to be seen as the central variable in local blood flow control by oxygen (Duling, 1978). Oxygen has been found to induce changes in the number of open capillaries (capillary density) and the velocity of flow through those vessels. As oxygen levels fall, capillary density and the velocity of flow increase. Zwiefach (1977) suggested that the arterioles and precapillary sphincters are controlled by different mechanisms. Duling (1978) attempted to clarify this when he reported that at low Po_2 values, precapillary sphincters are primarily affected while at higher Po_2 levels, the arterioles are affected. Blood flow within the immediate precapillary vessels is maintained within a narrow physiological range despite wide fluctuations in pressure. An increase in the oxygen tension of either blood or tissue will cause contraction of the microcirculatory vessels, reducing blood flow. However, at slightly lower than normal physiological ranges of Po_2, the arterioles are first to be affected. The drop in Po_2 will cause arterioles to begin to open to maintain tissue perfu-sion. It is not until the Po_2 decreases to a more critically low level that the precapillary sphincters respond. At this point blood flow to capillary beds is not sufficient; thus the precapillary sphincters open to provide vital blood flow.

The evidence supporting the role of oxygen in autoregulation is convincing. Vas-cular smooth muscle is the effector in local control processes related to oxygen avail-ability. Duling (1978) suggests that oxygen exerts indirect effects on smooth muscle by altering the rate of synthesis of some vasoactive tissue metabolite. The question of identifying this metabolite has not yet been answered.

Carbon dioxide and hydrogen ion are additional chemical mediators that influence blood flow regulation in the microcirculation. However, they do not provide the mecha-nism of control for autoregulation. An elevation of carbon dioxide creates vasodilation. Relaxation of vascular smooth muscle by hydrogen ion is the source of vasodilation

---

Mediators for microcirculatory regulation

Humoral

Catecholamines
 Epinephrine (C, D)
 Norepinephrine (C)
 Dopamine (C, D)
Amines
 Serotonin (C, D)
 Acetylcholine (D)
 Histamine (D)
Polypeptides
 Angiotensin (C)
 Kinins (D)
 Vasopressin (C)

Chemical

Hypoxemia (D)
Hydrogen ion (D)
Potassium (D)
Hypercapnea (D)
Hyperosmolarity (D)

C, Vasoconstriction; *D,* vasodilation.

---

produced by lactic acid, and the elevation of serum lactate is one metabolic alteration seen during shock. Duling (1978) hypothesizes that the mechanism in which carbon dioxide and hydrogen ion alter vascular tone is probably through an alteration in the flux of calcium through the membrane.

There are other humoral and chemical substances believed to play a role in the autoregulation of the microcirculation. However, no one substance has been found as a primary mediator. Histamine is a humoral mediator released from the mast cells of almost every body tissue in response to injury or antibody-antigen reactions. It is a vaso-active substance released from white blood cell–platelet microaggregates, which are pathological findings in adult respiratory distress syndrome, a complication of shock. Histamine is likewise found to play a role in the pathogenesis of septic shock. Histamine dilates larger venules in addition to increasing their permeability.

Another group of humoral substances that influence the integrity of the micro-circulation are the kinins. Kinins are polypeptides whose role in the pathophysiology of circulatory shock has been postulated on the basis of studies of shock caused by acute pancreatitis (Altura, 1978). Bradykinin is one member of that group which causes generalized vasodilation, hypotension, and an increase in capillary permeability. Altura (1978) has reported that kinins, which are liberated by proteolytic lysosomal enzymes, may play a role in tissue injury and anaphylaxis. The question remains: Even though the role of kinins in pathophysiological responses has been well substantiated, is there evidence for the role of these substances in blood flow regulation?

As a result of diminished renal perfusion the release of renin triggers the biochemical pathway that produces angiotensin II. Angiotensin II is believed to have a profound effect on the vessels of the microcirculation. Vasoconstriction appears to be the primary response, although many vessels dilate or oscillate between constriction and dilatation. This variation is believed to be a manifestation of autoregulatory and neural influences that modulate vasomotion.

The resistance of vascular beds can be raised or lowered from the basal state by adjustments in vascular smooth muscle tone. These alterations in resistance serve to control the quantity of blood delivered to the microcirculation as well as the pressure under which the blood is delivered. Oxygen and carbon dioxide are the most important of a number of substances that directly affect vascular tone. However, a substance that predominates in the control of autoregulation still has not been found. Future research may identify the mediator of control that has remained elusive to scientists.

FLUID EXCHANGE IN MICROCIRCULATION

The balance of fluid movement from the plasma to the interstitium is a function of the microcirculation. Zweifach (1977) has acknowledged that surprisingly few definitive data regarding the local regulatory mechanisms for balancing transcapillary fluid exchange under varying physiological states have been found. Maintenance of a balanced equilibrium for fluid exchange is vital to cellular survival. An interaction of mechanisms functions to prevent the dehydration or swelling of tissues as well as hypovolemia or hypervolemia within the vascular network. A disturbance in fluid exchange becomes the hallmark of shock, wherein a deficiency in perfusion and loss of fluid into tissue spaces results in the inadequate delivery of oxygen and substrates to the cells.

Starling's hypothesis

Starling (1896) developed a hypothesis to explain the dynamics of transcapillary fluid exchange:

$$M° = K_f [P_c - \pi_p l - (P_t - \pi_t)]$$

$M°$ = Fluid movement filtration/reabsorption
K_f = Filtration coefficient
P_c = Capillary hydrostatic pressure
$\pi_p l$ = Plasma osmotic pressure
P_t = Tissue hydrostatic pressure
π_t = Tissue osmotic pressure

His formula became universally accepted and unchallenged for many years. In fact, even today Starling's explanation for the balance of forces controlling transcapillary fluid movement remains a valid, workable concept. The hypothesis proposes that the balance of fluid between intravascular and extravascular compartments was the result of a filtration-reabsorption mechanism based on three factors: (1) hydrostatic pressure on each side of the capillary wall, (2) osmotic pressure of protein in the plasma and interstitial fluid, and (3) permeability characteristics of the microcirculatory vessel walls.

Starling's hypothesis assumes that blood entering the microcirculation at the arterial end is under a higher hydrostatic pressure (35 mm Hg) than at the venous end (15 mm Hg) (Fig. 3-6). The driving force of hydrostatic pressure tends to force fluid out of the capillaries and into the interstitial spaces. On the basis of capillary hydrostatic pressure fluid would move out of the vessels and into the interstitial space. The hydrostatic pressure of tissue is considered to be equal along the length of the capillary network (at a measurement of 0 to 2 mm Hg) and thus has little influence on net fluid exchange.

Colloid osmotic pressure is attributed to the concentration of plasma proteins, particularly albumin, which exerts two thirds or more of the total osmotic effect. If two solutions of different solute (protein) concentrations are separated by a membrane (capillary wall) that is permeable to water but does not allow for the passage of the solute, water will move from the solution of lower solute concentration (osmolality) to that of higher concentration (Fig. 3-7). Typically the plasma colloid osmotic pressure is 26 mm Hg, while tissue osmotic pressure is 1 mm Hg. The hypothesis described the interstitial fluid as a homogeneous fluid-filled compartment that exerted little effect on fluid movement. Thus the difference between plasma and interstitial osmotic pressure results in an effective colloid osmotic pressure of 25 mm Hg, which acts to draw fluid back into the capillary lumen.

Starling originally made the assumption of isoporosity of the capillary endothelium. All vessels were believed to have the same permeability characteristics. This concept simplified the explanation of the overall filtration and reabsorption balance. As a result of the discovery of the interaction between hydrostatic and osmotic forces, Starling proposed a net movement of fluid from capillary to interstitium on the arterial end by filtration. Midpoint along the capillary, hydrostatic and osmotic forces are approximately balanced, resulting in no net movement in either direction. At the venular side of the microcirculation, the dominance of osmotic pressure over hydrostatic pressure favors capillary resorption from the interstitial fluid.

Current theory explaining fluid exchange

Starling's model for fluid exchange was consistent with the basic understanding of how nutrients are delivered to tissues and wastes are removed. However, it represented only one of many possible sets of conditions. The model for fluid movement was based on a closed system that contained no variations in vessel size, geometric pattern of the vascular bed, vessel wall porosity, or lymphatic exchange. The mechanisms for regulation of local capillary blood flow demonstrate that vessel size does not remain constant; the

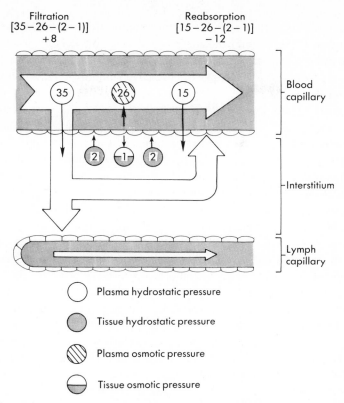

Filtration
$[35 - 26 - (2 - 1)]$
$+8$

Reabsorption
$[15 - 26 - (2 - 1)]$
-12

Blood
capillary

Interstitium

Lymph
capillary

○ Plasma hydrostatic pressure

● Tissue hydrostatic pressure

⊘ Plasma osmotic pressure

⊖ Tissue osmotic pressure

Fig. 3-6. Diagrammatic model of transcapillary fluid exchange. Starling's original hypothesis proposed that net filtration occurred on the arterial side while reabsorption occurred on the venous side. (From Intaglietta, M., and Zweifach, B.: Advances in Biological and Medical Physics **15:**111-159, 1974.)

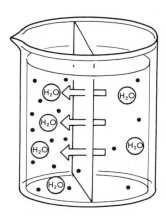

Fig. 3-7. Water containing different concentrations of solute separated by a semipermeable membrane. Osmotic forces cause movement of water toward the side of greater solute concentration.

appearance of vascular beds is not one of branching uniformity but rather of complex diverging channels. Physiologic findings made during this century have called for a revision of Starling's hypothesis. The mechanism by which the terminal vascular bed achieves a steady state of fluid exchange has been oversimplified, and additional variables must be considered.

One of the primary areas of controversy arises over the actual measurements of tissue hydrostatic and tissue colloid osmotic pressure. The strategic difficulty in gaining accurate measurements of these spaces has been the source of the problem. Diana and Fleming (1979) reported that tissue hydrostatic pressure varied considerably between -8 and $+6$ mm Hg. This range of 14 mm Hg disputes the validity of Starling's proposal that a constant hydrostatic tissue pressure exists. Likewise tissue colloid osmotic pressures have been found to range between $+1$ and $+10$ mm Hg. This increase in the value of tissue colloid osmotic pressure would lessen the influence of plasma osmotic pressure in reabsorption. Zweifach (1977) further confuses the question of fluid balance by reporting that the net drop in capillary hydrostatic pressure averages no more than 6 to 8 mm Hg. This would suggest that filtration would be the primary means of fluid exchange in the majority of vessels. Depending on the tissue environment, the balance of interstitial and intravascular pressures may favor venular filtration instead of reabsorption. This dramatically conflicts with Starling's hypothesis.

The venules possess large pores or gaps that allow for the direct passage of plasma into the interstitium. The status of pressures within the microcirculatory bed alone does not govern fluid movement. Fluid exchange has been associated with vasomotion. Zweifach (1977) reported that the absorption of fluid occurs primarily in capillaries where blood flow has come to a halt because of precapillary narrowing. Thus the amount of fluid reabsorbed is limited by the volume of plasma trapped in the static vessels. These findings suggest that absorption does not occur continuously but rather intermittently depending on the number of capillaries involved in vasomotion. Therefore filtration occurs at a continuous rate into the lymphatics within the interstitium, a point to be further explored.

The interstitial space is not the fluid-filled compartment Starling envisioned. It is a gel-like structure consisting of a ''colloid rich'' mucopolysaccharide phase and a ''colloid poor'' plasma protein phase. These phases of the interstitium provide a solid-seeming skeleton that gives the system its shape (Silberberg, 1979). The dynamics of large molecular and fluid movement in the interstitium are maintained in equilibrium between the two phases. The system possesses an osmotic buffering effect limiting excessive fluid shifts and thereby preventing edema. The protective mechanism against edema, being an open ended system, is also linked to the interstitium. The interstitium is drained continuously by the movement of fluid into the terminal lymphatics, a system largely ignored by Starling.

The lymphatics have been extremely difficult to study. Their thin, delicate endothelial channels are difficult to recognize in living organisms, being visible only through special dye techniques. The lymphatic capillary barrier is influential in fluid exchange.

The lymphatic capillaries have porous gaps that can be occluded. As a result of closure of these cell spaces the lymphatic wall becomes a semipermeable membrane across which concentration gradients develop (Intaglietta and Zweifach, 1974). Pressures in the lymphatics vary over a range of -1 to $+4$ cm H_2O (Intaglietta and Zweifach, 1974). Fluid in the terminal lymphatics is similar if not identical to the fluid of the interstitium. A reassessment of Starling's hypothesis would indicate that the extent of filtration may have been overestimated and lymph flow may play a more important role.

Protein concentration, being higher in plasma, exerts a higher osmotic potential there than in the interstitium. This acts to maintain an equilibrium whereby water tends to remain within the intravascular compartment. Protein can only leak out of capillaries; it cannot be reabsorbed. Since the capillaries are not completely impervious to protein, a finite concentration builds up in the interstitium. The body strives to maintain a steady

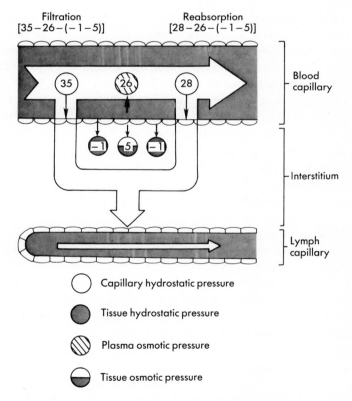

Fig. 3-8. Diagrammatic model of the revision of Starling's hypothesis, revealing filtration as the dominant force in transcapillary fluid movement. Flow through lymphatic capillaries plays a significant role in the ultimate return of plasma fluid to the intravascular space. (From Intaglietta, M., and Zweifach, B.: Advances in Biological and Medical Physics **15:**111-159, 1974.)

balance within the tissue environment, controlling the water and protein potentials. The protein acts as a resistance element to water flow, protecting the tissues from the sudden loss of pressure that Silberberg (1979) believes is an important reason for the presence of diffusable proteins in the interstitium. The lymphatics are essential for protein to be eventually returned to the plasma. Fluid is moved from the terminal lymphatics into the collecting system by means of pressure fluctuations, valvular action, and the vasomotor activity of the blood capillary system (Intaglietta and Zweifach, 1974). Ultimately the filtered plasma that enters the interstitium is returned to the capillaries.

Basic to Starling's hypothesis was the assumption that fluid exchange was the result of an interaction between hydrostatic and colloid osmotic pressures in both directions across vascular walls. Clearly filtration does occur at the arterial end as the result of a dominant hydrostatic force. However, the hydrostatic forces are variable, influenced by vasomotion, in which precapillary and postcapillary resistance fluctuates. On the venous side, fluid exchange is more complex. As a result of the large venous pores or gaps that permit the passage of plasma into the interstitium, osmotic effects are not manifested since a barrier to protein solute does not exist. Fluid exchange is most likely determined on the venous end by hydrostatic factors. It is highly unlikely that absorption can occur in the venous endothelium (Intaglietta and Zweifach, 1974). Fluid exchange by filtration likely occurs at the venous end of the microcirculation.

Fig. 3-8 represents a revision of Starling's hypothesis for fluid exchange. Proposed by Intaglietta and Zweifach (1974), it demonstrates that fluid originating from the capillary beds does not return by reabsorption through the tissues but instead filters into the terminal lymphatics. Eventually lymphatic fluid reenters the systemic circulation to restore a balance of fluid between intravascular and extravascular compartments. The question of fluid exchange is still not resolved. Starling's explanations for fluid exchange continue to be challenged and serve as stimuli for further research.

SUMMARY

The nurse must be able to make rational, intelligent, quick decisions when caring for a critically ill patient. Reflecting on a complex discussion of microcirculatory physiology may not be the nurse's first consideration while the patient is being assessed. However, possession of a thorough knowledge of physiological and pathophysiological variables improves the nurse's ability to anticipate assessment and therapeutic measures.

Knowledge of the initial ischemic shock response and the resulting vasoconstriction of arterioles and venules alerts the nurse to observe for cool extremities, pallor of the skin, and a reduced urine output. Recognizing the sensitivity of the lung to microcirculatory hypoperfusion, the nurse will initiate rigorous pulmonary hygiene to maximize the lung's existing defense mechanisms. Since the brain continues to receive the majority of cardiac output despite microcirculatory disruption in other organs, changes in the patient's level of responsiveness will signal a deteriorating condition. The gastrointestinal system is one that can be significantly affected by shock. The development of an edematous intestinal wall prevents absorption and creates the obvious problem of excess fluid loss.

An enlightened nurse is a better prepared nurse. The principles of normal physiology go hand in hand with the implications of pathophysiological alterations. A sound knowledge of physiology is mandatory for the nurse to provide the most comprehensive nursing care to a shock patient.

REFERENCES

Altura, B.M.: Humoral, hormonal and myogenic mechanisms in microcirculatory regulation. In Kaley, G., and Altura, B.M., editors: Microcirculation, vol. 2, Baltimore, 1978, University Park Press.

Baez, S.: Microvascular terminology. In Kaley, G., and Altura, B.M., editors: Microcirculation, vol. 1, Baltimore, 1977, University Park Press.

Bendayan, M., Sandborn, E., and Rasio, E.: Blood vessel structure: an intracellular tubular system in capillary endothelium. In Grayson, J., and Zingg, W., editors: Microcirculation, New York, 1976, Plenum Publishing Corp.

Bernick, S.: Histology of selected microvessels. In Kaley, G., and Altura, B.M., editors: Microcirculation, vol. 1, Baltimore, 1977, University Park Press.

Crone, C.: Autoregulation of the microcirculation, Acta Medica Scandinavica Suppl. **578:**15-18, 1975.

Dahlberg, B.: Transcapillary solute exchange in skeletal muscle after injury and during shock, Acta Physiologica Scandinavica Suppl. **472:**1-82, 1979.

Diana, J.N., and Fleming, B.P.: Some current problems in microvascular research, Microvascular Research **18:**144-152, 1979.

Duling, B.R.: Oxygen metabolism and microcirculatory regulation. In Kaley, G., and Altura, B.M., editors: Microcirculation, vol. 2, Baltimore, 1978, University Park Press.

Duling, B.R.: O_2, CO_2, and H^+ ion as local factors causing vasodilatation. In Vanhoutte, P.M., and Leusen, I., editors: Mechanisms of vasodilatation, Basle, Switzerland, 1978, S. Karger AG.

Hauck, G.: Physiology of the microvascular system, Angiolica **8:**236-260, 1971.

Intaglietta, M., and Zweifach, B.W.: Microcirculatory basis of fluid exchange, Advances in Biological and Medical Physics, **15:**111-159, 1974.

Krogh, A.: Anatomy and physiology of capillaries, New Haven, 1922, Yale University Press.

Mountcastle, V.B., editor: Medical Physiology, vol. 2, ed. 14, St. Louis, 1980, The C.V. Mosby Co.

Palade, G.E., Simionescu, M., and Simionescu, N.: Structural aspects of the permeability of the microvascular endothelium, Acta Physiologica Scandinavica Suppl. **463:**11-32, 1979.

Pappenheimer, J.R., Renkin, E.M., and Barrero, L.M.: Filtration, diffusion, and molecular sieving through peripheral capillary membranes, American Journal of Physiology **167:**13-45, 1951.

Robertson, R.P., and Porte, D., Jr.: Adrenergic modulation of basal insulin secretion in man, Diabetes **22:**1-8, 1973.

Rosell, S., and Belfrage, E.: Adrenergic receptors in adipose tissue and their relation to adrenergic innervation, Nature **253:**738-739, 1975.

Rosenblum, W.I.: Viscosity in vitro versus in vivo. In Kaley, G., and Altura, B.M., editors: Microcirculation, vol. 1, Baltimore, 1977, University Park Press.

Silberberg, A.: Microcirculation in inflammation. In Hauck, C., and Irwin, J.W., editors: Microcirculation and the extravascular space, Bibliotheca Anatomica **17:**54-65, 1979.

Sobin, S.S., and Tremer, H.M.: Three dimensional organization of microvascular beds as related to function. In Kaley, G., and Altura, B.M., editors: Microcirculation, vol. 1, Baltimore, 1977, University Park Press.

Soloman, A.K.: Characterization of biological membranes by equivalent pores, Journal of General Physiology **51:**335S, 1968.

Starling, E.H.: On the absorption of fluids from the connective tissue spaces, Journal of Physiology (London) **19:**312-316, 1896.

Vacek, L., and Braveny, P.: Effects of angiotensin II on blood pressure and on microvascular beds in mesentary, skin, and skeletal muscle of the rat, Microvascular Research **16:**43-49, 1978.

Wolff, J.R.: Ultrastructure of the terminal vascular bed as related to function. In Kaley, G., and Altura, B.M., editors: Microcirculation, vol. 1, Baltimore, 1977, University Park Press.

Zweifach, B.W.: Functional behavior of the microcirculation, Springfield, Ill., 1961, Charles C Thomas, Publisher.

Zweifach, B.W.: Mechanisms of blood flow and fluid exchange in microvessels: hemorrhagic hypotension model, Anesthesiology **41:**157-168, 1974.

Zweifach, B.W.: Introduction: perspectives in microcirculation. In Kaley, G., and Altura, B.M., editors: Microcirculation, vol. 1, Baltimore, 1977, University Park Press.

4 Oxygenation

ANNE GRIFFIN PERRY

The primary function of the respiratory system is to exchange respiratory gases, oxygen, and carbon dioxide between the body and the atmosphere. Adequate respiration requires the coordinated function of the circulatory, nervous, and pulmonary systems as well as the balance of blood chemistry. Any alteration requires the human organism to adapt to maintain the body's oxygen demands. In shock the patient has diminished cardiac output and lung perfusion, resulting in tissue hypoxia.

This chapter on oxygenation will assist the nurse in providing and maintaining adequate organ and tissue oxygenation for the patient in shock. The total process of oxygenation will be presented with emphasis on ventilation, perfusion, and diffusion, as well as the chemical and neural regulation of respiration. The final section of this chapter will include the goals and general principles for the care of the patient on a mechanical ventilator. The knowledge of the process of oxygenation and the principles of mechanical ventilation will provide the scientific rationales for the nursing therapies selected for the patient in shock.

STRUCTURE AND FUNCTION

Although it is not the purpose of this chapter to detail the total anatomic structure of the respiratory system, the nurse must have knowledge of the gross structure and general functioning of the following units of the respiratory system (Table 4-1). The functioning of the alveoli, pulmonary circulation, pleural space, and respiratory muscles are essential to the three major functions of the respiratory system: ventilation, perfusion, and diffusion. Adequacy of oxygen delivery is dependent on the amount of oxygen entering the lungs (ventilation), blood flow to the lungs and to the tissue (perfusion), adequacy of diffusion, and the capacity of the blood to carry oxygen.

The primary function of the lung is to transfer oxygen from the atmosphere into the alveoli and carbon dioxide out as a waste product. In addition, this organ filters toxic materials from the circulation, metabolizes some compounds (e.g., angiotensin I, bradykinin, and prostaglandins), and serves as a reservoir for blood (West, 1979). Each lung lies in a pleural space, which surrounds the lung except at the medial attachment. This medial structure is the hilum, which contains the mainstem bronchi and pulmonary vessels (Bushnell, 1981). Actually the pleural space is a potential space, the thickness of which is only a thin film of liquid lying between the outer layer of the lung (visceral pleura) and the inner cell layer of the chest cavity (parietal pleura). The purpose of this film is to allow for an easy gliding movement along the chest wall. However, a great deal

Table 4-1. Supporting structures of the respiratory system

Gross structure	Supporting structures	General function
Upper airway	Nasal cavity Nasopharynx Oropharynx	Warms, filters, and humidifies inspired air.
Lower airway	Larynx Trachea Bronchi Alveoli	Conductive structure that delivers oxygen to the alveoli.
Pulmonary circulation	Right ventricle Pulmonary artery Pulmonary arteriole Pulmonary capillary Pulmonary venule Pulmonary vein Left atrium	Carries nonoxygenated (venous) blood to the lung and delivers oxygenated (arterial) blood to the systemic circulation.
Lung	Right: upper, middle, and lower lobes Left: upper and lower lobes	Contains the structures of the lower airway and pulmonary circulation.

Respiratory muscles	Inspiratory
	  Diaphragm
	  External intercostals
	  Sternocleidomastoids
	  Scapular elevators
	  Anterior serrati
	  Scaleni
	  Erectus muscle of the spine
	Expiratory
	  Abdominals
	  Internal intercostals
	  Posterior inferior serrati
		Provides the physical mechanism for the passage of respiratory gases in and out of the body.

of force would need to be exerted to pull the pleura away from the chest wall (Wade, 1977). The vessels of the pulmonary circulation are also contained within the lung. Greater specifics on the pulmonary circulation will be contained in the section that discusses perfusion.

The alveoli are tiny air sacs at the terminal end of the lower airway. The alveolar wall is composed of the alveolar membrane, a network of anastomosing capillaries, and interstitial fluid containing collagen fibers (Bushnell, 1981). The exchange of respiratory gases, oxygen (O_2) and carbon dioxide (CO_2), takes place in the alveoli. A unique characteristic of these tiny air sacs is their ability to expand during inspiration. This expansion greatly increases the surface area, over which the diffusion of gases can occur. Within the large alveolar cell (type II cell) surfactant is manufactured. Surfactant, a phospholipid, prevents the collapse of the alveoli and enhances their expansion during inspiration.

Ventilation, perfusion, and diffusion provide adequate blood oxygenation. Then, through the mechanics of the cardiovascular system, the oxygenated blood is delivered to the body's organs and tissues.

VENTILATION

Pulmonary ventilation is the mechanical process involving the muscular and elastic properties of the lung and thorax, or simply the means of getting inspired air into the alveoli (Shapiro, Harrison, and Trout, 1979; Wade, 1977; West, 1979). For this to occur, the respiratory muscles and their innervation must be intact. The major inspiratory muscle is the diaphragm, which is innervated by the phrenic nerves that exit the spinal cord at the level of the third to fifth cervical vertebrae. Phrenic nerve innervation allows the diaphragm to descend on inspiration, thus increasing the lung volume. The remaining inspiratory muscle groups elevate the chest cage and expand the anterior-posterior diameter, which also increases the lung volume. The entire process of inspiration is an active one. For lung volume to increase, work must be generated by the inspiratory muscles. The work of breathing is accomplished by stretching elastic tissues of the chest wall and lungs, moving nonelastic tissues, and overcoming airway resistance. The stretching of elastic and nonelastic tissues of the chest wall and lungs occurs during the inspiratory cycle of respiration.

Expiration is a passive process that requires little or no muscle work. The process of expiration is dependent on the elastic recoil properties of the lung. This elastic recoil is produced by elastic fibers in the lung tissue and by the surface tension in the fluid film lining the alveoli (Bushnell, 1981). In addition, passive elastic recoil of the chest wall and abdominal musculature further enhances expiration.

Pressures and volumes

The process of moving gases into and out of the lungs is accomplished through pressures (Fig. 4-1). Intrapleural pressure is negative with respect to atmospheric pressure, which is 760 mm Hg at sea level. For air to flow into the lungs, the intrapleural pressure must become negative, thereby setting up a pressure gradient between the atmosphere and the alveoli that causes a suctioning of air into the lungs. In addition, intra-alveolar pressures become slightly negative with respect to atmospheric pressure, thus facilitating increased airflow into the air sacs. Once atmospheric air is introduced into the intrapleural space, the negative pull is abolished, resulting in a collapse of the lung (Wade, 1977) (Fig. 4-2).

The normal volumes within the lung (Table 4-2) are measured through pulmonary function testing. Some of these measurements can be recorded with a spirometer, which measures the volume of air entering or leaving the lungs (Fig. 4-3). Variations in the lung volumes can occur from varying health states (e.g., pregnancy, exercise, obesity, or obstructive and restrictive pathological conditions of the lung). Factors such as the amount of surfactant, compliance, and paralysis of respiratory muscles can affect normal pressures and volumes within the lungs as well.

Surfactant, the lipoprotein originating in the alveolar type II cells, is essential for ventilation. The overall role of surfactant is to decrease the surface tension of the alveolar lining, therefore equalizing the pressure within each alveolus during inspiration and expiration. The three physiological advantages of surfactant are the decrease of surface tension, which promotes lung compliance and decreases the work needed for expansion on inspiration; the maintenance of alveolar stability that reduces the risk of alveolar

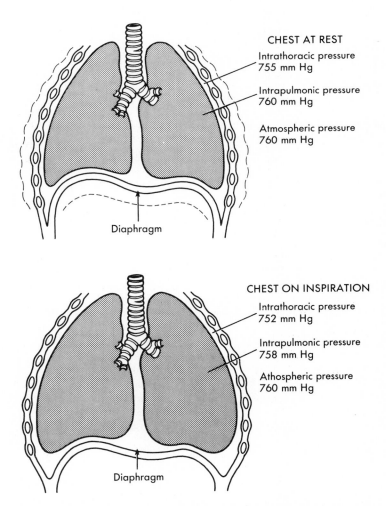

Fig. 4-1. Pressures within lungs and thorax at rest and during inspiration. (From Wade, J.F.: Respiratory nursing care, St. Louis, 1977, The C.V. Mosby Co.)

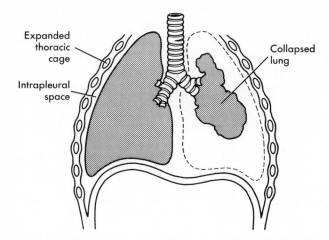

Fig. 4-2. Illustration of pneumothorax. Broken line shows position of normally expanded lung to demonstrate outward movement of thoracic cage, which occurs with pneumothorax. (From Wade, J.F.: Respiratory nursing care, St. Louis, 1977, The C.V. Mosby Co.)

Table 4-2. Normal lung volumes

Abbreviation	Volume	Definition	Normal volume
VC	Vital capacity	Maximal volume that can be expired after maximal inspiration	4,800 ml
IC	Inspiratory capacity	Maximal volume that can be inspired from resting expiratory level	3,600 ml
IRV	Inspiratory reserve volume	Maximal volume that can be inspired from end-tidal volume	3,100 ml
ERV	Expiratory reserve volume	Maximal volume that can be expired from resting expiratory level	1,200 ml
FRC	Functional residual capacity	Volume of gas in lungs at resting expiratory level	2,400 ml
RV	Residual volume	Volume of gas in lungs at end of maximal expiration	1,200 ml
TLC	Total lung capacity	Volume of gas in lungs at end of maximal inspiration	6,000 ml
V_T	Tidal volume	Volume of gas that passes into and out of the lungs in each respiratory cycle	500 ml

Modified from Comroe, J.H., Jr., et al.: The lung: clinical physiology and pulmonary function tests, ed. 2, Chicago, 1962, Year Book Medical Publishers, Inc.

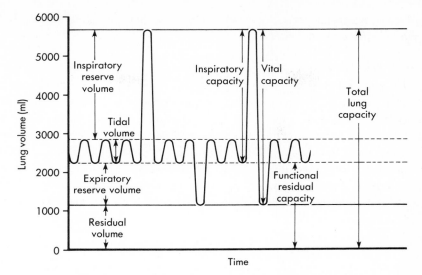

Fig. 4-3. Normal lung volumes measured by spirometry.

collapse; and the maintenance of dryness of the alveoli (West, 1979). The decrease or loss of this lipoprotein results in stiff lungs, atelectasis, and fluid-filled alveoli.

Pulmonary compliance is a measurement of the elastic properties of the lung. Decreased compliance occurs in conditions such as interstitial or pleural fibrosis, pulmonary edema, or pneumonia. These conditions decrease lung volume and cause the lung to become stiff and less distensible. Increased compliance occurs in emphysema and aging when the elastic fibers of the lung have been lost or damaged. Bushnell (1981) describes two types of compliance: static and effective. Static compliance is defined as the change in lung volume per unit change in airway pressure when the lungs are motionless. Effective compliance is obtained by dividing the tidal volume by the peak inspiratory pressure that is required to deliver the volume. The normal peak airway pressure for an adult lying supine is approximately 50 ml/cm H_2O (Bushnell, 1981). Effective compliance can be reduced by three processes: disease processes that make the lungs stiff (e.g., atelectasis, pulmonary edema), processes that occupy intrathoracic space (e.g., effusion or pneumothorax), and processes that decrease chest wall distensibility (e.g., obesity and abnormal spinal curvatures). Regardless of the factors that reduce pulmonary compliance, the effect is the same. Low pulmonary compliance increases the work of breathing.

Conditions that result in permanent or temporary paralysis of the respiratory muscles significantly alter the volume of gas exchanged during inspiration and expiration. The alterations leading to paralysis of the respiratory muscles can result from infections, such as Guillain-Barré syndrome or poliomyelitis; altered transmission of the nervous impulse, as in myasthenia gravis; and complete transection of the spinal cord at the level of the third to fifth cervical vertebrae.

Airway resistance

The relationship between pressure and flow is called airway resistance. In the healthy adult male, airway resistance across the tracheobronchial tree is about 0.5 to 2.5 cm H_2O/L/sec at flow rates of 0.5 L/sec (Bushnell, 1981). Current research has demonstrated that airway resistance is usually highest in medium-size bronchioles and lowest in the small bronchioles (West, 1979). In obstructive lung diseases resistance in the small bronchioles is greatly increased, which results in a further increase in airway resistance. Factors determining airway resistance are lung volumes, bronchial diameter, and density and viscosity. The lower the lung volume or bronchial diameter, the greater will be the airway resistance.

Alveolar ventilation

An important aspect of ventilation is alveolar ventilation. Alveolar ventilation is defined as the volume of gas entering the respiratory zone each minute, allowing for dead space.

$$V_T \quad - \quad V_D \quad \times \quad f \quad = \quad V_A$$

| Tidal volume | − Dead space volume | × Frequency of respiration | = Alveolar ventilation |

By definition, dead space is the volume of air that fills the conduction tubes but does not participate in gas exchange. The anatomical dead space consists of the conducting airways from the nose and mouth to the alveoli. Normally this volume is equal to 1 ml per each pound of body weight. Therefore a 170 lb man with healthy lungs would have an anatomic dead space of 170 ml. Alveolar dead space refers to the amount of gas that reaches the alveoli but does not participate in gas exchange. The reason for alveolar dead space can be two-fold: first, a volume of gas was delivered to an alveoli without a blood supply; second, the volume of gas was too great in relation to the blood flow to that alveoli. The total physiological dead space is a combination of the alveolar and anatomical dead space. In the individual with healthy lungs, the anatomical and physiological dead space are one.

There are regional differences in alveolar ventilation. Research has demonstrated that in normal subjects the dependent portion of the lung is best ventilated (West, 1979). During exercise, ventilation is increased throughout the lung because of an increase in tidal volume and the hyperinflation of the alveoli, which are normally closed. Hypoinflation is defined as an inadequate volume of air entering the alveoli as it relates to the metabolic needs of the body. Hyperinflation results when the volume of air entering the alveoli is greater than the metabolic needs of the body.

PERFUSION

The primary function of the pulmonary circulation is to move blood to and from the blood-gas barrier so that gas exchange is able to occur. The pulmonary circulation also serves as a reservoir for blood, so that the lung is able to increase its blood volume without causing large increases in the pulmonary artery or venous pressures. Finally, this circulatory system filters blood so that small thrombi are removed prior to their reaching the brain or other vital organs (West, 1977).

Pulmonary circulation

The blood flow begins at the pulmonary artery, which receives mixed venous blood from the right ventricle. The blood flow through this system is dependent on the pumping ability of the right ventricle, which has an output of approximately 5 to 6 L/min. The flow continues from the pulmonary artery through the pulmonary arterioles, pulmonary capillaries, pulmonary venules, and pulmonary veins and finally returns oxygenated blood to the left atrium.

Distribution

The pressures within the pulmonary circulatory system are low in comparison to pressures in the systemic circulatory system. The pulmonary systolic arterial pressure is between 20 and 30 mm Hg, the pulmonary diastolic pressure is less than 12 mm Hg, and the mean pulmonary pressure is less than 20 mm Hg (Daily and Schroeder, 1981). As a result of low pressure and low resistance, the walls of the pulmonary vessels are thinner than those in the systemic circulation and contain a smaller amount of smooth muscle, because the lung accepts the total cardiac output from the right ventricle and, except in the case of alveolar hypoxia, is not required to direct blood flow from one region to another.

The pulmonary capillaries receive approximately 75% of their blood flow during systole. The exact pressure within the pulmonary capillaries is uncertain. It is currently believed to range halfway between pulmonary arterial and venous pressures, approximately 4 to 12 mm Hg (Daily and Schroeder, 1981). However, when the pressure in these capillaries rises above 25 mm Hg, pulmonary edema can result. This is caused by the critical pressure elevation altering the hydrostatic forces in the pulmonary capillaries. As a result, fluid is driven across the capillary membrane into the interstitial space and the alveoli. Disease processes, such as left ventricular failure and mitral stenosis, which elevate the pressures in the pulmonary circulation, increase the risk for pulmonary edema.

In the healthy lung the distribution of blood flow is similar in pattern to the distribution of ventilation. This is demonstrated by the gradual decrease in blood flow from the base to the lung apex. As with ventilation, there are changes in perfusion that occur in exercise.

VENTILATION-PERFUSION RELATIONSHIPS

A balanced relationship between ventilation and perfusion must exist to ensure adequacy of gas exchange. An inadequate balance between ventilation and perfusion is responsible for most of the ineffective exchange of gases in pulmonary diseases. Normally about 2% of the blood in the systemic arteries bypasses the pulmonary capillaries.

This sets up a ventilation-perfusion inequality. However, this inequality is considered normal and is referred to as the physiological shunt. This physiological shunt accounts for the reason that the blood in the systemic arteries contains less oxygen per 100 ml than the blood that has equilibrated with alveolar air (Ganong, 1979).

Shunting

In a shunt blood enters the arterial system without going through ventilated areas of the lung (West, 1979). The amount of blood involved varies; the shunt may be normal or it may be worsened by diseases of ventilation (primarily lung diseases) or by diseases of perfusion (primarily cardiovascular diseases). Shunts can be caused by three categories of alterations: diffusion defects, alveolar hypoventilation, and ventilation-perfusion inequalities. The shunting, if severe enough, can result in hypoxemia.

One is able to measure the degree of hypoxemia caused by shunting by having the patient breathe 100% oxygen for 20 to 30 minutes through a closed system and then measuring the Pao_2. If only the physiological shunt is present, the Pao_2 should be 580 to 600 mm Hg. The rationale for inhaling 100% oxygen over a 20 to 30 minute period is that all the nitrogen gas is removed from the lung, and the alveoli are exposed to pure oxygen. If a large degree of shunting is present in a patient, hypoxemia results. This hypoxemia cannot be corrected by administering 100% oxygen because the shunted blood is never exposed to the higher oxygen concentrations in the alveoli. Therefore the hypoxemia continues to worsen since the cause of the ventilation-perfusion inequality has not been corrected. Usually the shunt does not result in increased $Paco_2$ because the central chemoreceptors are stimulated by the change in $Paco_2$ and respond by increasing the ventilation rate. This, in turn, reduces the $Paco_2$ of the unshunted blood until the $Paco_2$ is normal (West, 1979).

Effect of ventilation-perfusion inequalities on gas exchanges

The lung with ventilation-perfusion inequality is not able to transfer as much oxygen and carbon dioxide as a lung that is evenly ventilated and perfused. Fig. 4-4, *A*, demonstrates a lung unit with a normal ventilation and perfusion ratio. If the ventilation is obstructed (Fig. 4-4, *B*) and the blood flow remains the same, the ventilation-perfusion ratio is reduced. The result is a decreased oxygen level and elevated carbon dioxide level. Conversely, if the blood flow is obstructed (Fig. 4-4, *C*) and the ventilation is unchanged, the ventilation-perfusion ratio is increased, causing the oxygen level to become elevated and the carbon dioxide level to decline (West, 1979). It should be noted that as the ventilation-perfusion ratio is altered, the gas within the lung unit will approach the concentration of inspired gas or mixed venous blood.

Clinical assessment of ventilation-perfusion inequality is essential in caring for the patient in shock. To do this effectively, arterial blood gas samples must be obtained following 15 minutes of ventilation with 100% oxygen (forced inspiratory oxygen [Fio_2] = 1). The Pao_2 can provide some useful information in the evaluation of ventilation-perfusion inequalities. However, this value is readily affected by the level of ventilation,

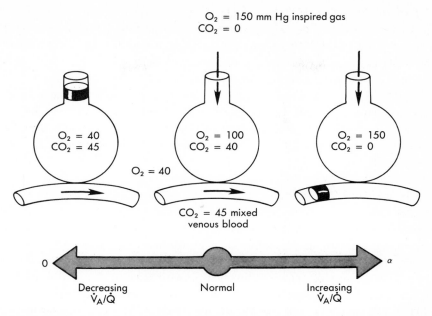

$O_2 = 150$ mm Hg inspired gas
$CO_2 = 0$

$O_2 = 40$
$CO_2 = 45$

$O_2 = 40$

$O_2 = 100$
$CO_2 = 40$

$O_2 = 150$
$CO_2 = 0$

$CO_2 = 45$ mixed
venous blood

0

Decreasing
$\dot{V}_A/\dot{Q}$

Normal

Increasing
$\dot{V}_A/\dot{Q}$

α

Fig. 4-4. Ventilation-perfusion ratios: decreased, normal, and increased. (From West, J.B.: Ventilation/blood flow and gas exchange, ed. 3, Oxford, 1977, Blackwell Scientific Publications, Ltd.)

shunts, or diffusion deficits. Therefore it is important to calculate the alveolar-arterial oxygen difference ($P[A - a]O_2$) to assess for any intrapulmonary shunting. This is calculated in two steps:

$$1. \ PaO_2 = (PB - PH_2O) \times FIO_2 - \frac{PaCO_2}{0.8}$$

$PB = 670$ mm Hg at sea level
$PH_2O = 47$ mm Hg with a body temperature of $37°$ C
$0.8 =$ Respiratory quotient, usually a constant value
$2. \ P(A - a)O_2 = PAO_2 - PaO_2$

Normally this value is 10 mm Hg for room air. As the concentration of inspired oxygen rises, so should the $P(A - a)O_2$ until, at 100% oxygen, this value is 100 mm Hg in the normal person who has healthy lungs (Harper, 1981). The specific advantage of the $P(A - a)O_2$ value is that it is more sensitive to the level of ventilation than the PaO_2 alone. Serial $P(A - a)O_2$ values provide a rough indication of potentially reversible lung disease. They are some of the most valuable measurements of respiratory failure, a common occurrence in severe shock. The $PaCO_2$ alone is of little value in evaluating the ventilation-perfusion inequality because the $PaCO_2$ is sensitive to the level of ventilation. Therefore the body is able to decrease the $PaCO_2$ by altering the ventilation depth and rate.

DIFFUSION

In order to meet tissue oxygen demands, diffusion of respiratory gases must also occur. Diffusion is the movement of molecules from an area of high concentration to an area of lower concentration. Diffusion through the tissues is governed by Fick's law of diffusion. Various texts describe this law, which states that the rate of transfer of a gas through a sheet of tissue is proportional to the tissue area and the difference in gas partial pressure between the two sides and inversely proportional to the tissue thickness (West, 1979). The transport of respiratory gases within the body is dependent on diffusion. The surface area (50 to 100 m^2) and the tissue thickness (6.5 μm) of the lung are ideal for the diffusion of gases.

Transport of oxygen

The oxygen delivery system in the body consists of the lungs and the cardiovascular system. The capacity of the blood to carry oxygen is influenced by the amount of dissolved oxygen in the plasma, the amount of hemoglobin, and the affinity of hemoglobin for oxygen.

A relatively small amount of oxygen, approximately 3%, is dissolved in the plasma, making this an obviously inadequate method for transporting oxygen to the tissues. Therefore an alternate, more efficient means of oxygen transport is needed. This alternate method is by way of the hemoglobin.

The hemoglobin molecule serves as the carrier for both respiratory gases. The hemoglobin molecule combines with oxygen to form oxyhemoglobin. The maximum amount of oxygen that can be combined with hemoglobin is called the oxygen capacity. Each gram of hemoglobin can combine with 1.39 ml of oxygen (West, 1979). Multiplying the total hemoglobin with this figure will provide the total oxygen-carrying capacity of hemoglobin.

The oxyhemoglobin molecule is easily dissipated, thereby allowing hemoglobin and oxygen to dissociate and freeing oxygen to enter the tissues. The oxygen-hemoglobin dissociation curve (Fig. 4-5) relates the percentage saturation to the arterial oxygen saturation. The characteristic shape of the curve has several physiological advantages. The flat upper portion of the curve demonstrates that if the Pao_2 decreases slightly, the unloading of oxygen to the tissues is slightly affected. Second, as the red blood cells take up oxygen along the pulmonary capillary, a large partial pressure difference between alveolar gas and blood continues, even when most of the oxygen has been transferred, and therefore the diffusion process is increased (West, 1979). Finally, the steep lower part of the oxygen-hemoglobin dissociation curve demonstrates that even when the peripheral tissues draw large amounts of oxygen, there will be only a small drop in capillary oxygenation. This helps to maintain the blood Pao_2 that promotes the diffusion of oxygen into the tissue cells.

There are various factors that can affect the affinity of hemoglobin for oxygen, thereby shifting the curve to the right or left. The variables that can shift the oxygen-hemoglobin dissociation curve include: carbon dioxide (CO_2), hydrogen ion concentra-

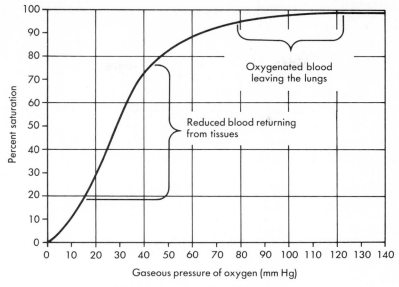

Fig. 4-5. Oxygen-hemoglobin dissociation curve.

Table 4-3. Factors that shift oxygen-hemoglobin dissociation curve

Direction	Variable	Rationale
Left shift	Decreased P_{CO_2} Increased pH Hypothermia Decreased 2,3-DPG	Alterations cause an interference with cellular respiration. Left shift results in decreased unloading of oxygen to the cells.
Right shift	Increased P_{CO_2} Decreased pH Hyperthermia Increased 2,3-DPG Exercise	Alterations in these variables require increased oxygen at the cellular level. Right shift results in increased unloading of oxygen to the cells.

tion (pH), 2,3-diphosphoglycerate (2,3-DPG), and exercise (Table 4-3). When the oxygen-hemoglobin dissociation curve shifts to the left, the oxygen saturation of hemoglobin will be higher than normal. Even though the affinity of hemoglobin for oxygen is higher, the release of oxygen at the tissue capillaries is decreased. This decrease in unloading interferes with cellular respiration, which results in tissue hypoxia. When the oxygen-hemoglobin dissociation curve shifts to the right, the hemoglobin's affinity for oxygen is less than normal; however, there is an increased unloading of oxygen at the tissue capillary. Factors producing a right shift are those alterations that require increased oxygen at the tissue level.

Transport of carbon dioxide

The discussion of the transport of respiratory gases cannot be limited to oxygen. The fate of carbon dioxide in the blood must also be understood. The carbon dioxide, which diffuses into the red blood cells, is rapidly hydrated into carbonic acid. This rapid hydration occurs due to the presence of carbonic anhydrase. The carbonic acid then dissociates into hydrogen (H^+) and bicarbonate (HCO_3^-) ions. The hydrogen ion is then buffered by hemoglobin and the bicarbonate ions diffuse into the plasma (Ganong, 1979).

$$CO_2 + H_2O \rightleftarrows H_2CO_3 \rightleftarrows H^+ + HCO_3^-$$

In addition, some of the carbon dioxide in the red blood cells react with amino acid groups, forming carbamino compounds.

$$Hb \cdot NH_2 + CO_2 \rightleftarrows Hb \cdot NH \cdot COOH$$

This reaction can occur rapidly without the presence of an enzyme. It must be remembered that reduced hemoglobin (deoxyhemoglobin) can combine with carbon dioxide more easily than with oxyhemoglobin; therefore the majority of carbon dioxide is transported by venous blood. The bicarbonate ion readily diffuses from the red blood cell into the plasma. Normally anions cannot cross the cell membrane because of the sodium-potassium pump. The chloride ion (Cl^-) makes this diffusion possible, because this cation will maintain the electrochemical neutrality of the cell. This shifting of bicarbonate ions into the plasma and chloride ions into the red blood cell is called the chloride shift.

Fate of carbon dioxide in the blood

In plasma

1. Dissolved
2. Formation of carbamino compounds with plasma protein
3. Hydration, H^+ buffered, HCO_3^- in plasma

In red blood cells

1. Dissolved
2. Formation of carbamino compounds
3. Hydration, H^+ buffered, 70% of HCO_3^- diffuses into plasma
4. Cl^- shifts into cells; mOsm/l in cells increases

From Ganong, W.F.: Review of Medical Physiology, ed. 9, Los Altos, Calif., 1979, Lange Medical Publications.

REGULATION OF RESPIRATION

The main purpose of respiratory regulation is to supply sufficient oxygen to the blood in the presence of varying demands (e.g., exercise, infection, or pregnancy). In addition, respiratory regulation promotes the exhalation of metabolically produced carbon dioxide, which is a determinant of acid-base status. The adequacy of this respiratory regulation is measured by arterial blood gases (Table 4-4).

Neural regulation

Synchronized inspiration and expiration can be regulated through either voluntary or automatic control. The center for voluntary control is located in the cerebral cortex and delivers impulses to the respiratory motor neurons by way of the corticospinal tract (Ganong, 1979). An individual voluntarily controls respiration to accommodate various activities such as speaking, eating, and swimming. The medulla contains the center for the automatic control of respiration that occurs continuously through sleeping and most waking activities. This neural regulation maintains the appropriate rhythm and depth of respiration, in addition to the balance between the lengths of inspiration and expiration.

Humoral regulation

The respiratory chemoreceptors are located in the medulla and the aortic and carotid bodies. Changes in the Pa_{CO_2}, pH, and Pa_{O_2} are identified by these chemoreceptors. These chemoreceptors then stimulate the neural regulators to adjust the rate and/or depth of ventilation to maintain Pa_{CO_2} at a constant level, to alter the effects of excess hydrogen concentration, and to raise the Pa_{O_2} (Ganong, 1979). This is an adaptive mechanism and cannot be utilized over long periods. In shock, patients have the potential for severe respiratory imbalances to which the body cannot adapt. One means of controlling these imbalances is through mechanical ventilation.

MECHANICAL VENTILATION

Patients in shock frequently require mechanical ventilation. The decision for utilizing mechanical ventilation takes place whenever the ventilatory function of the patient fails to maintain adequate pulmonary blood gas exchange. When mechanical ventilation is initiated, one must remember that first, this is a supportive, therapeutic

Table 4-4. Normal arterial blood gas values

Variable	Normal range*
Pa_{O_2}	95-100 mm Hg
Pa_{CO_2}	36-44 mm Hg
pH	7.36 to 7.44
O_2 saturation	97%
HCO_3^-	23 to 26 mEq/L

*Values obtained from a review of literature on arterial blood gases. These values may vary from one clinical setting to another.

measure, and not curative, and second, once the patient is placed on mechanical ventilation, the responsibility for adequate alveolar ventilation becomes that of the health care professional and not the patient. This section of the chapter will focus on the basics of mechanical ventilation, trouble shooting, the weaning of the patient from mechanical ventilation, and complications.

Mechanical ventilation provides movement of respiratory gases into and out of the pulmonary system. This mode of therapy is chosen only when ventilation can be improved or maintained through positive pressure (Shapiro, Harrison, and Trout, 1979). There are three mechanisms in which positive pressure ventilation facilitates gas exchange: First, mechanical ventilation provides the power to maintain ventilation. When, for whatever reason, the inspiratory muscles are unable to generate enough muscular energy for the normal inspiratory process, ventilation then becomes compromised. Second, mechanical ventilation can improve distribution of ventilation by altering inspiratory airway pressures and flow patterns. Finally, mechanical ventilation improves overall gas exchange by altering ventilatory patterns of inspiratory to expiratory ratios, ventilatory rate, or tidal volume (Shapiro, Harrison, and Trout, 1979).

Positive-pressure mechanical ventilators are time cycled, pressure cycled, or volume cycled. The ventilator divides the respiratory cycle into four units: inspiration, the inspiratory/expiratory changeover, expiration, and the expiratory/inspiratory changeover (Fuchs, 1979). The type of ventilator determines the inspiratory/expiratory changeover. Therefore inspiration ceases whenever a preset time (time-cycled ventilator), pressure (pressure-cycled ventilator), or volume (volume-cycled ventilator) has been attained. The expiratory cycle in a patient on mechanical ventilation most commonly occurs two ways: passive exhalation or exhalation against positive pressure (PEEP). The expiratory/ inspiratory changeover is determined by controlled or assisted ventilation. The controlled ventilation does not allow the patient to have any participation with the ventilator; the machine does everything. During assisted ventilation, the ventilator cycles inspiration in response to the patient's inspiratory effort (Fuchs, 1979). A ventilator capable of both modes of ventilation would be ideal; under certain conditions the patient could initiate ventilation, but the ventilator would guarantee that a minimum respiratory rate was maintained.

Connecting the patient-ventilator system

It is important that the nurse caring for the patient in shock recognize the potential for inadequate alveolar ventilation. To do this, the nurse must have expertise in the area of respiratory assessment so that the adequacy of oxygenation can be evaluated. Ideally placing a patient on mechanical ventilation should occur prior to cardiopulmonary collapse and subsequent resuscitation. Shapiro, Harrison, and Trout (1979) have identified four classifications of cardiopulmonary pathophysiology that may ultimately warrant mechanical ventilation (Table 4-5).

Once the decision has been made to place the patient on a ventilator, the practitioner must proceed to connect the patient to the ventilator system. Shapiro, Harrison,

Table 4-5. Classification of cardiopulmonary pathophysiology requiring medical ventilation

Classification	Assessment findings
Apnea	Absence of spontaneous ventilation
Acute ventilatory failure	Increased minute ventilation Decreased alveolar ventilation Progressive acidemia (pH $<$ 7.36) Progressive increased Pa_{CO_2} > 50 mm Hg
Impending acute ventilatory failure	Patient exhibiting increased work in breathing *Sequential* arterial blood gas values displaying decreasing alveolar ventilation: pH $<$ 7.36 Pa_{CO_2} > 50 mm Hg V_D/V_T > 0.60
Oxygenation	Poor Pa_{O_2} with room air, nasal oxygen, or mask oxygen: Pa_{O_2} $<$ 70 mm Hg $P(A - a)_{O_2}$ > 400 mm Hg

Data from Shapiro, B.A., Harrison, R.A., and Walton, J.R.: Clinical application of blood gases, Chicago, 1977, Year Book Medical Publishers, Inc.

and Trout (1979) established the following five steps as a general guideline for the safe and orderly progression to connecting the patient to the ventilator: (1) establishment of the airway and manual support of ventilation, (2) cardiovascular stabilization, (3) establishment of appropriate monitors and baselines, (4) establishment of ventilatory patterns, and (5) connection to the ventilator.

For correct mechanical ventilation an artificial airway by means of a cuffed endotracheal, nasotracheal, or tracheal tube must be inserted. A cuffed tube must be utilized to ensure that positive pressure is maintained and to protect the lungs from aspiration and subsequent aspiration pneumonia. Once the airway has been established, it is then necessary to manually support ventilation using a self-inflating Ambu bag with a one-way valve that is connected to an oxygen source.

Intubation and the initiation of positive pressure ventilation may further compromise the cardiovascular system in the shock patient. Most commonly these patients experience further hypotension and cardiac arrhythmias, which can be caused by decreased sympathetic tone and decreased venous return resulting in diminished cardiac output (Shapiro, Harrison, and Trout, 1979). The physiological stress of shock and the institution of positive pressure ventilation causes the sympathetic branch of the autonomic nervous system to receive much stimulation. Once the work of breathing is relieved, some of the stimulus to the sympathetic nervous system declines, thus reducing the amount of circulating catecholamines, and subsequent hypotension and cardiac arrhythmias may

Table 4-6. Guidelines for initial mechanical ventilator settings

Setting	Rationale
F_{IO_2}: 1:0	In shock patient, who is newly intubated, F_{IO_2} of 1.0 should be used for at least 20 minutes, at which point arterial blood gases as well as the alveolar-arterial ($P[A-a]O_2$) gradient should be determined. F_{IO_2} should then be adjusted to maintain PaO_2 between 60 and 100 mm Hg (Martz, Joiner, and Shepherd, 1979). *Note:* Frequently positive end-expiratory pressure (PEEP) will be used as a means of maintaining adequate PaO_2 levels without the risk of oxygen toxicity (see section on PEEP).
V_T: 15 ml/kg in a patient without history of restrictive lung pathology	Large tidal volumes with slower, controlled respiratory rates produce high alveolar ventilation without risk of atelectasis, and previously collapsed alveoli may be reinflated (Martz, Joiner, and Shepherd, 1979).
Frequency: 8 to 12 breaths/min	Conscious patients tolerate a slower frequency with a large tidal volume better than a lower volume (Shapiro, Harrison, and Trout, 1979).
Inspiratory/expiratory ratio: 1:1.5 or 1:2	Reduces the cardiovascular effects of mechanical ventilation (e.g., impaired venous return and cardiac output) (Wade, 1977). The inspiratory time should never exceed expiratory time.
Sensitivity: -2 cm H_2O	Sensitivity is the amount of inspiratory effort required to initiate an inspiratory cycle. The higher the sensitivity, the lower the patient effort required.
Sigh volume: 1.5 to 2 times V_T	Sigh mechanism is utilized to further expand alveoli and prevent alveolar collapse. In some cases, if PEEP is being utilized, the sigh mechanism may not be activated.

occur. Positive pressure ventilation also results in increased intrathoracic pressure, which leads to a decrease in venous return. In the shock patient this further compromises the cardiac output and can potentiate further cardiovascular decompensation.

Frequently the shock patient is already undergoing extensive hemodynamic and cardiovascular monitoring. If an arterial line is present, it is the nurse's responsibility to ensure patency of the line so that the adequacy of oxygenation can be continually evaluated through serial arterial blood gas values.

Prior to connecting the patient to the mechanical ventilator, the nurse must establish the ventilatory pattern and complete the initial ventilator settings. Although these settings will be readjusted according to the patients' physiological response to mechanical ventilation, Table 4-6 provides some guidelines for the initial settings.

The patient on mechanical ventilation requires meticulous nursing care. To ensure this, preestablished nursing goals can be readily individualized for a patient on a mechanical ventilator:

Maintain patent airway

Promote adequate oxygenation

Maintain fluid balance

Maintain adequate nutritional balance

Promote psychological adaptation to mechanical ventilator

Prevent concomitant infections

Prevent alterations in the musculoskeletal system

Provide pulmonary rehabilitation

The clinical picture of the patient with adult respiratory distress syndrome (Chapter 13) details the nursing interventions that are implemented to achieve these goals.

Trouble shooting

The nurse must continuously utilize assessment skills to evaluate the efficiency of the patient-ventilator system (Table 4-7). The continuity of assessment readily identifies the actual or potential problem that then is corrected. The nurse is responsible for obtaining and evaluating physiological data that determine the adequacy of oxygenation and ventilation. These values should be obtained 20 to 30 minutes after the initiation of mechanical ventilation, then every 30 to 60 minutes until the patient has stabilized, and finally every 4 to 8 hours depending on the patient's condition (Levy and Stubbs, 1978). In addition, there must be continual assessment of the shock patient for non-ventilator-related problems. These problems include the hazards of immobility, gastrointestinal bleeding, infection, and sensory alterations.

Increasing Pao$_2$

It is not uncommon for the mechanically ventilated shock patient to continue in a hypoxemic state that is refractory to high concentrations of inspired oxygen (Fio$_2$). When this occurs, the patient's ventilator settings are changed to accommodate positive end-expiratory pressure (PEEP). By definition, PEEP is the artificial maintenance of positive pressure at the end of expiration, which stops the expiratory flow when the alveolar pressure is above the atmospheric pressure. The overall purposes of PEEP are two-fold. Initially PEEP augments arterial oxygen saturation (Pao$_2$) in a patient with refractory hypoxemia. It is also believed that PEEP can reverse or improve the pathology responsible for the gas-exchange abnormality (Stevens, 1977). Therefore PEEP results in an increased Pao$_2$ without dangerously high Fio$_2$ concentrations, which could result in oxygen toxicity and further damage to the lung tissues; a decreased work of breathing; and improvement in ventilation-perfusion inequalities (Shapiro, Harrison, and Trout, 1979). Through the use of PEEP, the functional residual capacity (FRC) is increased because the lung volumes are increased at the end of expiration and the small airways and atelectatic alveoli are reopened. This will result in a decrease in the amount of shunting and an increase in the Pao$_2$ (Levy and Stubbs, 1978).

Nurses caring for patients who are being placed on PEEP must continually assess vital signs, central venous pressure, and/or pulmonary artery pressure to evaluate the ef-

Table 4-7. Nursing assessment of the patient-ventilator system

Assessment	Problem	Nursing intervention
Mental status		
Anxiety, restlessness, agitation	Response to the ICU environment	Reassure and teach patient and family about environment and equipment.
	$\downarrow$ Pao$_2$	Evaluate adequacy of ventilation system, patency of airway, and arterial blood gases (ABGs).
Disorientation, confusion	$\downarrow$ Pao$_2$, $\uparrow$ Paco$_2$, $\downarrow$ pH	Evaluate adequacy of ventilator system, patency of airway, and ABGs.
	Altered sleep patterns	Organize nursing care to provide for scheduled sleep periods.
Pulmonary status		
Dyspnea	Anxiety, $\downarrow$ Pao$_2$, $\downarrow$ Ventilation	Reassure and teach; evaluate ventilator settings and ABGs.
	Pneumothorax	Order immediate chest x-ray film.
Changes in respiratory rate	Tampering with ventilator settings	Evaluate or correct ventilator settings.
	Anxiety, altered metabolic needs (fever, muscle spasms, etc.)	Reassure and teach.
Diminished breath sounds	Decreased tidal volume, atelectasis	Evaluate and correct ventilator settings.
	Pneumonia, endotracheal tube displacement	Order immediate chest x-ray film.
	Pneumothorax	Order immediate chest x-ray film.
Secretions: thick, thin	Inadequate humidification, too much humidification, moisture accumulating in ventilator tubing	Increase humidity settings; decrease humidity settings. Remove moisture from ventilator tubing.
Air leak around artificial airway	Inadequate cuff inflation, ruptured cuff	Reinflate cuff; replace with new cuffed tube.
Asynchrony with ventilator	Anxiety, inadequate flow rate, inappropriate inspiration/expiration ratio	Reassure and teach; check ventilator settings. Immediately "bag" with Fio$_2$ of 1.0 until cause is identified and corrected.
	$\downarrow$ Pao$_2$, $\uparrow$ Paco$_2$	If unable to easily correct, obtain and evaluate ABGs.

Modified from Martz, K.V., Joiner, J., and Shepherd, R.M.: Management of the patient-ventilator system: a team approach, St. Louis, 1979, The C.V. Mosby Co.

Table 4-7. Nursing assessment of the patient-ventilator system — cont'd

Assessment	Problem	Nursing intervention
Cardiovascular status		
Diminished cardiac output	Changes in intrathoracic pressure from the ventilator that impair venous return, decreased perfusion due to cardiac output caused by shock	Evaluate hemodynamic parameters for perfusion; evaluate and adjust fluid balance.
New cardiac arrhythmias	↓ Pao_2, ↑ $Paco_2$, ↓ venous return	Evaluate adequacy of ventilator settings; check hemodynamic parameters for perfusion.
	Inaccurate use of antiarrhythmic drugs	Evaluate possible drug interactions and/or toxicity.
Arterial blood pressure		
Hypotension	↓ Venous return	Evaluate hemodynamic parameters for perfusion; decrease PEEP level.
Hypertension	Anxiety	Evaluate patient ventilatory system, ABGs; reassure.
	Imprecise use of pressors	Evaluate drug toxicity.
Fluid balance: decreased renal output	Diminished circulating blood volume	Evaluate hemodynamic parameters for perfusion; obtain serum electrolytes; evaluate parenteral fluid administration.

fects of continuous positive intrathoracic pressure on the cardiovascular system. Levy and Stubbs (1978) recommend that these values be monitored every 15 minutes until they are stable following the institution of PEEP or increases in the PEEP level. Shapiro, Harrison, and Trout (1979) have identified the therapeutic levels of PEEP in the adult as between 10 and 30 cm H_2O. The baseline assessments of the adequacy of oxygenation and ventilation should be reevaluated 20 to 30 minutes following the institution of PEEP or changes in the PEEP level. The use of PEEP is very effective in increasing arterial oxygen saturation levels, but the nurse must be aware of potential complications. These complications can occur in two categories: physiological and anatomical (Stevens, 1977). Physiologically there can be reduced cardiac output, which can increase the arterial-venous shunting, further decreasing the Pao_2. If the decrease in cardiac output cannot be reversed, the PEEP must be discontinued. Anatomical complications include pneumothorax, subcutaneous emphysema, and bronchial/tracheal rupture. If anatomical complications occur, PEEP can usually be continued with caution once the treatment for the anatomical complications has been instituted.

Weaning

Once the arterial oxygenation has been stabilized and the patient shows signs of clinical improvement, weaning from PEEP is initiated. The first stage of this weaning is accomplished by decreasing the FIO_2 delivered by the mechanical ventilator. The goal is to maintain the PaO_2 at 70 mm Hg with an FIO_2 of 40% or less (Shapiro, Harrison, and Trout, 1979). Once this goal has been achieved the level of PEEP is gradually reduced by 2 to 5 cm H_2O every 4 to 6 hours until the end-expiratory pressure is equal to atmospheric pressure and an adequate PaO_2 is maintained (Adams, 1979; Levy and Stubbs, 1978). While the weaning from PEEP is continuing, the nurse should monitor the patient's vital signs, central venous pressure, and/or pulmonary artery pressure every 15 minutes until they are stable with each decrease in PEEP level. The continuous monitoring is critical because hypoxia may occur within 1 minute following discontinuance of PEEP because of the rapid closure of small airways and alveoli (Kumar, Falke, and Giffin, 1970).

Following the discontinuation of PEEP, the patient may be completely weaned from the mechanical ventilator. One method for successful weaning is to utilize the intermittent mandatory ventilation (IMV) mode of ventilation. The benefit of the IMV mode is that it provides a gradual transition from mechanical ventilation to spontaneous breathing (Klein, 1975). However, before any weaning can be initiated, patient readiness must be determined. To do this one must evaluate the patient's ability to do the work of breathing by evaluating two areas. First, the vital capacity must be measured. The vital capacity is the maximum number of liters of air that the patient can exhale. If the patient has a vital capacity of 15 ml/kg or greater, weaning may begin because the patient is moving an adequate quantity of air for the exchange of respiratory gases (Klein, 1975). In addition, the inspiratory pressure must be determined. An individual needs a minimum inspiratory pressure of -20 cm H_2O to cough effectively. A pressure of -25 to -30 cm H_2O is needed for effective weaning from mechanical ventilation (Adams, 1979; Klein, 1975).

Once patient readiness for weaning has been determined, the nurse must continually assess the patient's tolerance to the weaning process. The IMV mode combines a constant rate of mechanical ventilation with continuous oxygen-enriched gas to allow spontaneous ventilation during the time intervals between mechanical (mandatory) breaths (Klein, 1975). Continual improvement in the respiratory assessment parameters provides the necessary physiological documentation to decrease the IMV rate 1 to 2 breaths/min and allow spontaneous ventilation to assume a greater proportion. It is necessary that the nurse evaluate the adequacy of oxygenation and ventilation, assess the cardiopulmonary status of the patient, and ensure a patent airway with each decrease in the IMV rate. An increased $PaCO_2$ during weaning indicates inadequate alveolar ventilation and the IMV rate may need to be increased and the weaning process may need to progress more slowly. A declining PaO_2 may require readjustment of the FIO_2 or even returning to PEEP. The use of the IMV mode of weaning is advantageous because it provides smooth transition from controlled to spontaneous ventilation without increasing the patient's anxiety or fatigue. The nurse is able to constantly evaluate the patient's tolerance to the weaning process and to implement appropriate nursing interventions.

Complications

While the use of the mechanical ventilator has life-saving value in some shock patients, a considerable number of complications may result. These complications fall into three categories: those associated with an artificial airway, those associated with ventilator function, and those associated with fluid and electrolyte balance (Levy and Stubbs, 1978; Petty, 1976).

The artificial airway selected may be the oral endotracheal, nasotracheal, or tracheal tube. If prolonged intubation is anticipated, the oral endotracheal tube is a poor selection because it is poorly tolerated in the semiconscious or conscious patient; it is difficult to stabilize; premature extubation is common; it may become occluded by the patient's biting, unless a bite-block is used; and the tube's curvature may occasionally cause difficulty in suctioning (Shapiro, Harrison, and Trout, 1979).

Hazards associated with the artificial airway may vary with different types of airways. However there are some universal problems that the respiratory care practitioner must be aware of. First, an artificial airway bypasses normal respiratory defenses that prevent bacterial contamination of the lower airway. Second, because the use of the artificial airway makes the vocal cords nonfunctional, the cough is no longer effective. Third, the patient is no longer able to communicate vocally. Finally, in the conscious patient, placement of the artificial airway can alter the patient's body image (Shapiro, Harrison, and Trout, 1979). Complications following the insertion of an artificial airway can occur with intubation, premature extubation, maintenance of airway patency, and too much pressure on the trachea from inflation of the cuff. The most common complication occurring with artificial airway placement is intubation of the right mainstem bronchus. Diagnosis of right mainstem bronchus intubation is confirmed by x-ray examination and is commonly associated with right-sided alveolar hyperventilation, left-sided atelectasis, or a pneumothorax. The pneumothorax when it occurs is frequently on the right side and is associated with tension (Petty, 1976). Premature extubation can be patient or staff initiated. One of the hazards with extubation of the endotracheal or nasotracheal tube is laryngospasm, which may impair immediate reintubation and require a tracheostomy. While a major goal of nursing is to maintain artificial patency through suctioning and pulmonary hygiene techniques, occlusion of the airway can still occur. The airway can become occluded when the cuff herniates over the distal portion of the tube, which requires immediate deflation of the cuff. The airway can also become occluded through kinking or impingement on the wall of the trachea, bronchus, or carina. If this is the cause, deflation of the tube or simple manipulation of the tube can correct the occlusion. Finally, complication from artificial airways can result from too much cuff pressure on the tracheal wall. Previously it had been recommended that deflation of the cuff for 5 minutes out of each hour would decrease the risk of tracheal necrosis. However, studies on anesthetized dogs have not demonstrated any advantage to this method by decreasing the risk of damage to the tracheal mucosa (Dunn, Dunn, and Moser, 1974; Powaser et al., 1976). Presently high volume–low pressure cuffs or the foam cuff is utilized in respiratory care. It is believed that these cuffs decrease the pressure on the tracheal mucosa and in turn decrease the risk of tracheal necrosis (Dunn, Dunn, and Moser, 1974; Geffin et al., 1971).

Complications occurring in the patient on mechanical ventilation can also result from problems associated with the ventilator. Inappropriate settings on the mechanical ventilator or patient asynchrony with the ventilator can result in alveolar hypoventilation or hyperventilation, which results in diminished tissue oxygenation. Patients undergoing PEEP have an increased risk of developing a pneumothorax, which can have deteriorating effects on tissue oxygenation and patient survival. Finally disastrous results can occur when there is a disconnection of the patient-ventilator system. One means of control for these complications is by continual assessment of the patient-ventilator system. Evaluation of ventilator settings and nursing respiratory assessment should be carried out at least hourly on these patients. The warning alarm on a mechanical ventilator should never be routinely turned off. This may be the only indicator to the nurse that the system is not working properly.

One major complication associated with the mechanical ventilator is oxygen toxicity. An FIO_2 greater than 40% is potentially dangerous if used for more than a few days (Petty, 1976). The patient with oxygen toxicity develops reduced lung compliance, atelectatic areas, and an increased risk of sepsis because of the decrease in lung macrophage activity (Petty, 1976; Shapiro, Harrison, and Trout, 1979). The use of PEEP has reduced the risk of oxygen toxicity by lowering FIO_2 levels and maintaining the opened airways at the end of inspiration.

Patients who are critically ill are at risk for developing secondary infections. Placement of these patients on mechanical ventilation further increases the risk of infection. The nurse can reduce this risk by instituting nursing interventions that prevent stasis of pulmonary secretions. To achieve this goal the nurse must develop an individualized routine for pulmonary hygiene for each patient and utilize aseptic techniques for removing secretions from the artificial airway of the critically ill shock patient.

Patients on mechanical ventilation are also at risk for fluid and electrolyte imbalances. Fluid overload can be caused by several factors: (1) the attachment of a patient to the mechanical ventilator inhibits the normal insensible fluid loss from the lungs, (2) utilization of humidified air increases the amount of fluid entering the body, and (3) poorly controlled administration of parenteral fluids can increase circulating fluid volume. Fluid overload places the patient at risk for increased pulmonary extravascular water, pulmonary edema, and severe respiratory distress (Levy and Stubbs, 1978). Fluid deficit can be caused by too little humidification delivered by the ventilator, unreplaced body fluid loss, and poorly controlled parenteral fluids. This fluid deficit can result in thickened bronchial secretions and, in some cases, diminished cardiac output. The nurse must utilize the skills of physical assessment to continuously monitor fluid balance. In addition to intake and output recordings, daily weights must be obtained, hemodynamic parameters must be continuously monitored, and skin turgor, mucosal membrane hydration, and the consistency of bronchial secretions must be evaluated. This data will give the nurse an objective basis for the evaluation of fluid status.

While caring for the shock patient on a mechanical ventilator the nurse utilizes the knowledge of the process of oxygenation to provide the scientific rationales for the nursing therapies selected for respiratory care. The nursing therapies are directed toward ensuring adequate alveolar ventilation. To effectively accomplish this, the nurse must have knowledge of the basics of mechanical ventilation, special features of the ventilator, trouble shooting, weaning the patient from mechanical ventilation, and complications. The nurse also needs the necessary assessment skills to monitor the patient-ventilator system frequently and to document the adequacy of oxygenation and ventilation of the shock patient requiring mechanical ventilation.

REFERENCES

Adams, N.R.: The nurse's role in systematic weaning from a ventilator, Nursing '79 **9:**35-41, 1979.

Boyce, B.A.: Respiratory care terminology. Part I, NLN Clinical Newsletter **1:**1-6, 1976.

Bushnell, S.S.: Respiratory intensive care nursing, ed. 2, Boston, 1981, Little, Brown & Co.

Brigham, K.L., and Newman, J.H.: The pulmonary circulation, Basics of RD **8:**1-6, 1979.

Daily, E.K., and Schroeder, J.S.: Techniques in bedside hemodynamic monitoring, ed. 2, St. Louis, 1981, The C.V. Mosby Co.

Dunn, C.R., Dunn, D.L., and Moser, K.M.: Determinants of tracheal injury by cuffed tracheostomy tubes, Chest **65:**128-134, 1974.

Fitzgerald, L.M.: Mechanical ventilation, Heart & Lung **5:**939-950, 1976.

Fuchs, P.C.: Understanding continuous mechanical ventilation, Nursing '79 **9:**26-33, 1979.

Galich, R., and Goertzen, E.W.: Tracheal protection in assisted ventilation: a survey, Laryngoscope **82:**131-138, 1972.

Ganong, W.F.: Review of medical physiology, ed. 9, Los Altos, Calif., 1979, Lange Medical Publications.

Geffin, B., et al.: Stenosis following tracheostomy for respiratory care, Journal of the American Medical Association **216:**1984-1988, 1971.

Halloway, N.M.: Nursing the critically ill adult, Menlo Park, Calif., 1979, Addison-Wesley Publishing Co., Inc.

Harper, R.W.: A guide to respiratory care, Philadelphia, 1981, J.B. Lippincott Co.

Klein, E.F.: Weaning from mechanical breathing with intermittent mandatory ventilation, Archives of Surgery **110:**345-347, 1975.

Kumar, A., Falke, K.J., and Giffin, B.: Continuous positive pressure ventilation in acute respiratory failure. Effects on hemodynamics and lung function, New England Journal of Medicine **283:**1430, 1970.

Lake, K.B., and Van Dyke, J.J.: Prolonged nasotracheal intubation, Heart & Lung **9:**93-96, 1980.

Levy, M.M., and Stubbs, J.A.: Nursing implications in the care of patients treated with assisted mechanical ventilation modified with positive end-expiratory pressure, Heart & Lung **7:**299-306, 1978.

Martz, K.V., Joiner, J., and Shepherd, R.M.: Management of the patient-ventilator system: a team approach, St. Louis, 1979, The C.V. Mosby Co.

Mathewson, H.S.: Respiratory therapy in critical care. St. Louis, 1976, The C.V. Mosby Co.

Powaser, M.M., et al.: The effectiveness of hourly cuff deflation in minimizing tracheal damage, Heart & Lung **5:**734-741, 1976.

Petty, T.L.: Complications occurring during mechanical ventilation, Heart & Lung **5:**112-118, 1976.

Shapiro, B.A., Harrison, R.A., and Walton, J.R.: Clinical application of blood gases, Chicago, 1977, Year Book Medical Publishers, Inc.

Shapiro, B.A., Harrison, R.A., and Trout, C.A.: Clinical application of respiratory care, ed. 2, Chicago, 1979, Year Book Medical Publishers, Inc.

Stevens, P.M.: Positive end expiratory pressure breathing, Basics of RD **5:**1-6, 1977.

Wade, J.F.: Respiratory nursing care, ed. 2, St. Louis, 1977, The C.V. Mosby Co.

Waldron, M.W.: Oxygen transport, American Journal of Nursing **79:**272-275, 1979.

West, J.B.: Ventilation perfusion relationships, American Review of Respiratory Disease **116:**919-941, 1977.

West, J.B.: Respiratory physiology: the essentials, ed. 2, Baltimore, 1979, The Williams and Wilkins Co.

PART TWO

MANAGEMENT OF THE PATIENT IN SHOCK

5 Classification of shock

LINDA NIEDRINGHAUS

CLASSIFICATION SYSTEMS FOR SHOCK

The clinical syndrome known as shock can originate from many causes and involves many complex physiological mechanisms. Shock is not a single disease entity with well-defined symptoms that can be treated by a single therapeutic medical or nursing approach. Rather, shock is a complex syndrome of cardiopulmonary, hemodynamic, and vascular changes that reduce cellular perfusion and oxygen transport. This common physiological denominator, reduced cellular perfusion, can be initiated by a loss of circulating fluid volume, pump failure, or widespread vasodilation.

Because of the possible underlying differences in the cause of shock, medical and nursing therapies to treat shock will differ. A mode of treatment suitable for one variety of shock may be entirely inappropriate for another. A rigid approach to clinical management is unrealistic. Effective treatment depends on a thorough knowledge of the exact physiological and biochemical disturbances that exist in a particular patient at a particular time. Several classification or nomenclature systems have been developed to aid physicians and nurses in the recognition and diagnosis of the various types of shock. These classification systems are valuable in that they help to explain the causes or indicate the treatment of shock.

Hardaway (1968, 1979) has developed three classification systems for shock. These classification systems have been used and expanded by clinicians to establish the diagnosis of shock and to organize the treatment approach for each patient. These three classification systems will be discussed.

Classification of shock by cause

The etiology of shock serves as the basis for this classification system. This method is simple, direct, and easy to use. It suggests what assessments need to be made and what medical and nursing management will be necessary to promote recovery. This classification system encompasses three general types of shock: (1) *hypovolemic shock,* in which blood or plasma has been lost from the circulation to the exterior of the body or into the tissues, (2) *cardiogenic shock,* in which the pumping action of the heart is inadequate, and (3) *vasogenic or low-resistance shock* in which widespread vasodilation increases the capacity of the circulation so that the existing blood volume, even if it is normal, becomes inadequate. This method of classifying the various types of shock

91

Classification of shock according to cause

Type of shock	Cause/description
Hypovolemic	
Hemorrhagic shock	Blood loss caused by minor tissue trauma; can be caused by gastrointestinal bleeding, bleeding disorders, or gunshot or knife wounds.
Traumatic shock	Blood loss plus major tissue injury; occurs with severe damage to muscle or bone; seen with battle casualties and car accidents; leakage of myoglobin into the circulation can cause renal damage.
Burn shock	Plasma loss as burn exudate from burned body surfaces; increased hematocrit and hemoconcentration are seen.
Dehydration shock	Fluid loss caused by prolonged vomiting, diarrhea, or intestinal fistulas or obstruction; also can occur with metabolic disorders such as adrenal insufficiency and diabetic ketoacidosis.
Cardiogenic	Cardiac pump failure caused by myocardial infarction, heart tamponade, or pulmonary embolism; because of inadequate cardiac output, tissue perfusion remains inadequate in spite of normal blood volume.
Vasogenic	
Septic shock	Massive vasodilation caused by endotoxin from gram-negative bacteria; this toxin is liberated in the body in large amounts in certain infections.
Anaphylactic shock	Severe allergic, antigen-antibody reaction that releases histamine, causing increased capillary permeability and widespread dilation of arterioles and capillaries.
Neurogenic shock	Loss of sympathetic control of resistance vessels resulting in dilation of arterioles and venules that increases the vascular space and renders the circulating blood volume ineffective; hypotension caused by spinal anesthesia is an example of this phenomenon.

---

according to cause has gained widespread use in the clinical area. Each of the types of shock will be discussed, briefly.

Hypovolemic shock. Hypovolemic shock is the most common type of circulatory shock. Profound hemorrhage is the usual precipitating factor of this type of shock, but it can also occur in patients who become severely dehydrated. Because hemorrhage is more closely associated with trauma, hypovolemic shock is more prevalent in the younger active age groups. Volume loss can also be the result of the loss of plasma that occurs with burns. Third-space fluid loss caused by peritonitis and intestinal obstruction can be another cause of hypovolemic shock.

If the hypovolemic shock is caused by a loss of plasma through burned tissue, blood viscosity becomes markedly increased and promotes the development of venous stasis in the presence of an already compromised blood flow. Capillary damage and increased capillary permeability from the thermal assault cause a shift of plasma from the intravascular compartment to the interstitial space. Loss of plasma protein from the intravascular system reduces plasma osmotic pressure, which limits the return of fluid to the capillary.

If the hypovolemic shock is caused by intestinal obstruction, the following series of events creates a loss of plasma volume. Increased intestinal capillary hydrostatic pressure causes a shift of plasma from the capillaries into the intestinal lumen where it is trapped and unavailable for circulation through the intravascular system. After several hours the patient becomes dangerously hypovolemic and demonstrates signs of decreased cardiac output and hypoperfusion of the peripheral circulation (Groër and Shekleton, 1979).

Cardiogenic shock. Cardiogenic shock occurs when the heart is unable to pump enough blood to meet the body tissue's need for oxygen. The most common precipitating factor of cardiogenic shock is a massive myocardial infarction. Cardiogenic shock can also develop as a result of severe congestive heart failure caused by coronary artery disease, valvular problems, or myocardial disease. In addition, cardiogenic shock can occur following open-heart surgery when the heart becomes unable to meet the body's need for oxygen and the cardiac output becomes extremely low. Heart disease is the leading cause of death in the United States, and cardiogenic shock is the second most common form of circulatory collapse. This form of shock is prevalent in the middle and older age groups (Zschoche, 1981).

Cardiogenic shock associated with myocardial infarction is very likely to be fatal. The mortality of cardiogenic shock associated with myocardial infarction continues to be high in spite of aggressive treatment. Cardiogenic shock is more likely to be a complication when 40% or more of the left ventricle is damaged. However, cardiogenic shock does not appear to be related to heart failure. The two seem to be completely different diseases. Treatment for heart failure is ineffective in the treatment of cardiogenic shock (Groër and Shekleton, 1979).

Vasogenic shock. The third type of shock in this classification system is vasogenic shock, which is caused by widespread vasodilation from decreased vasomotor tone. Blood volume remains within normal limits, but the capacity of the vessels is increased. This increased capacity of the vessels without a corresponding increase in blood volume leads to a decreased venous return that results in diminished cardiac output. Two common types of vasogenic shock are septic shock and anaphylactic shock.

One form of vasogenic shock is *septic shock,* which is caused by a widespread overwhelming infection with gram-negative or gram-positive organisms, fungi, yeasts, or possibly viruses. Septic shock is the third most common form of shock. It occurs in all age groups and is most frequently seen in postoperative patients. Because this shock is caused by an overwhelming infection, the very young, the old, and the debilitated are most commonly affected. Patients with indwelling catheters, burns, chronic debilitating diseases, or postpartum infections risk developing septic shock. Early symptoms of septic shock are related to the underlying infection and widespread vasodilation. These symptoms may include fever, mental confusion, tachycardia, tachypnea, and reduced urine output.

Another form of vasogenic shock is *anaphylactic shock,* which is the result of an antigen-antibody reaction. The release of histamine, serotonin, and bradykinin affects the local blood vessels directly, causing vasodilation and increased capillary permeability. Slow-reacting substances are also released, causing constriction of the bronchioles. Hypotensive, shocklike symptoms are caused by the widespread vasodilation and by the leakage of plasma from the intravascular circulation (Price and Wilson, 1978).

If the reduction in vasomotor tone occurs at the level of the vasomotor center in the medulla, the resulting generalized vasodilation would be called *neurogenic shock.* This form of shock can develop with the use of spinal anesthesia, with spinal cord injury, or with direct damage to the medulla. Altered function of the vasomotor center in response to low blood sugar and drugs such as tranquilizers, narcotics, or sedatives can lead to neurogenic shock.

Clinical classification of shock

The same types of shock can be classified clinically; the organizing factor is the patient's blood pressure and other clinical signs that can be assessed at the bedside. This classification system uses descriptive terms that are helpful in understanding the causes, symptoms, and progression of the various types of shock.

The clinical classification system defines two broad categories of shock: (1) *hypotensive shock* and (2) *normotensive or hypertensive shock.* Hypotensive shock, the first category, is further divided into (a) shock with cold skin, and (b) shock with warm skin. This classification system is more complex. For example, septic shock appears in both of the classification categories, shock with cold skin and shock with warm skin (see Chapter 9). The reader should remember, in this classification system the clinical *symptoms* of the state of shock, not the *cause,* are the organizing factors.

The second broad category in this classification system is normotensive or hypertensive shock. This category is further divided into compensated shock, overcompensated shock, epinephrine shock, shock associated with vasoconstrictor drugs, and shock associated with pheochromocytoma. Many authors would argue that epinephrine shock is not a specific type of shock but rather a compensatory response of the endocrine system to hypotension. The shock state associated with pheochromocytoma (a tumor of the adrenal medulla) is caused by the release of epinephrine that increases peripheral resistance to the point that local flow to various capillary beds is severely restricted. Again,

---

Clinical classification system for shock

Hypotensive shock

Cold skin: low cardiac output, arterioles constricted
  Hypovolemic shock
    Hemorrhage
    Third-space loss
  Normovolemic shock
    Septic shock
  Cardiogenic shock
Warm skin: high cardiac output
  Severe septic shock
  Vasodilated shock
    Spinal anesthesia
    Vasodilating drugs

Normotensive or hypertensive shock

Compensated: hemorrhage insufficient to lower blood pressure
Overcompensated: intensive catecholamine response to hemorrhage that raises blood pressure
Epinephrine shock: intense vasoconstriction caused by epinephrine
Vasoconstrictor administration: high blood pressure caused by aggressive administration of exogenous vasoconstrictor drugs
Pheochromocytoma: high blood pressure caused by endogenous release of catecholamines from the adrenal medulla

---

many authors do not consider this condition to be one of the classic forms of shock but rather classify it as an acute endocrine problem.

Classification of shock by severity

Shock may also be classified by severity or stages of development. These stages or phases of shock are a series of pathological changes that unfold in dramatic sequence if medical and nursing interventions are delayed or inappropriate. These stages do not progress at the same speed for all patients; some patients go through their episode of shock or circulatory failure more rapidly than others. Therefore there are no arbitrary time periods for each of the stages.

Shock can be divided into four stages. Each stage is demonstrated by specific changes in the microcirculation as well as clinical manifestations that can be assessed at the bedside. The first three stages of shock are reversible; the last stage is not.

Classification of shock by severity

Stage of shock	Characteristics
Early reversible shock	Vasoconstriction, poor venous return, drop in blood pressure; reversed by infusions of blood or other fluids.
Late reversible shock	Sluggish capillary blood flow, beginning lactic acidosis; reversed by infusions of fluid in excess of amount of blood or fluid lost.
Refractory shock	Stagnation of blood flow, beginning coagulation alterations; can be reversed by aggressive medical and nursing management to replace fluids and support failing organ systems.
Irreversible shock	Cellular necrosis and multiple organ failure; failure of resuscitation measures to restore blood pressure, cardiac output, and oxygen consumption.

Stage I: Early reversible shock. In the early phase of shock, elevated catecholamines cause vasoconstriction of the microcirculation. Poor venous return to the left ventricle leads to a drop in the arterial blood pressure. These two factors, vasoconstriction and poor venous return, cause a decrease in the rate of flow through the tissue capillaries. During the early reversible shock phase, the only clinical symptom may be a small drop in the arterial blood pressure caused by poor venous return. Changes in the blood pressure are not predictable. The arterial pressure may remain normal or be elevated. At this stage, shock is easily treated by small infusions of blood or other fluids.

Stage II: Late reversible shock. During late reversible shock, capillary flow is extremely slow and a fall in pH along the capillary is caused by anaerobic metabolism and lactic acid production. This stage is characterized by capillary and venule dilation, which produces expansion of the vascular space. At this point, fluid replacement must exceed the amount of blood or fluid lost because of expansion of this vascular space. Once the compensatory responses to shock are exhausted, the arterial blood pressure will fall. This stage is reversible if adequate amounts of fluid are given.

Stage III: Refractory shock. In refractory shock, stagnant, acid blood, produced by sepsis or tissue injury, begins to coagulate, causing the red blood cells and platelets to occlude the capillaries. When occlusion stops perfusion in the capillaries completely, cells nourished by these capillaries begin to die. Endogenous fibrinolysin begins to lyse the blood that has clotted. (Blood that is still circulating is incapable of clotting.) This collection of physiological alterations is known as disseminated intravascular coagulation. A complete description of this clinical picture is presented in Chapter 14. This phase of shock responds poorly to routine fluid replacement since the patient's condition is usually complicated by severe trauma, infection, heart failure, kidney failure, or delay in treatment. While this stage is difficult to treat, it is refractory and will respond to aggressive medical and nursing management. Large volumes of fluid given with the benefit of hemodynamic monitoring will save the patient. Frequently vasodilators will be required since catecholamine levels may remain high as the body attempts to compensate. Vasodilators will be given only when the blood volume is adequate as demonstrated by hemodynamic monitoring (Chapter 6).

Stage IV: Irreversible shock. In irreversible shock, cells nourished by the compromised microcirculation have died, producing tissue necrosis in vital organs such as the kidney, liver, heart, and lungs. Large areas of necrosis can result in multiple organ failure that leads to death. Fortunately, considerable necrosis can be tolerated without organ failure or death. If these natural safety margins are decreased by renal, liver, or heart disease, a much smaller amount of cellular death will be sufficient to cause organ failure.

Research has been unable to explain why some patients survive shock and others do not. Some die, and others recover when the compensatory mechanisms, aided by appropriate treatment, gradually return the circulation to normal. In some patients recovery is impossible no matter how vigorous the approach to treatment. Patients appear to reach a stage in which there is no longer any physiological response to vasopressor drugs and in which, even if the blood volume is returned to normal, cardiac output remains depressed. Peripheral resistance falls, the heart slows, and the patient eventually dies.

Disagreement exists as to the cause of this phenomenon of irreversible shock. A number of physiological changes appear to combine to produce this stage. For example, prolonged cerebral ischemia, produced by maldistribution of blood flow, leads to depression of the vasomotor and cardiac center in the medulla. This depression causes slowing of the heart rate and vasodilation. Blood pressure drops further causing a further reduction in cerebral blood flow and further depression of the vasomotor and cardiac centers. Thus a vicious cycle known as a positive feedback mechanism is created in which the low flow state produces an even further reduction in flow (Ganong, 1977).

Another example of a dangerous positive feedback mechanism is the development of myocardial depression in severe shock states. The coronary blood flow is reduced because of hypotension and tachycardia even though the coronary vessels are dilated. This reduced coronary blood flow produces acidosis, which leads to further depression of myocardial function. If this depression of the myocardium is prolonged, the heart muscle may be so severely damaged that cardiac output cannot be restored to normal in spite of vigorous blood volume expansion with fluids.

Changes in splanchnic circulation also occur as a patient approaches the irreversible shock stage. The precapillary sphincters of the mesentery, which were constricted as a result of early compensatory mechanisms, now dilate while the venules remain constricted. Blood can enter the capillaries but stagnates in these vessels, so that tissue hypoxia continues. As capillary hydrostatic pressure rises, fluid leaves the vascular system, and capillary walls lose their integrity and slough cells. Hemorrhage occurs as whole blood is lost to the tissues. As a result, stagnant hypoxia in the gastrointestinal tract destroys the barriers that prevent the entry of bacteria into the circulation from the intestinal tract. Intestinal bacteria gain access to the systemic circulation causing widespread septicemia.

Although the irreversible stage of shock is fatal, all efforts at fluid, cardiac, and respiratory resuscitation are continued. Irreversible shock is considered a laboratory diagnosis, not a clinical one.

THE COMMON DENOMINATOR: REDUCED CELLULAR PERFUSION

Regardless of the classification of shock, the principle physiological defect remains the same: reduced cellular perfusion. Although the fundamental pathophysiology of the early stages of hypovolemic, cardiogenic, and vasogenic shock differs, the pathophysiological and metabolic changes of the later stages are similar among the various types of shock.

Cellular changes

The cellular effects of reduced perfusion have been studied extensively. Hypotension and hypoxia cause a shift from aerobic to anaerobic cellular metabolism. This metabolic shift causes an increase in lactic acid production, which reduces cellular pH. A sharp decrease in systemic oxygen consumption reflects this shift from aerobic to anaerobic metabolism.

Because anaerobic metabolism is less efficient in meeting the energy requirements of the cell, stores of the high-energy phosphate compound, adenosine triphosphate (ATP), are depleted. The mitochondria, the intracellular organelles that produce ATP, begin to swell and their function becomes impaired (Baue, 1976). The ultimate consequence of reduced mitochondrial activity is reduction in the tissue levels of ATP as well as the intracellular chemical messengers derived from ATP (Zschoche, 1981).

At the same time the mitochondria are undergoing alterations caused by reduced cellular perfusion, the membrane transport system of the cell is beginning to fail. Active transport of sodium and potassium through the cell membrane is greatly diminished. As a result, sodium and chloride accumulate inside the cell, and potassium is lost. In addition, water is drawn to the inside of the cell and the cell begins to swell. Alterations in sodium and potassium ions across the cell membrane reduce the resting membrane potential of the cell and result in a decreased amplitude of the cell's action potential. Depolarization times and repolarization times are prolonged (Baue, 1976).

Another organelle that is affected during shock is the lysosome. These intracellular organelles contain hydrolytic enzymes that cause damage to the inside of the cell. Research evidence has indicated that the enzymes are able to get out of the cell and cause damage to neighboring cells and organs (Baue, 1976). The primary site of lysosomal enzyme release has been identified to be the gastrointestinal tract.

The progression of cellular alterations occurring during early septic shock is somewhat different from the progression of cellular alterations that occurs during hypovolemic and cardiogenic shock. In the latter two forms of circulatory collapse, hemodynamic alterations precede metabolic changes. In septic shock cellular alterations precede and may actually cause the cardiovascular abnormalities. The reason for these pathophysiological differences between septic shock and other forms of circulatory collapse is still unknown. Speculation on this difference centers on the combined effects of vasoactive toxins, endotoxin, and other substances such as histamine and kinins that are present during septic shock (Zschoche, 1981).

Metabolic changes

Several metabolic changes occur during shock to compensate for the reduced cellular perfusion. Changes in circulating hormone levels are dramatic and account for many of the observable clinical symptoms that accompany shock. The release of epinephrine and norepinephrine has been discussed in an earlier section. These hormones account for the early compensatory mechanism in shock of tachycardia and increased myocardial contractility.

Serum cortisol concentration rises rapidly during the first 12 hours of shock and decreases thereafter. Growth hormone levels as well as serum glucagon levels increase. The serum insulin level remains normal or is decreased. This decrease in insulin, accompanied by an increase in the level of circulating epinephrine, cortisol, and glucagon, leads to the hyperglycemia of shock.

Despite the elevated levels of glucose in the blood, the reduction of cellular perfusion during shock decreases the delivery of glucose to the cell. The decrease in the amount of circulating insulin also impairs the transport of glucose into the cell. Research evidence exists to indicate a tissue insulin resistance that persists for as long as 1 week after recovery from shock. These multiple factors alter the cell's ability to utilize glucose during circulatory collapse, despite its availability in the blood.

Levels of circulating fatty acids are reduced during the shock state. Not only is serum free fatty acid concentration reduced, but also free fatty acid turnover and lipolysis are diminished. Since utilization of both fat and glucose is impaired during shock, the cellular fuel of choice is protein. Muscle mass progressively decreases as muscle protein is broken down and used for fuel. In early septic shock, serum levels of glucose insulin, and free fatty acids remain elevated instead of declining as in other forms of shock. As septic shock progresses, the metabolic alterations resemble those of hypovolemic and cardiogenic shock.

The cellular and metabolic changes of shock are reflected in the many clinical parameters used to evaluate and treat patients (Chapter 6). In summary, the primary clinical symptoms of a patient who is developing shock are tachycardia, cold, clammy skin, hypotension, and oliguria. In addition, a reduction in cardiac output, oxygen consumption, and cellular pH occurs. This developing hypotension, hypoxia, and acidosis lead to mental deterioration.

SUMMARY

This brief introduction demonstrates that shock may occur as a complication of numerous and diverse pathological states including hemorrhage, trauma, dehydration, cardiovascular emergencies, septicemia, and anaphylaxis. It is impossible to offer a single precise etiological and functional definition. Classification systems have been developed to bring order to the diverse terminology, concepts, and facts about shock that the health profession has accumulated.

Four types of shock, hypovolemic, cardiogenic, septic, and anaphylactic, are discussed in this section on management of the patient in shock. The classification system that identifies the various types of shock by cause has been chosen because this system is simple, logical, and descriptive.

REFERENCES

Baue, A.E.: Metabolic abnormalities of shock, Surgical Clinics of North America **56:**1059-1071, 1976.

Berk, J.L., Sampliner, J.E., Artz, J.S., and Vinocur, B.: Handbook of critical care, Boston, 1976, Little, Brown & Co.

Ganong, W.F.: Review of medical physiology, ed. 8, Los Altos, Calif., 1977, Lange Medical Publications.

Groër, M.E., and Shekleton, M.E.: Basic pathophysiology: a conceptual approach, St. Louis, 1979, The C.V. Mosby Co.

Guyton, A.G.: Textbook of medical physiology, ed. 5, Philadelphia, 1976, W.B. Saunders Co.

Hardaway, R.M.: Clinical management of shock, Springfield, Ill., 1968, Charles C Thomas, Publisher.

Hardaway, R.M.: Monitoring of the patient in a state of shock, Surgery, Gynecology and Obstetrics **148:** 339-345, 1979.

Hechtman, H.B.: Adequate circulatory responses or cardiovascular failure, Surgical Clinics of North America **56:**929-943, 1976.

Jahre, J.N.: Medical approach to the hypotensive patient and the patient in shock, Heart & Lung **4:** 577-587, 1975.

O'Donnell, T.F., and Belkin, S.C.: The pathophysiology, monitoring and treatment of shock, Orthopedic Clinics of North America **9:**589-609, 1978.

Price, S.A., and Wilson, L.M.: Pathophysiology, clinical concepts of disease process, New York, 1978, McGraw-Hill Book Co.

Zschoche, D.A., editor: Mosby's comprehensive review of critical care, ed. 2, St. Louis, 1981, The C.V. Mosby Co.

6 Hemodynamic monitoring of the patient in shock

ANNE GRIFFIN PERRY

Recent advances in critical care have resulted in invasive monitoring techniques to evaluate venous pressures, arterial pressures, left and right heart function, and overall cardiac performance. Regardless of the specific pressures or the system being monitored, each of these techniques requires cannulization of a blood vessel or cardiac chamber. The more sophisticated monitoring systems also incorporate a transducer and amplifier system. Invasive hemodynamic monitoring of the shock patient enables the nurse to do the following:

1. Obtain data on immediate changes in hemodynamic status.
2. Obtain data necessary to estimate overall cardiac performance.
3. Have immediate access to arterial, venous, and mixed venous blood samples for laboratory studies and, in some selected cases, for the administration of drugs.
4. Obtain data to construct ventricular function curves based on left ventricular filling pressures, thereby determining optimum filling pressures for specific patients (Walinsky, 1977).

This chapter will discuss hemodynamic monitoring and its application for the patient in shock. Diagnostic and therapeutic utilization of hemodynamic monitoring will be explored. Initially, summaries of venous pressure monitoring, intra-arterial pressure monitoring, monitoring with a balloon-tipped catheter, and assessments of systolic performance will be discussed. This will be followed by a section on the hemodynamic alterations that are present in various types of shock and the respective response to therapeutic measures.

For the patient in shock, it is essential that the hemodynamic status be continuously evaluated so that subtle changes can be recognized and treated. Perhaps most important is the information that this monitoring provides regarding the adequacy of the therapeutic measures that are implemented in various types of shock.

VENOUS PRESSURE MONITORING

The development of the balloon-tipped flow-directed catheter has decreased the frequency of central venous pressure (CVP) monitoring as a sole indicator of hemodynamic stability. The overall weakness of this monitoring system is its inability to be a reliable measure of left ventricular function.

Strictly defined, the CVP is the force exerted by the blood against the right atrium (Haughey, 1978). This measurement will reflect the pressure in the great veins as blood returns to the heart from the systemic circulation (Daily and Schroeder, 1981). The CVP line is useful in the administration of drugs, especially potent antibiotics that can be caustic to peripheral veins; the administration of total parenteral nutrition (hyperalimentation); the administration of large volumes of fluids and/or blood and its components; the evaluation of heart function in relation to blood volume; the determination of a patient's fluid volume requirements; and the insertion of a cardiac pacing wire if it should become necessary (Murray and Smallwood, 1977). The normal CVP value ranges from 5 to 12 cm H_2O.

Indications

Literature notes that the CVP has been most beneficial in monitoring patients' hydration status, patients' postoperative status, the status of patients who are actively bleeding, and hemodynamic responses to a fluid challenge (Daily and Schroeder, 1981). Also, in the early phase of diagnosis and treatment of the patient in shock, the greatest value of the CVP is monitoring the fluid challenge. This challenge is useful in the differential diagnosis of hypovolemic shock and cardiogenic shock, especially when a medical history is not obtainable. The result of the fluid challenge monitor will indicate if the shock is caused by depleted extracellular volume (hypovolemic shock) or the result of an inadequate myocardial pump (cardiogenic shock). There are various methods for conducting a fluid challenge. Most commonly 200 ml of fluid is given intravenously over 30 minutes and the CVP is monitored continually. If the intravascular volume is normal, the CVP will rise. In normovolemic shock, such as cardiogenic shock, the left ventricular end-diastolic pressure should also be monitored by means of a Swan-Ganz catheter during the fluid challenge. In the hypovolemic shock patient, the CVP usually rises after the initial fluid challenge and then rapidly falls. CVP monitoring during the fluid challenge is helpful for diagnostic as well as therapeutic purposes. However, the nurse should not minimize the need for total physical assessment of the patient. Focusing only on selected hemodynamic parameters diverts the attention of the health care team from the patient to the evaluative equipment.

Equipment

A CVP is obtained by a central venous catheter (CVC) that is inserted into a large vein. The subclavian vein is most frequently used. Other veins utilized are the internal jugular, external jugular, saphenous, and femoral veins. The CVC is then progressed through the venous system until it reaches the right atrium. Proper placement of the catheter must be validated through a chest x-ray film. Haag (1979) noted that the catheter tip should be placed just above the superior cavoatrial junction in the superior vena cava.

The insertion of the catheter and validation of its placement are a physician's

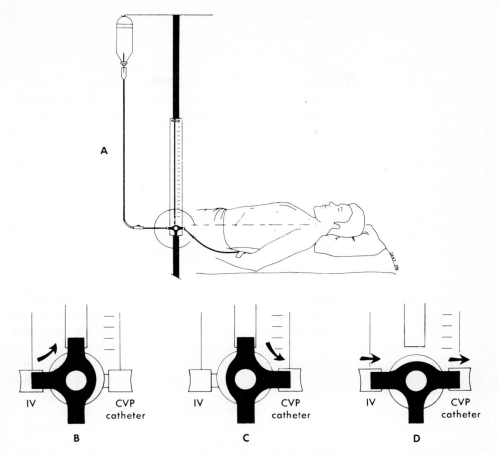

Fig. 6-1. Procedure for measuring CVP with manometer. **A,** Manometer and IV tubing in place. **B,** Turn stopcock so that manometer fills with fluid above level of expected pressure. **C,** Turn stopcock so that IV is off and fluid in manometer flows to patient. Obtain a reading after fluid level stabilizes. **D,** Turn stopcock to resume IV flow to patient. (From Daily, E.K., and Schroeder, J.S.: Techniques in bedside hemodynamic monitoring, ed. 2, St. Louis, 1981, The C.V. Mosby Co.)

responsibility. However, the nurse is responsible for proper connection of the intravenous line to the manometer and the zeroing of the manometer. The zeroing is done by establishing external reference points. The most common method is to have the patient assume the supine position and to measure 5 cm down from the top of the chest at the fourth intercostal space. This point will be at the midaxillary line. This external reference point must be clearly marked so that subsequent CVP measurements will have the same zero point (Fig. 6-1). Failure to do this can result in inaccurate information regarding a patient's hydration status and/or the physiological responses to the administration of large volumes of parenteral fluid.

Abnormal venous pressure recordings

Frequent problems associated with the CVP are poor fluctuation of the fluid in the manometer, infection at the catheter insertion site, and increased risk of an air embolism. Poor fluctuation can be the result of incorrect manipulation of the stopcock, clot formation at the tip of the CVC, displacement of the CVC itself, or a kink in the distal portion of the CVC.

Once poor fluctuation of the fluid in the manometer has been observed the nurse should first check the intravenous solution, the tubing, and the stopcock. There should be fluid present in the intravenous fluid bag, and the intravenous tubing should be patent and free of kinks. The nurse should also note that the stopcock is in the correct position (Fig. 6-1), thereby permitting the fluid to flow from the manometer to the CVC. If these items are correct, the fluid level should fall rapidly and fluctuate during respirations.

Complications

If poor or absent fluid fluctuation remains, the nurse may need to aspirate the CVC because of the presence of a small clot. This aspiration should be done with a tuberculin syringe. Either the catheter or the stopcock should be aspirated with normal pressure until a blood return is present on aspiration (Murray and Smallwood, 1977). It is important to stress that these catheters should not be irrigated with force because of the risk of releasing a large clot into the circulation, thereby increasing the risk of emboli.

Other problems associated with a CVP, such as a kink in the catheter tubing and/or infection, are common problems associated with various hemodynamic monitoring systems. A discussion of these common complications will be presented with the discussion of the balloon-tipped flow-directed catheter.

In summary, CVP monitoring reflects the venous return of the great veins to the right ventricle. This filling pressure is dependent on right ventricular compliance, venous tone, and, most importantly, blood volume. A singular CVP value provides little information about the patient's response to treatment. The critical factor in CVP monitoring is the observation of serial CVP measurements of the patient in shock.

INTRA-ARTERIAL PRESSURE MONITORING

It is difficult to reliably assess the systemic blood pressure of patients in shock by utilizing the cuff method. Because of the diminished cardiac output and subsequent decreased tissue perfusion, it becomes nearly impossible to auscultate Korotkoff's sounds. True, palpation may provide information about the mean arterial blood pressure, but this becomes progressively ineffective over long-term monitoring (Daily and Schroeder, 1981). The use of an intra-arterial line in these patients provides continuous assessment of the arterial blood pressure and immediate access to arterial blood for arterial blood gas determinations, which are useful in determining the metabolic status of the patient. The intra-arterial line aids in the determination of the shock pathology by monitoring the physiological response to treatment modalities such as volume replacement in hypovolemic shock, afterload reduction in cardiogenic shock, and vasoconstrictors in anaphylactic and septic shock.

Indications

Patients in shock receive large doses of vasoconstrictors and, in some selected cases, doses of potent vasodilators as well. To accurately monitor the blood pressure in these patients, it is necessary that an arterial line be inserted. Various arteries may be used for insertion of the catheter. However, it must be remembered that the further the site is from the aorta, the higher the systolic pressure will be because of the amplification effect in the arterial system during systole. For example, the recorded peak systolic pressure may be as much as 15 to 20 mm Hg higher than the actual systolic pressure (Daily and Schroeder, 1981). The radial artery is the best and most common artery selected. While this artery is small and the actual passing of the catheter may be difficult, it is easy to locate and keep clean with minimal blood loss.

Prior to the insertion of the catheter into the radial artery, the Allen test should be performed on the arm in which the catheter will be placed. The purpose of this test is to validate the adequacy of ulnar collateral circulation to the hand when the radial artery is occluded. The test is performed by compressing both the ulnar and radial arteries while the patient repeatedly makes a fist, then releasing the ulnar artery. If the hand fails to blush, blood supply from the ulnar artery is insufficient (Zschoche, 1981). In this case the radial artery should not be cannulated. The results of this test should be documented in the patient's record prior to the insertion of the radial arterial catheter.

Arterial catheters may be placed into the brachial and femoral arteries as well. As with the radial artery, it is important to validate the presence of arterial circulation to the distal portion of the extremity. Both of these arteries are readily palpable and easy to cannulate. However, it is difficult to control bleeding and to maintain cleanliness at the catheter insertion site. In critical situations the patient's physiological status may provide the only rationale for arterial line site selection. In the patient with severe shock, the femoral artery may be the only accessible site, and the nurse must then take measures to ensure the patency of the arterial line, to maintain cleanliness of the site, and to control bleeding from the insertion site.

Equipment

Once cannulation of the artery has taken place, the catheter is connected to the monitoring system. Although each system may vary as to operation and components, there are common pieces of equipment present in the varying systems. These include stopcocks, an arterial catheter attached to low-compliance tubing, a transducer, and an

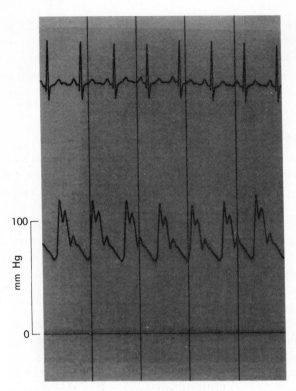

Fig. 6-2. Normal arterial waveform pattern. (From Daily, E.K., and Schroeder, J.S.: Techniques in bedside hemodynamic monitoring, ed. 2, St. Louis, 1981, The C.V. Mosby Co.)

intravenous fluid bag attached to pressure. The intra-arterial pressures are then displayed on an oscilloscope. It is important that the arterial monitoring system be zeroed routinely to ensure accuracy in the arterial pressures obtained from one reading to another.

Waveform patterns

The normal waveform of an arterial pressure pattern should be sharp, have a clearly represented dicrotic notch, and display a diastolic phase (Fig. 6-2). Flattening of the waveform can be the result of various factors and requires immediate attention by the nurse. If flattening of the waveform occurs, the nurse should institute measures to return the waveform to the correct pattern. Ideally, dampening or flattening can be prevented by providing a constant or intermittent flush system within the arterial system. The flush solution should be heparinized in a ratio of 1 unit of heparin per 1 ml of fluid in patients who do not have a history of coagulation problems (Swan and Ganz, 1975;

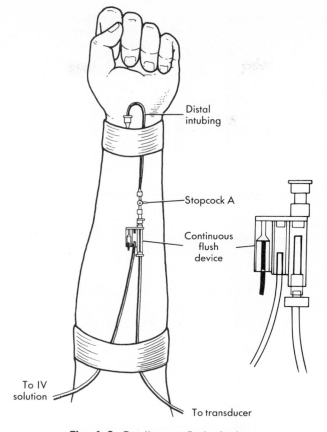

Distal
intubing

Stopcock A

Continuous
flush
device

To IV
solution

To transducer

Fig. 6-3. Continuous flush device.

Lantiegne and Civetta, 1978). It is essential to have a continuous flush device (Fig. 6-3) that will flush the arterial line with 3 to 5 ml of fluid every hour in the adult patient. A fast-flush device is also present on most arterial line set-ups. This permits the nurse to flush the arterial line if necessary.

The patient in shock may have frequent arterial blood samples drawn from the arterial line. This is certainly acceptable providing that measures to ensure the patency of the system following the withdrawal of the blood sample are implemented. The nurse must assume responsibility for the protection of the arterial line. Many clinical agencies discourage house officers from obtaining the arterial blood. This is done because the physician may be unfamiliar with the set-up of the arterial line and incorrectly withdraw the sample, thereby risking the patency of the monitoring system or causing severe blood loss by the patient.

Causes of flattening of arterial pressure waveforms

1. Presence of a clot in the arterial catheter
2. Drop in the pressure of the intravenous solution resulting in backflow into the tubing
3. Presence of a kink in the catheter
4. Air bubbles in the transducer dome
5. Catheter resting against the arterial wall
6. Inadequate flow of fluid through the arterial tubing
7. Improper position of the stopcocks

Trouble shooting arterial lines

1. Assess the position of all stopcocks.
2. Assess the position of the extremity into which the catheter was inserted.
3. Withdraw 5 to 8 ml of arterial blood from the system and discard.
4. Flush the arterial line using the pigtail fast-flush device present in most arterial line set-ups.
5. Assess the transducer domes.
6. Zero the arterial monitoring system.
7. Return all stopcocks to their correct positions.
8. Assess the waveform.

Obtaining arterial blood samples

1. Turn off the alarm.
2. Clean the "exit" port with alcohol.
3. Close the stopcock to the transducer.
4. Aseptically withdraw 3 to 5 ml of blood from the exit port and discard; because this specimen is diluted with the flush solution, blood chemistry studies of this sample are inaccurate.
5. Aseptically withdraw the desired amount needed for the specimen. NOTE: For blood gases be sure any air is expelled from the syringe.
6. Close the stopcock to the exit port; flush the system.
7. Turn on the alarm.
8. Assess the arterial line system for proper waveform.

Complications

Although the presence of an arterial line provides continuous evaluation of the blood pressure of the patient in shock, it is certainly not without hazards. Some of these complications can be prevented or reversed by following the steps outlined in Table 6-1. Unfortunately, some complications may necessitate the removal of the arterial catheter to avoid permanent damage to the cannulated extremity. The presence of a cold extremity, with or without the absence of distal pulses, indicates impaired circulation to the distal tissues. The arterial line must be removed and continuous assessment of the circulation to the extremity must take place. In rare instances surgical removal of a thrombus is necessary to avoid loss of the extremity.

Once any erythema, edema, or pain is noted at the catheter insertion site, an infection must be suspected. Because of the invasive technique, these patients are at risk for septicemia and, although the arterial line may be discontinued at this time, the nurse should send the tip of the arterial catheter for bacteriological examination. In addition, any temperature elevations should be evaluated, and if necessary, cultures of sputum, urine,

Table 6-1. Complications of arterial lines

Arterial line complication	Prevention
Decreased or absent distal pulse, or cold extremity	1. Assessment of adequate collateral circulation (e.g., Allen test) prior to arterial line insertion. 2. Routine assessment of (a) quality of pulse, (b) color, and (c) temperature in distal extremity. 3. Proper withdrawal of blood samples from arterial line.
Exsanguination	1. Use of Luer-Lok connections throughout the system. 2. Use of alarm that indicates interruption of the system. 3. Routine assessment of patency and functioning of system.
Infection	1. Sterile technique used during (a) initial arterial line insertion and (b) changing of the dressing every 24 hours. 2. Application of antibiotic ointment to insertion site. 3. Changing the fluid and tubing in the system every 24 hours. 4. Routine assessment for erythema, edema, or excessive tenderness at insertion site.
Flattened waveform caused by (a) air in system, (b) blood on transducer dome, (c) kink in tubing, or (d) thrombus at catheter tip.	1. Maintain 300 mm Hg pressure on intravenous bag. 2. Check all stopcocks and connections. 3. If thrombus is suspected, aspirate clot and discard before flushing. 4. Flush system routinely.

blood, and wounds, if present, should be obtained. The risk of infection is reduced by changing the dressing over the insertion site and the intravenous solution and tubing every 24 hours. This procedure is carried out with sterile technique, and an antibiotic ointment is applied to the insertion site.

The arterial line provides the nurse with a continuous assessment of blood pressure. The experienced, competent nurse is aware of the potential hazard of this monitoring system. However, correct usage of the system and complete assessment of the patient in shock will permit the nurse to utilize the system to its fullest value.

MONITORING WITH BALLOON-TIPPED FLOW-DIRECTED CATHETERS

The development of the balloon-tipped flow-directed catheter has led to further advances in hemodynamic monitoring of the critically ill. The Swan-Ganz catheter provides guidelines for therapy in patients requiring rapid-acting vasodilators or inotropic agents, circulatory assistance, hemodialysis, and mechanical ventilation (Lalli, 1978).

Indications

The indications for use of this catheter vary; however, a review of the literature identified common physiological alterations that may require insertion of such a monitoring catheter. This catheter enables the nurse to obtain data on left ventricular function for diagnostic purposes and the evaluation of treatments. In addition, this catheter provides ready access to arterial and mixed venous blood samples for laboratory studies.

The balloon-tipped flow-directed catheter contains two, three, or four lumens. The type of catheter selected depends on the expected range of function. All catheters measure

---

Indications for Swan-Ganz catheter

Shock
  Cardiogenic
  Hypovolemic
  Anaphylactic
  Septic
Adult respiratory distress syndrome
Pulmonary embolism
Cardiac bypass surgery
Multiple trauma
Myocardial infarction

pulmonary artery (PA) and pulmonary capillary wedge pressures (PCWP)* and permit access to arterial and mixed venous blood samples by means of the PA lumen. The most sophisticated is the four-lumen catheter (Fig. 6-4). This catheter has a thermistor port, balloon port, right atrial (RA) (proximal) port, and a PA (distal) port. The thermistor port is essential if cardiac output or cardiac index determinants are necessary. The balloon port is used to insert 0.6 to 0.8 cc of air to obtain the PCWP. The RA and PA ports are used to obtain right atrial and pulmonary artery pressure readings, respectively. If both of these pressures are desired, each of the last two ports can be attached to one trans-ducer (Fig. 6-5). Although continuous monitoring of these values is impossible, the turning of two stopcocks readily makes either pressure tracing available. If it is necessary to have both pressure tracings displayed simultaneously, two transducers must be used. In a busy unit it may not be realistic to utilize available equipment in this manner.

Equipment

Prior to the insertion of the catheter by the physician, the nurse has the prime responsibility to properly prepare the necessary equipment and to explain the procedure to the patient and family. Since each critical care unit has its own Swan-Ganz catheter insertion procedure, the step-by-step process will not be included in this text. Patient

---

*The pulmonary capillary wedge pressure may also be abbreviated as PCW, PAWP, and PAW. We will use *PCWP* for pulmonary artery wedge pressure.

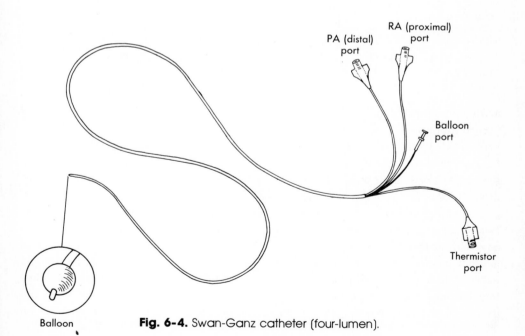

Fig. 6-4. Swan-Ganz catheter (four-lumen).

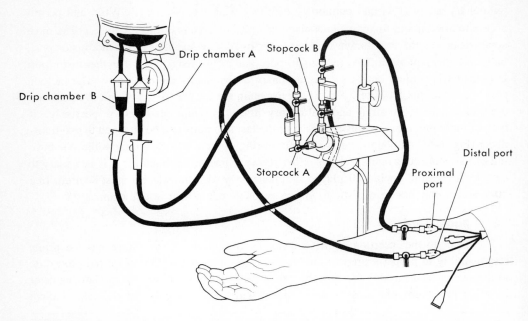

Fig. 6-5. Setup showing use of one transducer and one IV pressure bag for two monitoring lines. Drip chamber *A* is inserted into outlet port of IV bag and delivers IV fluid to distal port of quadruple lumen catheter. Drip chamber *B* is inserted into the medication port of IV bag and delivers fluid to proximal port of the catheter. In this illustration stopcock *A* is turned off to transducer; pressure monitored is through system *B*, proximal port of catheter (RA). To monitor pressures at distal port (PA or PCW), turn stopcock *B* off to transducer and open stopcock *A* to transducer. (From Daily, E.K., and Schroeder, J.S.: Techniques in bedside hemodynamic monitoring, ed. 2, St. Louis, 1981, The C.V. Mosby Co.)

and family preparation is essential. Frequently, constraints of time, critical illness, and limited staff leave this area untouched. It is important that the patient and/or family members know why the catheter is being inserted, the procedure involved, restraints on activities, who will take care of the catheter, and when to notify the nurse if there is inflammation, pain, bleeding, or numbness. Providing this information can help to decrease some of the anxiety and increase appropriate cooperation of the patient.

The physician assumes the responsibility for aseptically inserting the catheter. Before actual insertion of the balloon-tipped catheter, the integrity of the balloon must be tested. Common practice is to inflate the balloon with 0.8 cc of air while the balloon is submerged in sterile water or saline. The presence of any air bubbles in the solution indicates leakage from the balloon, and another catheter should be selected. The most frequent sites of catheter insertion are the internal jugular vein, the subclavian vein, and the antecubital vein (Woods, 1976; Pego and Luria, 1979). The site of catheter insertion

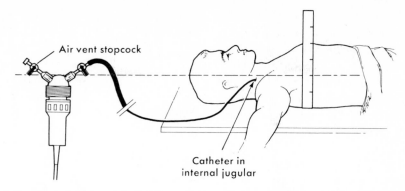

Air vent stopcock

Catheter in
internal jugular

Fig. 6-6. Patient's midchest position is measured, marked, and used as an anatomical reference point for placement of transducer. (From Daily, E.K., and Schroeder, J.S.: Techniques in bedside hemodynamic monitoring, ed. 2, St. Louis, 1981, The C.V. Mosby Co.)

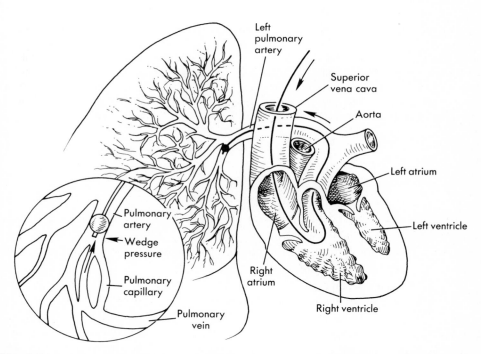

Left
pulmonary
artery

Superior
vena cava

Aorta

Left atrium

Left ventricle

Pulmonary
artery

Wedge
pressure

Pulmonary
capillary

Pulmonary
vein

Right
atrium

Right ventricle

Fig. 6-7. Location of Swan-Ganz catheter in pulmonary artery. Inset shows wedge position.

should be well planned so that catheter patency can be ensured, cleaning of the entry site can be accomplished, distal extremity circulation is not impaired, bleeding can be controlled, and patient mobility is maintained.

Before any pressure measurements may be obtained, the transducer must be level to the patient's right atrium (Fig. 6-6) and the monitoring equipment must be calibrated. Daily and Schroeder (1981) recommend that the stopcock be opened to room air and the zero dial on the monitor be set and calibrated. If the stopcock is not open to air, a buildup of pressure within the transducer will give a false reading.

The location (Fig. 6-7) of the catheter within the pulmonary artery permits the nurse to obtain PA pressure and PCWP readings. The PA waveform (Fig 6-8) is represented with a systolic and diastolic phase. The systolic phase occurs during right ventricular ejection after the opening of the pulmonic valve. As the blood is ejected from the chamber, there is a gradual decrease in pressure until the pulmonary valve closes. Closure of this valve is indicated by the dicrotic notch on the PA waveform and indicates the beginning of the diastolic phase. In the patient with normal lungs and mitral valve, the PA diastolic (PAD) pressure is closely correlated to the left ventricular end-diastolic pressure (LVEPD) and is useful as an index of left ventricular function. The rationale for

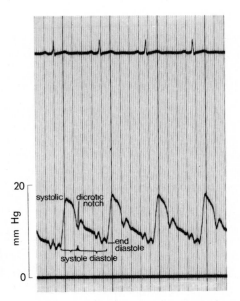

Fig. 6-8. Normal pulmonary artery wave form, showing phases of systole, dicrotic notch (pulmonic valve closure), and diastole. Normally PA end-diastolic pressure closely represents LVEDP. (From Daily, E.K., and Schroeder, J.S.: Techniques in bedside hemodynamic monitoring, ed. 2, St. Louis, 1981, The C.V. Mosby Co.)

this follows: At the end of diastole, the mitral valve is still open and pressure between the left ventricle and left atrium are equal. Since there are no valves in the pulmonary venous system, the pressure also equilibrates in the pulmonary vasculature; therefore PAD pressure is equal to LVEDP.

Waveform patterns

Because of the placement of this catheter in the pulmonary vessels, there is the potential for PA waveform variation in response to respiration and the respective changes in intrathoracic pressure. Whenever possible, PA values should be recorded at the end of expiration. In patients who are being mechanically ventilated, the ventilator should be disconnected while the values are being obtained unless the patient is on PEEP. Patients with changes in pulmonary circulation or pulmonary diseases will have elevated PA pressures.

The PCWP is obtained by inflating the balloon (Fig. 6-8), which occludes a branch of the pulmonary artery. When this occurs, the catheter only records the pressure in the more distal pulmonary capillaries and venous systems. The PCWP is often equivalent to the PAD pressure, and frequently these two values are used interchangeably. The PCWP reflects the movement of fluid from the vascular bed to the interstitial and alveolar spaces of the lung (Afifi et al., 1974). Pulmonary congestion results with a PCWP greater than 20 mm Hg, and severe pulmonary edema occurs when the PCWP is greater than 30 mm Hg (Bleifeld, Hanrath, Mathey, and Merx, 1974). Normally the PCWP should be less than the PA pressure. Table 6-2 indicates normal values for the PA and PCWP values. The PCWP waveform (Fig. 6-9) should indicate a significant fall in pressure as the bal-

---

Causes of elevated PA pressures

1. Increased pulmonary blood flow:
   Left to right shunts caused by atrial and/or septal defects
2. Increased pulmonary vascular resistance (PVR)
   Pulmonary diseases
   Pulmonary hypertension
3. Increased venous pressure
   Mitral stenosis
   LV failure
4. Mechanical ventilator
   PEEP settings

From Daily, E.K., and Schroeder, J.S.: Techniques in bedside hemodynamic monitoring, ed. 2, St. Louis, 1981, The C.V. Mosby Co.

loon is inflated. Elevations in PCWP occur in the presence of cardiac or fluid alterations. The balloon-tipped flow-directed catheter has enhanced the application of sound physiological principles for the care of the patient in shock. The catheter permits the determination of filling pressures of the right and left ventricle as well as cardiac output. These physiological parameters, as well as cardiac rate and rhythm, arterial pressures, and arterial blood gas values, provide continuous information on cardiopulmonary function of the shock patient. Continued monitoring with these catheters provides objective physiological data concerning the effectiveness of treatment. Although the procedures for invasive monitoring have become more efficient, the complication rate has remained low. However, it is essential that the practitioner continually assess for and prevent these complications.

Complications

The use of balloon-tipped flow-directed catheters in the shock patient has increased greatly in recent years. Although complications are rare, the critically ill patient is at risk for the most common problems associated with these catheters. For each of these potential complications, the nurse must be aware of the specific problem, the pertinent assessment findings, causes of the problem, prevention, and the appropriate nursing interventions.

Waveform distortions. Waveform distortions are common problems with balloon-tipped catheters. Some of these are problems associated with the monitoring sys-

Table 6-2. Normal PA pressure values

Pressure	Normal values
Pulmonary artery systolic (PAS)	20 to 30 mm Hg
Pulmonary artery diastolic (PAD)	<12 mm Hg
Pulmonary artery mean (PAM)	<20 mm Hg
Pulmonary artery wedge (PCW)	4 to 12 mm Hg

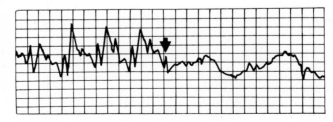

Fig. 6-9. Normal wave form for shift of PA reading to PAW reading. (Arrow indicates balloon inflation.)

tem excluding the catheter, and others are primarily associated with catheter placement or functioning. Waveform distortions can be a damped pressure tracing (Fig. 6-10, *A*), catheter fling (excessive vibration of catheter tip) (Fig. 6-10, *B*), inappropriate high or low pressure readings (Fig. 6-10, *C*), or respiratory variations (Fig. 6-10, *D*). It is important that the nurse recognize the distortion and, if possible, alleviate the cause (Table 6-3). Some of the causes, such as air in the system, improper transducer position, and blood on the transducer dome, may be easily corrected with no patient risk, and monitoring can continue. However, catheter malposition and wedging must be readily recognized and corrected. It is not uncommon that the catheter itself must be removed and replaced if continued monitoring is desired. Failure to recognize and/or treat a malpositioned catheter or wedging can put the patient at risk of pulmonary complications.

Causes of elevated PCWP

Left ventricular failure
Mitral stenosis
Mitral insufficiency
Constrictive pericarditis
Volume overload

From Daily, E.K., and Schroeder, J.S.: Techniques in bedside hemodynamic monitoring, ed. 2, St. Louis, 1981, The C.V. Mosby Co.

Problems associated with balloon-tipped flow-directed catheters

Waveform distortions
Cardiac arrhythmias
Pulmonary complications
  Infarction
  Embolism
  Pulmonary artery rupture
Balloon rupture
Infections
  Localized
  Endocarditis

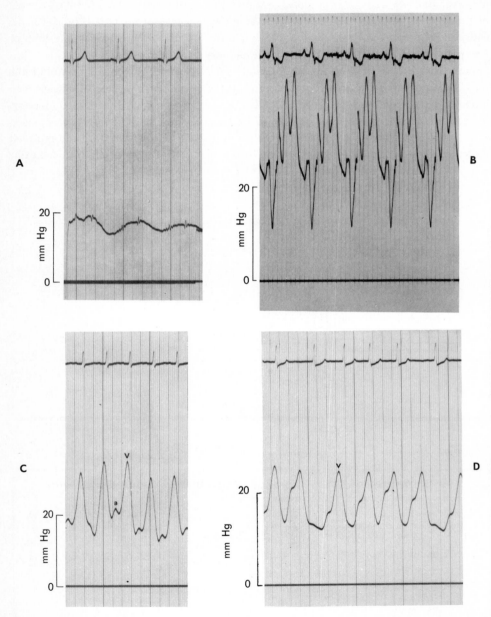

Fig. 6-10. Pulmonary artery wave form distortions. **A,** Damped pressure tracings. **B,** Catheter fling. **C,** Abnormally elevated (PCW) pressure reading in patient with mitral stenosis. **D,** Variation with respirations. (From Daily, E.K., and Schroeder, J.S.: Techniques in bedside hemodynamic monitoring, ed. 2, St. Louis, 1981, The C.V. Mosby Co.)

Table 6-3. Waveform distortions

Problem	Cause	Prevention	Action
Damped pressure tracing	Blood on transducer dome	Maintain proper connection and flush system.	Irrigate until blood is removed from dome.
	Transducer no longer calibrated	Check calibration each shift; check transducer placement with RA level; keep transducer catheter connection tight.	Recalibrate and position transducer at RA level. Secure all stopcocks and connections.
	Air in system	Set up monitoring system carefully, making sure all connections are secure.	Check security of system; flush air bubbles out; recalibrate if necessary; aspirate clot; flush with heparinized fluid until waveform appears normal; *Do not flush* unless clot is aspirated; Recalibrate if necessary.
	Clot at catheter tip	Adequately heparinize continuous drip solution; routinely fast flush system.	
	Malposition of catheter tip against artery wall	Check for adequate suturing of catheter at insertion site.	Instruct patient to cough; extend patient's arm to a 90° angle to his body and gently flush (Lali, 1978); obtain x-ray film if waveform remains damped.
Catheter fling	Wedging of catheter		
	Excessive catheter movement	May be unavoidable.	Reposition catheter; purposely damp waveform with mean switch and record only mean pressure (Daily and Schroeder, 1981).
Inappropriate high or low pressure readings	Transducer level inappropriate	Maintain transducer at RA level.	Reposition transducer.
	Loose connections	Check for proper setup of system.	Check and tighten all connections.
	Improper stopcock sequence	Utilize correct stopcock sequence.	Flush system, recalibrate, and obtain pressure using correct stopcock sequence.

As a result of technological advances, hemodynamic monitoring with balloon-tipped flow-directed catheters can be accomplished accurately and safely. The nurse is not only responsible for maintaining the system but is also responsible for identifying problems and selecting the appropriate interventions. These balloon-tipped flow-directed catheters have increased physiological monitoring of the critically ill patient.

Cardiac arrhythmias. The design of the catheter shaft and its protective tip assist in reducing the frequency of cardiac arrhythmias (Walinsky, 1977; Woods, 1976). The most common arrhythmias include atrial premature contractions (APCs) or ventricular premature contractions (VPCs), which result from three common causes. Initially arrhythmias can be induced by irritation of the endocardium or cardiac valves as the catheter passes through the heart (Lalli, 1978). Kinking or knotting of the catheter further increases the risk of arrhythmia. Finally, displacement of the catheter from the pulmonary artery into the right ventricle frequently results in ventricular arrhythmias (Nichols, 1979).

Although it may be impossible to prevent these arrhythmias from occurring, the nurse should initially examine the catheter for kinks prior to insertion. If the arrhythmias are caused by displacement of the catheter into the right ventricle, and this is adequately documented by appropriate waveform changes, it is essential that this be recognized and the physician be notified. The balloon will need to be reinflated and the catheter advanced into the pulmonary artery. As in any situation with critically ill patients, continual monitoring of the electrocardiogram (ECG) and ready access to emergency drugs and a defibrillator are essential.

Pulmonary complications. Pulmonary complications are frequent and varied. Table 6-4 provides a ready reference guide to the types of pulmonary complications. Pulmonary infections are usually small, asymptomatic, and detectable by comparing before and after chest x-ray films (Foote, Schabel, and Hodges, 1974). The frequency of pulmonary infarcts becomes increased if irrigation fluid is injected at increasing pressures to correct damped waveforms (Swan and Ganz, 1975). To decrease the risk of these infarctions, the pulmonary artery waveform should be continuously monitored. The inflation time of the balloon should be limited to 2 minutes or less (Swan, 1975).

Critically ill patients are predisposed to thrombus formation. The physiological alteration itself can impair the normal clotting mechanism. It is important to note that the very nature of critical illness first restricts mobility and second requires placement of invasive catheters for nutritional support as well as hemodynamic monitoring. The literature documents the fact that inactivity increases a patient's risk of thrombus formation and the subsequent development of coagulation imbalances. The introduction of a catheter into the blood vessel increases the risk of small thrombi formation. A small thrombus at the tip of the Swan-Ganz catheter can result in a medical emergency if this embolus migrates into the pulmonary circulation. Prevention of emboli through the provision of appropriate mobility and adequate heparinization of the flush solution is essential in the critically ill patient.

Balloon rupture. The longer the balloon-tipped catheter is in place, the greater is

Table 6-4. Pulmonary complications

Problem	Assessment	Cause	Prevention	Intervention
Infarction	Initially asymptomatic Pleural pain, sudden dyspnea, hemoptysis, syncope, bloody pleural effusion Chest x-ray film showing consolidation (Harrison et al., 1981)	Prolonged wedging or overinflation of balloon; thrombus formation at catheter tip (Lali, 1978)	Deflate balloon completely after obtaining value and leave deflated; continually assess waveform for unexplained wedging; inflate balloon to volume indicated by manufacturer; make sure catheter is sutured in place.	Double check for balloon inflation; if wedging is documented, withdraw catheter 1-2 cm and gently flush; check for PA waveform; *do not* forcefully flush catheter lodged in a wedge position; if wedging remains, notify physician and obtain chest film.
Embolism	Substernal chest pain Cough, hemoptysis Dyspnea Rapid, thready pulse Syncope Sudden death (Harrison, 1981)	Predisposing factors: inactivity, postoperative status, coagulation abnormalities; migration of thrombus from catheter tip (Lali, 1978)	Check for adequately heparinized flush solution; flush catheter syringe every hour with heparinized solution.	If clotting at the tip of the catheter is suspected, *never* flush; gently aspirate (Lali, 1978); pulmonary embolism may necessitate removal of catheter itself.
Pulmonary artery rupture	Cough, hemoptysis Rales	Migration of catheter into small artery branches; overdistention of arterial walls; inflation of balloon under high pressure	Avoid overdistention of balloon; slowly inflate balloon; validate position of catheter on chest x-ray film; assess waveform for PA position	Remove catheter; inspect for thrombus (Daily and Schroeder, 1981).

the risk for balloon rupture because the latex membrane of the balloon absorbs lipoproteins from the blood, which decrease the elasticity of the balloon (Lalli, 1978; Nichols, 1979). Also, balloon rupture occurs more frequently when the inflation volumes exceed the manufacturer's recommendation. Rupture of the balloon places the patient at risk for air embolism and embolism formation caused by fragmentation of the balloon. Either of these can produce dyspnea, vascular collapse, weak thready pulse, and loss of consciousness (Nichols, 1979). Precautionary measures should be used to prevent these emboli. For example, carbon dioxide can be used as an inflation medium in patients suspected of having an intracardiac shunt (Lalli, 1978; Nichols, 1979). Also proper care and inflation of the balloon can decrease the risk of rupture and subsequent adverse sequelae.

Infections. Because of the invasive nature of the monitoring catheter, there is an increased risk of infection. The infection can be localized or systemic. Localized infections are associated with irritation of the insertion site. This risk can be decreased by using sterile technique during catheter placement as well as during subsequent dressing changes. It is considered routine practice to change the dressings and apply a topical antibiotic ointment at least every 24 hours, more frequently if the dressing becomes saturated with blood or intravenous fluid. Although rare, endocarditis has been reported to have occurred in patients with balloon-tipped flow-directed catheters (Pace and Horton, 1975).

As with any diagnostic or therapeutic procedure, the practitioner must be aware of potential complications. Nursing interventions should be selected that are directed toward obtaining correct hemodynamic values as well as preventing complications. The critically ill patient needs to be continually assessed by the knowledgeable and experienced practitioner. Immediate recognition of any undesired effects of treatment can affect the prognosis of the patient. The nurse is the professional who has the responsibility of recognizing these problems and implementing appropriate action.

HEMODYNAMIC ALTERATIONS PRESENT IN SHOCK

During clinical evaluation of the patient with diminished tissue perfusion and poor cardiopulmonary functioning, it is necessary to monitor areas of oxygen uptake, transport, and delivery. Present state-of-the-art monitoring strives to document the ongoing changes in physiological parameters in the critically ill patient and to provide for diagnosis and evaluation of therapeutic modalities in the shock patient (Vij, Babcock, and Magilligan, 1981). The prognosis of shock in a patient, whether it is cardiogenic, hypovolemic, anaphylactic, or septic in origin, depends on the data and accuracy of hemodynamic monitoring.

Continuous monitoring of these values can identify physiological trends in response to fluids, inotropic agents, vasoconstrictors, or vasodilators in the patient in shock. The clinical pictures of specific shock states and the treatment modalities are discussed at length in subsequent chapters of this text. However, it is important to identify physiological parameters to monitor the cardiovascular system and the respiratory system.

Table 6-5. Physiological parameters for cardiovascular function

Value	Formula	Units
Cardiac output (CO)	Thermodilution method via Swan-Ganz catheter	L/min
Cardiac index (CI)	$\dfrac{CO}{BSA}$	L/min/m²
Stroke index (SI)	$\dfrac{CI \times 1,000}{hr}$	ml/m²
Pulmonary vascular resistance (PVR)	$\dfrac{(PAMP - PCWP)\ 79.9}{CO}$	Dyne/sec/cm⁵/m²
Systemic vascular resistance (SVR)	$\dfrac{(MAP - CVP)\ 79.9}{CO}$	Dyne/sec/cm⁻⁵/m²

BSA, Body surface area; *CVP,* central venous pressure; *PAMP,* pulmonary artery mean pressure; *PCWP,* pulmonary artery wedge pressure; *MAP,* mean arterial pressure.

Cardiovascular parameters

The balloon-tipped flow-directed catheter provides information on left and right ventricular filling and total cardiac performance. In addition to the PA pressure and PCWP readings, these catheters provide more physiological data that determine prognostic indicators and evaluate therapy of the patient in shock (Table 6-5). Cardiac function is evaluated by (1) preload, which is monitored using left-sided filling pressure (PCWP) and right-sided filling pressure (CVP) and (2) afterload, which is monitored using pulmonary (PVR) and systemic vascular resistance (SVR), heart rate, and cardiac contractility (Vij, Babcock, and Magilligan, 1981). Some other parameters used to assess cardiac function are cardiac output (CO), cardiac index (CI), and stroke index (SI).

The major regulator of cardiac output is tissue oxygen need. In the shock patient this value provides the health team with information about the efficiency of the cardiac pump in the delivery of oxygen to the tissues. The cardiac index evaluates tissue oxygen need according to body surface area (BSA). The BSA can be obtained from a standard height and weight nomogram.

Respiratory parameters

The respiratory system is primarily involved with oxygen uptake and the transport of gases to the blood. Although the operation of this system is complex, the final phase of the inspiratory-expiratory cycle is the delivery of oxygen from the alveoli to the arterial blood, which is measured by the alveolar-arterial gradient $(P[A - a]O_2)$ (Chapter 4). This is an essential variable in monitoring the efficiency of gas exchange and is an early indicator of progressive respiratory failure (Del Guercio and Kazarian, 1977). In addition, practitioners need to monitor the dead space, tidal volume (V_D/V_T) ratio and correlate this to the $(P(A - a)O_2$. This is important in the presence of large shunting to correct the

Table 6-6. Physiological parameters for respiratory function

Value	Formula	Units
Minute ventilation	$V_T \times$ Respiratory rate	L/min
Alveolar ventilation	$(V_T - V_D) \times$ Respiratory rate	ml/min
Oxygen transport	$CI \times Cao_2 \times 10$	$ml/min/m^2$
Oxygen consumption	$CI \times a - vDo_2 \times 10$	$ml/min/m^2$

$a - vDO_2$, Arteriovenous oxygen difference; CaO_2, oxygen content of arterial blood; CI, cardiac index; VD, dead space volume; VT, tidal volume.

cause of the shunt, rather than continue unsuccessful attempts of raising arterial oxygenation (Pao_2) by increasing the inspired oxygen content (Fio_2). The patient on ventilatory support will also need flow studies for the health team to determine minute ventilation on and off the ventilator, as well as alveolar ventilation, oxygen transport, and oxygen consumption (Table 6-6).

The patient in shock must have coordinated functioning between the cardiovascular and pulmonary systems to ensure adequate oxygen uptake, transport, and delivery. Without this coordination, shock becomes increasingly more progressive, and anaerobic metabolism ensues. Mixed venous oxygen tensions (Pvo_2) and serum lactate levels have been identified as prognostic indicators of shock. A Pvo_2 of less than 40 mm Hg has proven to be a reliable indicator of cardiopulmonary deterioration, which is not obvious by physical assessment (Armstrong et al., 1978). Elevation in serum lactate levels greater than 13% increases morbidity (Del Guercio and Kazarian, 1977). As the Pvo_2 falls, anaerobic metabolism becomes significant, causing further increases in serum lactate levels; the oxygen delivery to the tissues obviously worsens; the patient in shock deteriorates clinically; and death results.

Hemodynamic alterations

Monitoring the patient in shock requires the nurse to assess the functioning of the cardiovascular pump and the respiratory system, and to monitor areas of oxygen uptake, transport, and delivery. Cardiac output is impaired in all types of shock. In hypovolemic shock the cardiac output is diminished by hemorrhage and fluid depletion. The patient in cardiogenic shock has diminished cardiac output as a result of an inadequate cardiac pump. In anaphylactic and septic shock cardiac output is diminished by systemic vasodilation and subsequent pooling of blood in the capillaries, which impairs venous return.

REFERENCES

Afifi, A.A., et al.: Prognostic indexes in acute myocardial infarction complicated by shock, The American Journal of Cardiology **33**:826-832, 1974.

Armstrong, P.W., and Bargre, R.S.: Hemodynamic monitoring in critically ill patients, Heart & Lung **9**:1060-1062, 1980.

Armstrong, R.F., et al.: Continuous monitoring of mixed venous oxygentension (Pvo_2) in cardiorespiratory disorders, Lancet **1**:632-634, March, 1978.

Aubin, B.A.: Arterial line: a review, Critical Care Quarterly **1**:757-764, 1979.

Bleifeld, W., Hanrath, P., Mathey, D., and Merx, W.: Acute myocardial infarction V: left and right ventricular haemodynamics in cardiogenic shock, British Heart Journal **36:**822-834, 1974.

Bolognini, V.: The Swan-Ganz pulmonary artery catheter: implications for nursing, Heart & Lung **3:**976-981, 1974.

daLuz, P., Weil, M.H., and Shubin, H.: Current concepts on mechanisms and treatment of cardiogenic shock, American Heart Journal **92:**103-113, 1976.

Daily, E.K., and Schroeder, J.S.: Techniques in bedside hemodynamic monitoring, ed. 2, St. Louis, 1980, The C.V. Mosby Co.

Del Guercio, L.R., and Kazarian, K.K., Monitoring the patient in shock, Hospital Physician **13:**12-17, 1977.

Fingeras, J., et al.: Relationship between pulmonary hemodynamics and arterial pH and carbon dioxide tenson in critically ill patients, Chest **70:**466-472, 1976.

Foote, G.A., Schabel, S.I., and Hodges, M.: Pulmonary complications of the flow-directed balloon-tipped catheters, New England Journal of Medicine **290:**927-931, 1974.

Gernert, C.F., and Schwartz, S.: Pulmonary artery catheterization, American Journal of Nursing **78:**1182-1185, 1978.

Haag, G.: Central venous catheter and monitoring, Critical Care Quarterly **2:**51-56, 1979.

Haas, J.M.: Understanding hemodynamic monitoring: concepts of preload and afterload, Critical Care Quarterly **2:**1-8, 1979.

Haughey, B.: CVP lines: monitoring and maintaining, American Journal of Nursing **78:**635-638, 1978.

Lalli, S.M.: The complete Swan-Ganz, *RN* **41:**64-78, 1978.

Lantiegne, K.C., and Civetta, J.M.: A system for maintaining invasive pressure monitoring, Heart & Lung **7:**610-621, 1978.

Murray, J., and Smallwood, J.: CVP monitoring: side stepping potential perils, Nursing '77 **7:**42-47, 1977.

Nichols, W., et al.: Complications associated with balloon-tipped, flow-directed catheters, Heart & Lung **8:**503-506, 1979.

Pace, N.C., and Horton, W.: Indwelling pulmonary artery catheters, Journal of the American Medical Association **233:**893-894, 1975.

Pego, R.F., and Luria, M.H.: Left sub-clavian vein puncture for insertion of Swan-Ganz catheters, Heart & Lung **8:**507-510, 1979.

Pennington, L.A., and Smith, C.: Leveling when monitoring central blood pressures: an alternative method, Heart & Lung **9:**1053-1959, 1980.

Qvist, J., et al.: Hemodynamic responses to mechanical ventilation with PEEP: the effect of hypervolemia, Anesthesiology **42:**45-55, 1975.

Sears, M.F., and Heise, C.: Troubleshooting the Swan-Ganz catheter, Heart & Lung **9:**303-305, 1980.

Smith, R.N.: Invasive pressure monitoring, American Journal of Nursing **78:**1514-1521, 1978.

Swan, H.J., and Ganz, W.: Use of the balloon flotation in critically ill patients, Surgical Clinics of North America **55:**1501, 1975.

Swan, H.J.: The role of hemodynamic monitoring in the management of the critically ill, Critical Care Medicine **3:**83-89, 1975.

Vij, D., Babcock, R., and Magilligan, D.J.: A simplified concept of complete physiologic monitoring of the critically ill, Heart & Lung **10:**75-82, 1981.

Walinski, P.: Acute hemodynamic monitoring, Heart & Lung **6:**838-844, 1977.

Walrath, J.M.: Stopcock: bacterial contamination in invasive monitoring systems, Heart & Lung **8:**100-103, 1979.

Woods, S.L.: Monitoring pulmonary artery pressures, American Journal of Nursing **76:**1765-1771, 1976.

Woods, S.L., and Marsfield, L.W.: Effect of body position upon pulmonary artery and pulmonary capillary wedge pressures in noncritically ill patients, Heart & Lung **5:**83-89, 1976.

Zschoche, D.A.: Mosby's comprehensive review of critical care, ed. 2, St. Louis, 1981, The C.V. Mosby Co.

7 Hypovolemic shock

LINDA NIEDRINGHAUS

Hypovolemic shock is the result of an inadequate circulating plasma volume and is generally associated with a plasma volume deficit of at least 15% to 25%. This deficit in plasma volume may be caused by hemorrhage or a loss of plasma to the third space as seen in patients with burns, peritonitis, or intestinal obstruction.

Hypovolemic shock can be subdivided into categories according to the cause of the plasma deficit. The use of terms such as *hemorrhagic shock, traumatic shock, surgical shock, burn shock,* and *dehydration shock* is helpful to the nurse because there are important features that are unique to each type. However, the underlying problem of all these categories of hypovolemic shock is an inadequate circulating plasma (blood) volume. The physiological effects, adaptive responses, precipitating causes, assessment, and objectives of medical and nursing management of hypovolemic shock will be presented.

PHYSIOLOGICAL EFFECTS OF INADEQUATE PLASMA VOLUME

All of the physiological effects of a plasma volume deficit are related to the drop in cardiac output associated with hypovolemia. A decreased blood volume caused by hemorrhage, or a plasma loss caused by third-space loss, decreases the venous return to the heart. As venous return falls, left ventricular filling falls, and cardiac output is decreased.

This decrease in cardiac output results in inadequate cellular perfusion and increased anaerobic glycolysis. Large amounts of lactic acid are produced, resulting in lactic acidosis. In severe cases, serum lactate levels can rise from the normal value of 1 mmol/L to 9 mmol/L (Ganong, 1977). Elevated serum lactate levels depress the myocardium, decrease vascular responsiveness to the catecholamines, and may induce coma.

Decreased tissue perfusion causes functional abnormalities of the white blood cells, impaired phagocytosis, and bacterial lysis, as well as delayed hypersensitivity reactions to antigens. A reduction in the number of clotting factors and thrombocytes can occur (Hechtman, 1976). These alterations create a situation in which the patient is more susceptible to infection and hemorrhage.

A decreased cardiac output and corresponding decreased cellular perfusion lead to damage of entire organs. There is a depression of liver function as evidenced by an increase in bilirubin in the blood (Baue, 1976). Liver enzyme activity is decreased as well as detoxification of chemicals and toxins.

Urine output decreases when the cardiac output drops. Because of decreased

Subcategories of hypovolemic shock	
Subcategory	**Etiology/description**
Hemorrhagic	Blood loss plus minor tissue trauma; can be caused by gastrointestinal bleeding, bleeding disorders, and gunshot and knife wounds.
Traumatic	Blood loss plus major tissue injury; occurs with severe damage to muscle or bone; seen with battle casualties and car accidents; leakage of myoglobin into the circulation can cause renal damage.
Surgical	Also known as wound shock; can be caused by various combinations of external hemorrhage, bleeding into the tissues, and dehydration during or following surgical procedures.
Burn	Hypovolemia caused by loss of plasma as burn exudate from burned body surfaces; increased hematocrit and hemoconcentration are seen. Myoglobin leakage may cause renal damage.
Dehydration	Hypovolemia caused by loss of body water and electrolytes; can occur with prolonged vomiting, diarrhea, or intestinal obstruction or fistulas; seen in diabetic ketotic and nonketotic hyperosmolar states.

blood flow to the kidneys, the glomerular filtration rate drops and urine production diminishes in an effort to conserve body fluids. The blood urea nitrogen (BUN) level will increase as a result of a decreased glomerular filtration rate. Hypovolemia will produce little or no change in the serum creatinine levels. A rising BUN with a stable creatinine level is indicative of a blood volume deficit (Graber, 1979).

Decreased perfusion of the intestines leads to necrosis of the intestinal mucosa so that *Escherichia coli* can gain access to the mucosa and circulatory system. If such organisms gain access to the general circulation, a septic shock can develop concurrently with hypovolemic shock.

ADAPTIVE RESPONSES

When blood volume is reduced and venous return is decreased, the arterial baroreceptors are stretched to a lesser degree, and sympathetic outflow to the heart and peripheral vessels is increased. This sympathetic outflow will result in an increased heart rate and increased peripheral resistance in an effort to sustain the arterial blood pressure. Vasoconstriction is generalized. Only the vessels of the brain and heart are spared. Vasoconstriction is most marked in the skin and accounts for the coolness and pallor of the patient in hypovolemic shock.

The baroreceptor response is the first response initiated by the cardiovascular system to the drop in the plasma volume. Other adaptive responses are made by the cardiopulmonary and endocrine systems (Condon and Nyhus, 1978).

Cardiopulmonary system responses

When the cardiac output is falling, increased sympathetic stimulation to the adrenergic receptors in the heart will increase its rate and force of contraction, thereby increasing its output. Although metabolic acidosis is compensated initially by increasing the rate of ventilation to augment carbon dioxide elimination, profound acidosis combined with hypoxia will lead to myocardial depression, irritability, and susceptibility to arrhythmias. Again, the patient is in danger of developing another form of shock. In this case, the patient is at risk for cardiogenic shock in addition to the hypovolemic shock that is already present.

Endocrine responses

An initial response to a plasma volume deficit is an increased secretion of antidiuretic hormone (ADH) by the posterior pituitary gland. ADH causes an increased retention of water by the kidney tubule. This conservation of water helps to expand the circulating plasma volume, thereby increasing venous return and cardiac output. A surge of adrenocorticotropic hormone (ACTH) by the anterior pituitary gland in response to the stress of a decreased plasma volume increases the circulating level of cortisol and aldosterone. These two hormones promote renal retention of sodium and water and renal excretion of potassium. The urine output will decrease below 30 ml/hour.

Increased secretion of the catecholamines epinephrine and norepinephrine causes vasoconstriction, thereby maintaining the blood pressure by decreasing the volume of the vascular space. Fluid is mobilized from the interstitial space to the intravascular space. The plasma volume is increased, and cardiac output increases in an effort to compensate for the initial hypovolemia.

Hyperglycemia develops during shock because of the formation of excessive glucose (gluconeogenesis and glycogenolysis) by cortisol and epinephrine. Recent studies have demonstrated that insulin secretion is depressed during shock. This suppression of insulin would account for the elevated blood glucose levels during the shock state (Liddell, Daniel, MacLean, and Shizgal, 1979).

Metabolic responses

During shock, the utilization of glucose by glycolytic and citric acid pathways to form energy is disrupted. Without oxygen, pyruvate is transformed anaerobically into lactic acid, which accumulates and causes acidosis. Amino acids and fatty acids that normally enter oxidative pathways for energy production also accumulate in shock, compounding the metabolic acidosis. The oxygen deficit, combined with the developing acidosis, interferes with cell membrane function. Intracellular potassium is lost as sodium and water move into the cell causing cellular edema. These metabolic alterations can occur in any body cell deprived of adequate oxygen and are the basis for the widespread cellular and organ damage seen in patients who develop hypovolemic shock.

CAUSES

The reader will recall that hypovolemia (plasma volume deficit) results from an actual loss of blood caused by hemorrhage or from a loss of plasma to the third space where it is unavailable for circulation. The circulating plasma volume can also be depleted by excessive vomiting, diarrhea, or gastrointestinal drainage. Hemorrhage can result from injury, surgery, gastrointestinal bleeding, or bleeding disorders. Third-space fluid loss can result from serious burns or bowel obstructions. A few of the conditions that produce hypovolemic shock will be discussed.

Hemorrhage

Trauma can lead to blood loss and extensive tissue damage. Two examples of injuries that can lead to hypovolemic shock are abdominal injury and pelvic fracture. Any patient involved in an automobile, industrial, or sports accident should be considered to have an abdominal injury until it is proven otherwise. Early assessment by the nurse would include checking for pain, localized tenderness, or abdominal wall rigidity by gentle palpation. All narcotics or other analgesics should be withheld until the decision concerning the need for surgery has been made.

Another assessment that should be made following an abdominal injury is observation for abdominal distention. The girth of the abdomen should be measured as soon as the patient is brought to the emergency room so that further objective measurement can be compared to this baseline data. Abdominal distention is an ominous sign. It is caused by hemorrhage of the liver, the spleen, or a major vessel. The absence of bowel sounds may also occur. These patients will need an exploratory laparotomy to locate and stop the source of hemorrhage. Of course, vigorous fluid resuscitation as described below will be begun before surgery to counteract the hypovolemia resulting from internal hemorrhage. An abdominal tap may be done to check for blood in the peritoneal cavity before surgery.

Pelvic fractures are frequently accompanied by a large blood loss because of the vascularity of the marrow of the pelvic bones. Pelvic fractures are difficult to immobilize by splinting, and surrounding tissues do little to tamponade the bleeding. Lacerations of the bladder, urethra, and rectum can occur as a consequence of pelvic fractures and contribute to the blood loss. Damage to the aorta and pelvic vessels also occurs with pelvic fracture. Again, treatment is to replace the blood loss to prevent hypovolemic shock and to locate and control the source of bleeding.

Hemorrhage can occur within the first few hours after surgery when the blood pressure returns to normal and washes away insecure clots from untied vessels. Postoperative hemorrhage can also be caused by the slipping of a ligature. Capillary hemorrhage is characterized by a slow ooze, venous hemorrhage bubbles out quickly, and arterial hemorrhage is bright red and spurts with each heart beat. Postoperative hemorrhage will not always be evident and can go unnoticed even when the nurse is most vigilant in checking vital signs and dressings. The bleeding may be concealed in a body cavity such as the thoracic or peritoneal cavity. Furthermore the signs of hemorrhage after an operation are often masked by the effects of the anesthetic or the shock state itself.

When hemorrhage is beginning, the baroreceptor response will elevate the blood pressure so that the patient's blood pressure will remain relatively normal. More subtle assessments of skin color and temperature, pulse, pulse pressure, presence of thirst, and respiratory rate need to be made. When postoperative hemorrhage is suspected, the wound should be inspected and reinforced with sterile dressings if necessary. Fluid replacement should begin and the patient should be prepared for a return to the operating room if it is deemed necessary by the physician.

Upper gastrointestinal bleeding refers to bleeding from the esophagus, stomach, or duodenum. Lower gastrointestinal bleeding refers to bleeding in the intestine and rectum (below the ligament of Treitz). Massive gastrointestinal hemorrhage occurs most frequently from the upper gastrointestinal tract. Esophageal bleeding may be caused by ruptured esophageal varices. Gastric or duodenal ulcers account for 85% of all cases of upper gastrointestinal bleeding. Lower gastrointestinal bleeding may be the result of ruptured hemorrhoids or invasion of mucosal vessels by a neoplastic growth.

The prime objectives of the initial therapy for gastrointestinal bleeding are to replace the lost blood and to determine the source of bleeding so that the hemorrhage can be stopped. A nasogastric tube with suction can be used to remove old blood from the stomach and to provide a means of early warning of recurrent gastrointestinal bleeding. If bleeding from esophageal varices persists, balloon tamponade with the triple-lumen Sengstaken-Blakemore tube may be necessary.

Arterial infusion of vasopressin may be necessary if bleeding continues. Vasopressin is a potent sympathomimetic agent that causes vasoconstriction in the distal branches of the perfused vessel. Care must be used in monitoring the arterial pressure during vasopressin infusion to prevent marked elevation in systemic blood pressure. Vasopressin infusion of the superior mesenteric artery will stop bleeding of esophageal or gastric varices. Vasopressin infusion of the left gastric or gastroduodenal artery will stop gastric hemorrhage. Vasopressin infusion controls gastric mucosal hemorrhage in approximately 80% of patients. This procedure involves catheterization of the left gastric artery followed by infusion of vasopressin at the rate of approximately 0.2 units/min for 24 hours, followed by 0.1 units/min for another 12 to 16 hours. An infusion pump is used to provide accuracy of administration. If these methods are not successful, surgery will be necessary to stop the bleeding. Usually, bleeding that requires five units of blood or more in 24 hours to maintain circulatory stability is indicative of the need for surgical exploration (Costrini and Thomson, 1977).

Bleeding disorders that lead to hemorrhage can be related to platelet disorders or to defects in the coagulation factors. Platelet disorders are known as thrombocytopenia. This disorder results from a decrease in platelet production or an increase in the peripheral utilization of platelets.

Defects in coagulation factors may be caused by inherited disorders such as hemo-

---

Platelet and coagulation factor disorders that can lead to hypovolemic shock

Platelet disorders	**Coagulation factor disorders**
Decrease in production	Hemophilia
Aplastic anemia	Plasma factor deficiencies caused by:
Marrow infiltration	Vitamin K deficiency
by cancer	Antibiotics
Myelosuppressive drugs	Biliary obstruction
Ionizing radiation	Liver disease
Viral infections	Disseminated intravascular coagulation
Nutritional deficiencies	Primary fibrinolysis
Vitamin B_{12}	Anticoagulation therapy
Folate	
Iron	
Increase in utilization	
Infections	
Drugs	
Thiazide diuretics	
Ethanol	
Estrogen	
Transfusions with stored blood	

---

philia or by acquired disorders such as plasma factor deficiencies, disseminated intravascular coagulation (DIC), primary fibrinolysis, or exogenous anticoagulation therapy (Chapter 14).

Plasma factor deficiencies may include vitamin K–related deficiencies of factors II, VII, IX, and X related to long-term antibiotic therapy, biliary obstruction, dietary deficiency, or acute stress. Liver disease also results in deficiency of these factors as well as factor V.

Third-space loss

Hypovolemia can occur with conditions other than hemorrhage. When a significant portion of the extracellular fluid volume or the circulating plasma volume is trapped in the interstitial spaces or a body cavity, this fluid is unavailable to the rest of the body for immediate use, even though it has not left the body. This loss leads to a plasma volume deficit and has been called the third-space syndrome or third-space loss. Third-space losses other than those caused by massive burns are usually slow to form, and symptoms develop over a period of days rather than minutes or hours.

The severity of third-space fluid loss depends on the clinical condition. Significant third-space loss is produced by burns. Within 12 to 18 hours after thermal injury, isotonic

---

Clinical conditions that may lead to a third-space fluid loss and hypovolemic shock

Rapid loss of fluid rich in protein
    Peritonitis
    Burns
    Crush injuries
    Sepsis
    Portal or iliac thrombosis
Slow loss of fluid lower in protein
    Intestinal obstruction
    Pleural effusion
    Portal hypertension (ascites)
    Gastric dilation
    Liver disease (decreased protein synthesis)

---

fluid containing plasma, protein, and sodium is sequestered in the burn wound. This loss of fluid produces an extracellular fluid volume deficit that must be corrected immediately to prevent hypovolemic shock that will occur when fluid shifts from the vascular compartment to replenish the extracellular space.

The amount of fluid loss depends on the depth and extent of the burn injury. An accurate estimate must be made of the percentage of the total body surface burned because appropriate fluid replacement is dependent on the accuracy of this estimate. An estimate can be made by using the rule of nines for adults. Persons younger than 10 years have a larger head and neck surface and smaller lower extremities when compared to an adult. Therefore the Lund and Browder chart is more frequently used. This chart estimates body surface area in relationship to age (Condon and Nyhus, 1978).

Fluid replacement is the most important aspect of initial care of burned patients. Because of the specific nature of the care required following a burn injury, the reader is encouraged to consult references specific to the nursing management of the burned patient.

Following gastrointestinal obstruction, large amounts of fluid, electrolytes, and protein can be lost into the lumen of the bowel and the peritoneal cavity depending on the area of obstruction and vascular involvement. The accumulation of fluid and gas within the obstructed bowel results in an increased intraluminal pressure that causes regurgitation of bowel contents into the stomach in an effort to reduce the pressure.

Normal intraluminal pressure in the resting gut is from 2 to 4 mm Hg. During obstruction, pressure may go as high as 40 to 70 mm Hg, interfering with blood and lymph flow in the mucosa. Ischemia and necrosis of the mucosa occur as submucosal vessels are occluded. Interference with lymph drainage produces edema and further decreases the absorptive capacity of the mucosa. Fluid is sequestered in the bowel lumen, and bacterial growth is enhanced. After a few hours of obstruction, the bowel is filled with fluid feces, plasma, and even blood from the breakdown of the mucosal wall. Absorption of coliform endotoxin into the bloodstream produces septic shock. Therefore the shock state becomes one of mixed septic and hypovolemic shock.

Accumulation of protein-rich fluid in the visceral and parietal peritoneum occurs during peritonitis because of the presence of infection in the peritoneal space. As the inflammatory process continues, considerable edema occurs as fluid is sequestered in the inflamed tissues. If a significant fluid shift occurs, the circulating plasma volume will be reduced, leading to signs of hypovolemia such as tachycardia and cool, pale extremities.

In liver disease, increased pressure in the portal system leads to ascites, a collection of protein-rich fluid in the abdominal cavity. Furthermore, protein synthesis by the liver is altered, leading to a low protein content of the plasma and consequent leakage of fluid into the interstitial spaces where it is trapped and unavailable for use by the rest of the body.

NURSING ASSESSMENT

Patients admitted from the emergency room following injury, postoperative patients admitted following surgery, and medical patients who are recovering from burns, gastrointestinal hemorrhage or obstruction, dehydration, liver disease, or peritonitis may be in danger of developing hypovolemic shock and should be assessed accordingly. Assessment is begun by reviewing the patient's reasons for hospitalization and all of the medical and surgical treatments received since admission.

If the patient was injured, the nature of that injury, the amount of tissue damage, and the estimated blood loss will be recorded on the emergency room record. Emergency procedures and treatments will be recorded on this record also. Operating room and recovery room records can be reviewed to determine blood and fluid losses during and following surgery. In addition, these records are a source of information about previous blood and fluid transfusions.

These written documents serve as an initial data base to alert the nurse to those patients who are in danger of developing hypovolemic shock. Verbal reports should be given by nurses who are transferring patients to the intensive care unit from other divisions within the hospital. Physical assessment of the patient will indicate if shock is actually developing and will determine if immediate medical and nursing intervention is necessary.

Clinical signs

Skin. A patient who is developing hypovolemic shock will have a cool, pale skin because of widespread vasoconstriction. This vasoconstriction is an adaptive measure the body uses to shunt the decreased blood volume to areas of most importance, such as the heart and brain. Capillary refill time in the nailbeds will be sluggish because of vasoconstriction. The skin will be clammy and moist from increased perspiration. An outpouring of catecholamines (epinephrine and norepinephrine) from the adrenal medulla causes this increase in perspiration.

Thirst. If the patient is conscious, he will ask for water since plasma volume depletion leads to stimulation of the thirst center in the hypothalamus. Thirst will not be as easy to assess in infants, the elderly, or confused patients.

Urine output. Urine output in hypovolemia will fall below 25 to 30 ml/hour (Condon and Nyhus, 1978). This is caused by widespread vasoconstriction that reduces blood flow to the kidneys. This reduced blood flow decreases the glomerular filtration rate so that less urine is produced. At the same time, increased circulating levels of hormones such as ADH and aldosterone promote water and sodium retention by the kidney tubule.

Level of consciousness. As the volume deficit develops following hemorrhage or fluid loss, the patient will have an initial increase in the level of consciousness and awareness, will appear alert, will experience the feeling of impending doom, will be anxious, and will even attempt to get out of bed. These symptoms are caused by cerebral stimulation by the catecholamines. If the blood volume is not replaced the patient will become sluggish and eventually lapse into unconsciousness.

Pulse rate. Tachycardia is one of the early signs of a circulating volume deficit. Resting heart rates in excess of 100 should be investigated. High pulse rates in conjunction with hypotension and a narrowing pulse pressure should be reported to the physician.

Respirations. Respirations will increase in depth and rate as the lungs attempt to improve blood oxygenation and simultaneously improve right heart filling in hypovolemia. Increased respirations improve right heart filling by the repeated creation of a negative intrathoracic pressure, which draws blood into the right atrium.

Blood pressure. A brief initial rise in blood pressure may occur as a result of adaptive vasoconstrictor activity in response to a decreasing blood volume. If an accurate flow chart of the blood pressure readings is kept, a gradual drop in systolic and diastolic pressures can be observed. Systolic blood pressures less than 90 to 100 mm Hg in a previously normotensive patient, or a decrease of 20 to 30 mm Hg in a previously hypertensive patient, are indicative of shock. The pulse pressure is the difference between the systolic and diastolic pressures. When blood pressure changes are caused by a blood loss, the systolic pressure falls more rapidly than the diastolic pressure. This results in a decreased pulse pressure. In hypovolemic shock, the pulse pressure falls to less than 20 mm Hg.

When the patient is raised to an upright from a supine position, a drop in systolic blood pressure of more than 10 mm Hg and an increase in the pulse rate of more than 20 beats/minute indicates a decrease in circulating blood volume of as much as 20% to 25% (Costrini and Thomson, 1977).

Hematocrit. Measurements of hematocrit are not a sensitive indicator of acute blood loss because of fluid shifts from the extravascular space that occur following hemorrhage. Hematocrit values 6 to 8 hours following the hemorrhage are more reliable. Hypovolemia caused by third-space fluid losses will result in false elevated hematocrit levels. These increased hematocrit readings are observed with burn injuries.

Hemodynamic values. If the patient's fluid volume is being monitored by a central venous catheter, the development of a worsening fluid volume deficit will be indicated by a CVP that falls below 5 cm H_2O. This central venous catheter will become important during therapy because it will be used to measure the adequacy of fluid replacement.

If a Swan-Ganz catheter is in place in the pulmonary artery, the PCWP will reflect the left atrial pressure, which indicates the adequacy of left ventricular filling prior to each heartbeat. The PCWP will be decreased (normal range is 4 to 12 mm Hg) if a fluid volume deficit is developing. The CVP and the PCWP will not be available for assessment unless the patient is already in the intensive care unit and is being monitored. If hemodynamic monitoring is available, data should be used to complete assessment of the adequacy of the patient's circulating plasma volume (O'Donnell and Belkin, 1978).

The patient going into hypovolemic shock will not exhibit all of these signs. Perhaps only one or two will be visible. Careful, repeated assessments of the patient at risk for hypovolemic shock are necessary to identify impending shock. The nurse is in the position to observe the patient constantly, discover the first evidence of hypovolemia, and initiate therapy before the irreversible stages of shock are reached. A ready summary of the nursing assessment of the patient developing hypovolemic shock is provided in the box on p. 136.

MEDICAL MANAGEMENT

Restoration of the circulating plasma volume is the most important aspect of care for the patient in hypovolemic shock. The amount of fluids and the speed at which they are infused will be dictated by the severity of the loss and the clinical status of each patient.

Blood volume should be expanded as rapidly as possible; circulatory overload is rare if the CVP is kept below 15 cm H_2O, and the PCWP below 18 mm Hg. The choice of fluid for volume replacement remains controversial and will be discussed. The importance of adequate volume expansion cannot be overemphasized, but first priority in the treatment of hypovolemic shock is the establishment of an open airway and maintenance of oxygenation.

Airway and oxygenation

Rapid losses of blood and severe head or chest injuries can compromise respiratory function (both ventilation and oxygenation). If so, an adequate airway must be established and effective oxygenation of the blood must be assured before fluid resuscitation can begin.

If the patient is having difficulty exchanging air, signs of stridor, retraction, wheezing, or cyanosis will be present. The oropharynx must be cleared of clotted blood, mucus, vomitus, or dentures. An airway will be inserted and oxygen started by mask. The patient should be allowed to sit up if he makes an effort to do so, since this position helps to maintain an open airway. Intubation of alert patients is difficult and impractical. Close observation and frequent suctioning are necessary to keep the airway open. A tracheostomy may be necessary if upper airway obstruction cannot be corrected and will

---

Summary of major findings from the nursing assessment of the patient suffering from hypovolemic shock

Finding	Cause
Skin pale, cool, and moist	Vasoconstriction and increased perspiration caused by sympathetic outflow of epinephrine.
Thirst	Stimulation of the thirst center in the hypothalamus by plasma volume deficit.
Collapsed neck veins	Plasma volume deficit.
Urine output below 30 ml/hour	Decreased glomerular filtration caused by volume deficit, increased ADH and aldosterone.
Anxious, hyperactive behavior	Increased circulating catecholamines stimulate cerebral cortex.
Lethargy, coma	Decreased cerebral perfusion.
Increased pulse	Increase in sympathetic stimulation of heart in effort to increase cardiac output.
Increased respirations	Attempt to increase oxygenation of body tissues; attempt to reverse acidosis from increased lactic acid production.
Hypotension	Decreased cardiac output as a result of decreased venous return.
Decreased pulse pressure	Blood loss causes systolic pressure to fall more rapidly than diastolic pressure.
Postural hypotension	Plasma volume deficit.
Decreased hematocrit	Loss of RBCs through hemorrhage.
Increased hematocrit	Loss of plasma to the third space.
CVP below 5 cm H_2O	Decreased right atrial pressure from plasma volume deficit.
PCWP below 10 mm Hg	Decreased left ventricular filling pressure from plasma volume deficit.

---

have to be done if the patient has a direct injury to the trachea or larynx. If a patient is comatose following hemorrhage or injury, intubation with a cuffed endotracheal tube reduces the possibility of aspiration and allows for the use of mechanical ventilation to maintain arterial oxygen tensions between 70 and 120 mm Hg and carbon dioxide tensions below 60 mm Hg (Berk, Sampliner, Artz, and Vinocur, 1976).

Fluid replacement

Fluid volume replacement is the first line of defense in prevention of the complications of shock. Since the normal distribution of body fluids is deranged in shock

Fluids used for resuscitation from hypovolemic shock	
Type of fluid	**Indication for use**
Crystalloid Lactated Ringer's	Used initially while blood is being crossmatched; if blood loss is below 1500 ml, may be the only fluid necessary.

Albumin
  Buffered saline albumin (5%)
  Salt-poor albumin (25%)
	Given to restore plasma albumin levels to normal, restore plasma volume, and promote urinary excretion.

Plasma
  Fresh frozen plasma
  Fresh plasma
  Plasmanate
	Used when hypovolemia is caused by plasma loss rather than hemorrhage; fresh frozen plasma is given to replace coagulation factors washed out by massive transfusions of whole blood.

Dextran Dextran 40 or 75 (Gentran 40 or 75, Rheomacrodex, Macrodex)	Used to expand plasma volume in emergency situations in which there is rapid hemorrhage; can produce prolonged intravascular expansion; use must be monitored.

Blood
  Whole blood
  Packed red cells
	Whole blood is given if hematocrit is less than 30%; packed red cells are used if a high CVP and myocardial failure limit fluid therapy.

states, volume loading is required to compensate for the circulation of those tissues and organs that were compromised (Berk, Sampliner, Artz, and Vinocur, 1976). This means that the administration of blood, plasma expanders, and fluids must continue after the initial plasma volume deficits have been corrected.

Following severe hypotension from massive hemorrhage, volume replacement should be given rapidly enough to maintain the systolic pressure above 100 mm Hg and the mean arterial pressure above 80 mm Hg (Berk, Sampliner, Artz, and Vinocur, 1976). The CVP and PCWP are also used to evaluate the adequacy of fluid replacement. Fluid should be given rapidly enough to raise the CVP to 15 cm H_2O to maximally stretch the ventricular fibers and augment stroke volume. If PCWP monitoring is available, the PCWP can be elevated to above normal levels, as high as 16 to 20 mm Hg in the shock state, to obtain maximal stroke output. These pressures can be maintained until termination of the shock state. The amounts of fluid to be infused often call for several intravenous lines in addition to those lines being used for monitoring. A minimum of two lines, one central and one peripheral, are necessary. Infusion pumps and controllers such as the IVAC 530 Peristaltic Infusion Pump, the IVAC 230 Controller, and the Abbott/ Shaw LifeCare Pump will provide a more accurate flow rate than the usual gravity and clamp system.

Fluid selection

Opinions vary concerning the amount and type of fluids that should be used for fluid replacement (Pruitt, 1979). One major criterion is the presence of a dramatic, observable hemodynamic response to the rapid fluid infusion that indicates improvement in the patient's condition. In other words, there should be an increase in the patient's mean arterial pressure, CVP and PCWP, as well as an increase in urine output following the initiation of infusions. All of these events signal that the plasma volume deficit is being corrected.

The following fluids may be used singly or in combination to replace the plasma volume deficit of hypovolemic shock. The selection of fluids will depend on the cause of the volume deficit and the clinical status of the patient.

Crystalloid solutions. Initial volume replacement with normal saline or Ringer's lactate provides effective intravascular expansion. Several liters can be given while blood is being crossmatched for the patient who has hemorrhaged. If the blood loss has been less than 1000 to 1500 ml, resuscitation with Ringer's lactate solution alone may be adequate. If blood loss has been greater than this or is continuing, repeated transfusion with whole blood will be necessary (Baue, 1976).

Diffusion of noncolloid salt solution out of the intravascular space is relatively rapid, so that up to four times the amount of blood lost must be infused as crystalloid solution to restore the circulating plasma volume. Salt-free crystalloid solutions (dextrose in water) are never given for primary resuscitation. When these solutions are given to a patient in the acute shock state, water is retained because of the action of ADH. Severe water intoxication (hypoosmolality) may result.

Albumin. Human serum albumin is readily available and is free of the risk of hepatitis. It is an effective plasma expander and is used to restore colloidal osmotic pressure and to prevent edema. Albumin is easily metabolized and spares muscle protein from catabolism. Albumin will remove edema fluid from the interstitial space by drawing the fluid into the vascular space. This fluid shift to the vascular space allows more water to become available for urinary excretion. As water is excreted, the plasma albumin concentration increases, cycling water from interstitial fluid to plasma to urine. If albumin transfusions are used, the dosage amount and rate will be selected to restore albumin levels to normal (3.5 to 4.8 gm/100 ml).

Current research has documented the transudation of albumin into the pulmonary interstitium and the development of the adult respiratory distress syndrome (ARDS) when large volumes of albumin are administered during fluid resuscitation (Weaver et al., 1978). Impaired salt and water excretion following albumin administration for hypovolemic shock has also been documented (Lucas, Ledgerwood, and Higgins, 1979). Albumin has also been indicated as the cause of serum protein changes following its administration for hypovolemic shock (Lucas, Bouwman, Ledgerwood, and Higgins,

1980). All of these effects of albumin may lead to a central volume overload that requires the administration of diuretics and digitalization. In addition, albumin therapy is expensive. Further research in the use of albumin for hypovolemia is indicated. See Chapter 12 for a discussion of ARDS.

Plasma. Plasma and plasma protein fraction (Plasmanate) may be given without crossmatching. Plasma infusions are used when the volume deficit is the result of plasma losses instead of hemorrhage. Plasma losses occur with burns, peritonitis, and bowel obstruction. The risk of hepatitis is present when plasma is used. This risk can be reduced by the use of single donor units but cannot be entirely eliminated. Plasma protein fraction carries no risk of hepatitis and is preferred for most clinical situations.

Fresh frozen plasma provides coagulation factors for patients with clotting abnormalities. It should be administered also whenever ongoing multiple transfusions are being given. Repeated transfusions wash out the coagulation factors. Normally, 1 unit of fresh frozen plasma is added for every 4 to 5 units of blood that is transfused (Weaver et al., 1978).

Dextran. Clinical dextran and low molecular weight dextran expand the intravascular volume, decrease blood viscosity, and improve flow throughout the microcirculation. The use of low molecular weight dextran has become controversial because of its association with the occurrence of renal tubular damage. This form of renal failure is caused by the hyperosmolar urine formed if dextran is excreted in an inadequate volume of urine. No more than 1L of dextran solution should be given each day. Dextran is metabolized from the circulation slowly and will provide volume expansion for some time.

Blood. Major losses of whole blood should be replaced with whole blood, packed red cells, and plasma substitute (albumin, Plasmanate, or fresh frozen plasma). If the hematocrit is below 30%, whole blood should be used. If the hematocrit is above 30%, plasma expanders may be used. Packed red cells should be used when the CVP is high or myocardial failure limits the amount and speed of fluid resuscitation (Berk, Sampliner, Artz, and Vinocur, 1976).

It is possible to provide adequate volume expansion initially with crystalloid solutions until crossmatching can be accomplished. The use of matched blood is recommended to prevent reactions caused by blood group incompatibilities. Transfusions should be continued until the hematocrit level stabilizes at 35%. Each transfusion should increase the hematocrit by 2 to 3 points.

Massive transfusions (in excess of 20 units) expose the patient to many complications. Banked blood becomes acidic, and hyperkalemic and loses many of its coagulation factors. Massive transfusions carry a higher risk of allergic reactions and also the potential for development of ARDS from the entrapment of fibrin and other aggregates in the blood. A microaggregate filter is always used to transfuse blood to prevent this syndrome.

NURSING MANAGEMENT

The patient who is resuscitated from hypovolemic shock by the use of massive fluid infusion still remains a critically ill patient and requires supportive nursing management. Although blood pressure has been restored to normal, the period of hypovolemic shock exposed many vital organs to ischemia and possible failure. Supportive therapy and constant nursing observation of vital signs and physical appearance and behavior as well as laboratory values are necessary to ensure survival.

Once adequate oxygenation and volume replacement have been accomplished, the following must be carried out in a systematic manner for the patient who is recovering from the stresses of hypovolemic shock.

Respiratory care

To prevent pulmonary complications, a program of respiratory care is started. Adequate oxygenation of all tissues is ensured when the airway remains open. The patient is stimulated to cough frequently. If this is impossible because of loss of consciousness, or if the patient is too weak or feeble, frequent suctioning of the oropharynx or trachea to remove secretions will be necessary. The patient is kept in a semiprone position by turning from side to side frequently. The chest, arms, and hips are supported with pillows to keep the patient in this position.

The respiratory therapist or physical therapist can assist the nurse with chest physical therapy and postural drainage. Gravity is an invaluable aid in the removal of secretions from the airway and lungs. Humidification of inspired air is also important. If the patient is receiving oxygen by mask or cannula, humidified oxygen will elevate alveolar oxygen concentration to about 35% to 40% (Berk, Sampliner, Artz, and Vinocur, 1976). The nasopharyngeal catheter should not be used if the patient is comatose or a mouth-breather, since adequate humidification is not possible.

If the patient has a tracheostomy, humidified oxygen can be delivered through a T-adaptor. Sterile technique is used for suctioning. Gloves are worn anytime the inner cannula is cleaned or changed. Dressings and tracheostomy ties are kept pristine clean to prevent infection.

Cardiovascular support

Impaired myocardial performance develops in patients with hypovolemic shock because of the increased work load associated with tachycardia, limited coronary blood flow, and reduced myocardial oxygenation (Belloni, 1979). For younger patients, correction of the plasma volume deficit by the initial fluid replacement is enough to increase myocardial performance and cardiac output. Older patients or those suffering from varying degrees of cardiac disease may need inotropic agents such as digitalis, isoproterenol (Isuprel), and dopamine (Intropin) to improve contractility of the left ventricle. Patients who develop signs of cardiac failure, pulmonary edema, or rising CVP and PCWP after the initial volume replacement is complete are candidates for digitalization. See Table 7-1 for a summary of drugs used for shock.

Hypokalemia should be corrected before digitalization to prevent digitalis toxicity (Chapter 8). Diuretics such as furosemide (Lasix) and ethacrynic acid (Edecrin) will be ordered if symptoms of pulmonary edema develop in relationship to plasma volume over-

Table 7-1. Drugs that might be needed following fluid resuscitation for hypovolemic shock*

Drug	IV dose	Indications
Cardiotonics		
Digoxin	0.5-1 mg initially 0.125-0.25 mg daily	Used to increase contractility of left ventricle.
Isoproterenol (Isuprel)	2-4 μg/min 1-4 mg in 250 ml = 4-16 μg/ml	Used to increase cardiac rate and force; stop if heart rate above 120/min.
Dopamine (Intropin)	2-30 μg/kg/min 200 mg in 500 ml = 400 μg/ml	Low dose has inotropic effect and causes vasodilation of renal vessels; high dose increases heart rate and peripheral vasoconstriction.
Vasodilators		
Phentolamine (Regitine)	5 mg slowly	Alpha blocker that produces widespread vasodilation.
Chlorpromazine (Thorazine)	5 mg slowly	Produces vasodilation; main side effect is hypotension.
Nitroprusside (Nipride)	0.5-0.8 μg/kg/min 50 mg in 500 ml D_5W = 100 μg/ml	Produces arterial vasodilation and and reduces afterload; potent drug requires continuous monitoring with an arterial line.
Steroids		
Dexamethasone (Decadron)	1-3 mg/kg	Acts as vasodilator; improves cardiac output and stabilizes lysosomal membrane.
Methylprednisolone sodium succinate (Solu-Medrol)	30 mg/kg	Action same as above; prolonged use of both drugs may cause stress ulcers; blood and urine glucose must be monitored.
Diuretics		
Mannitol 20%	12.5-25 gm	Promotes osmotic diuresis if fluid overload occurs following fluid therapy.
Furosemide (Lasix)	40-320 mg	Loop diuretic that promotes salt and water excretion by kidney tubule; corrects fluid overload.
Ethacrynic acid (Edecrin)	50-100 mg	Actions same as above.
Miscellaneous		
Sodium bicarbonate	Dose based on estimation of base deficit and serum pH	Used to reverse acid-base imbalance.
Cimetidine (Tagamet)	300 mg every 6 hr	Acts as a histamine H_2 receptor antagonist to block the release of hydrochloric acid by the gastric mucosa; prevents formation of stress ulcers.

*Drug dosages are guides only. Actual dosage schedules will be determined according to patient requirements.

load from too rapid administration of blood or plasma expanders. The therapy for fluid overload will be discussed below.

The cardiovascular system can suffer other assaults during the hypovolemic shock state or during the period following resuscitation. The combination of hypoxia and acidosis can lead to cardiac arrhythmias. Continuous ECG monitoring will be necessary to detect arrhythmias. Digitalis may be ordered for atrial arrhythmias and lidocaine for ventricular arrhythmias. Nursing management during this stage involves accurate administration of all therapeutic drugs ordered for the patient.

Maintenance of vascular tone

Profound vasoconstriction from the sympathetic nervous system response to hypoperfusion worsens the hypovolemic shock state. Vasodilating drugs such as phentolamine (Regitine), nitroprusside (Nipride), and chlorpromazine (Thorazine) provide increased tissue perfusion, thereby decreasing tissue hypoxia and acidosis. It is essential that blood volume be restored *before* the vasodilating drugs are used and that fluid therapy continue during their administration. Without these precautions, the blood pressure may drop dangerously because of the widespread opening of peripheral capillary beds in response to these drugs.

Vasoconstricting drugs are not being used today for the treatment of hypovolemic shock. Their use in the initial stages of hypovolemia would only aggravate the sympathetic vasoconstrictor response that is already present. Volume restoration, not artificial elevation of the arterial pressure by vasoconstrictors, is the usual way of treating plasma volume deficit.

Steroids are used in hypovolemic shock when response by the patient to volume replacement is not immediate. Steroids appear to increase tissue perfusion by capillary vasodilation. Additional benefits of steroids are improved oxygen and micronutrient uptake by body cells, increased conversion of lactic acid to glycogen, and lysosomal stabilization. Dexamethasone (Decadron) and methylprednisolone sodium succinate (Solu-Medrol) are given to reverse the effects of prolonged hypotension and hypovolemia. A newer group of drugs, the prostaglandins, is currently being evaluated for possible use in hypovolemic shock to increase cardiac output and provide vasodilation to ischemic tissues (Machiedo and Rush, 1979).

The patient is kept warm but not hot to promote vasodilation. One or two lightweight blankets will conserve body heat and promote vasodilation of peripheral vessels. Overheating should be avoided because overheating will contribute to the serious metabolic effects of shock by increasing cellular demands for oxygen. Additional strain would be placed on the cardiorespiratory system to supply this oxygen.

Correction of acid-base imbalance

The metabolic acidosis that develops during the hypoperfusion stage of hypovolemic shock can be corrected by the administration of buffering agents such as intravenous sodium bicarbonate. An initial dose of 1 mEq/kg of body weight can be given in emergencies, followed by 1 mEq/kg of body weight every 10 minutes. Serial blood gas measurements must be done before, during, and after bicarbonate therapy to evaluate the patient's response to therapy and to prevent the development of acidosis (Foster, 1976).

Respiratory acidosis can develop during hypovolemia especially if ventilation is depressed. It can be corrected by endotracheal suctioning and adequate ventilation. Sometimes a mechanical ventilator must be used if voluntary respiratory volume exchange is not adequate and acidosis persists. In this event, astute nursing care and observations are necessary to ensure that ventilator support is adequate (Chapter 4).

Correction of fluid overload

During the first 12 to 36 hours following hemorrhage or injury, the hypovolemic patient urgently needs volume loading to maintain the circulating plasma volume, arterial pressure, and tissue perfusion. After this rapid administration of crystalloid and electrolyte solutions, fluid is rapidly translocated to the interstitial space where it is sequestered, leading to symptoms of edema and pulmonary congestion. Therapy to reverse the life-threatening condition of fluid overload must begin at once.

If symptoms of fluid overload develop, the extravascular fluid compartment can be reduced by restoring plasma albumin concentration. The administration of albumin will restore albumin levels to normal, as well as increase the colloidal osmotic pressure and plasma volume without overexpanding the interstitial space. Albumin will draw water from the interstitial space into the vascular space (Chapter 3). As the plasma volume is expanded, more water is available for urinary excretion. As water is excreted, the plasma albumin concentration increases, thus drawing more water into the vascular space to be excreted as urine.

If the urinary output still does not increase following albumin administration, diuretics may be used if the CVP is rising and the pulse and blood pressure are normal. Osmotic diuretics such as mannitol, a monosaccharide that is filtered but not reabsorbed by the kidney tubule, will induce excretion of water that helps to maintain renal tubular flow and patency. Because mannitol acts as a plasma expander, the CVP is monitored closely throughout administration. Concentrated solutions of glucose (20%) can also be given to produce osmotic diuresis.

If there is no response to mannitol or concentrated glucose solution infusion, diuretics such as furosemide (Lasix) and ethacrynic acid (Edecrin) can be given intravenously. These diuretics act by inhibiting tubular reabsorption of sodium. The patient's CVP, arterial pressure, and hourly urine outputs must be monitored closely to prevent excessive fluid losses in response to diuretic therapy. Nursing management includes careful, systematic administration of drugs followed by close observation of responses and possible side effects.

If diuretic administration is ineffective in promoting urinary excretion of excessive fluid, it may be necessary to resort to hemodialysis or peritoneal dialysis to reduce fluid excess, high serum potassium concentration, urea, and other metabolic breakdown products. Acute renal failure, a frequent complication of hypovolemic shock, is discussed in Chapter 13.

Maintenance of nutritional status

Patients in shock require additional calories and protein to meet basal energy needs. The body's limited carbohydrate reserves are rapidly exhausted, and protein reserves in muscles are broken down to supply the energy required for body metabolism during periods of stress. If the patient is able to eat, small frequent feedings of high-protein, high-calorie foods such as malts, milkshakes, cheese, cottage cheese, and custard will provide needed calories and protein. Perhaps the patient could be encouraged to increase nutritional intake with one of the commercial liquid diets (Isocal, Meritene, Sustacal, or Vivonex). These diets can be used to supplement the patient's hospital diet or can provide a temporary sole source of nutrition if necessary. These diets are tolerated better if served cold and taken slowly.

If the patient is unable to swallow, a Levine or feeding tube may be used to ensure positive nitrogen balance. Food prepared in a blender is preferred, but the commercial liquid diets described above are gaining widespread use because of their ease of storage and administration. Tube feedings should be allowed to drip by gravity and should not be given in a bolus or forced by a syringe. Rapid feeding may result in gastric reflux that will produce aspiration of gastric contents in patients with weak gag and cough reflexes. If an infusion pump is used, caution should be taken to see that the patient does not become immobilized and afraid to move for fear of dislodging the feeding tube or equipment.

Feeding tubes are not used indefinitely because of the danger of the development of a tracheoesophageal fistula. Prolonged use may also result in acid reflux and subsequent esophageal stricture. If prolonged tube feedings are necessary, a gastrostomy or jejunostomy tube should be used.

If the patient's recovery is complicated by gastrointestinal obstruction, ileus, or fistulas, total parenteral nutrition (TPN) through a central venous catheter is indicated. TPN is also used for patients who were already nutritionally depleted. The solutions used for TPN are calculated to provide from 2000 to 3000 calories per day. Glucose solutions are the principal calorie source. A 50% glucose solution provides 1000 calories for each 500 ml infused (Costrini and Thomson, 1977). This solution can be infused at a constant rate by use of an infusion pump over a 24-hour period. Amino acids are added to the glucose solution to provide for nitrogen requirements. Usually 80 to 160 gm of protein in the form of crystalline amino acid (Freamine) is given with the glucose solution to provide a total of 3 L/day. Insulin may be ordered at the rate of 1 unit of insulin for every 4 to 6 gm of glucose that is infused. The insulin dose is ordered by the physician based on frequent blood and urinary glucose and blood osmolarity studies (Berk, Sampliner, Artz, and Vinocur, 1976). In addition, the patient requires the following electrolyte replacements, which can be added to the parenteral solutions: sodium (160 mEq), potassium (100 mEq), calcium (4.5 mEq), and magnesium (8 mEq). One ampule of multivitamins is added to the solutions each day.

TPN can be hazardous and requires continual nursing care and observation. To prevent infection, dressings should be changed every 48 hours using strict sterile technique (Costrini and Thomson, 1977). The parenteral nutrition line should not be used for measurement of the CVP or for the "piggybacking" of other intravenous fluids. The patient should be monitored frequently for temperature elevation, hyperglycemia (measured by keto-diastix on urine), and signs of fluid overload such as pulmonary rales, dyspnea, and rapid pulse. Any of these signs is reported to the physician at once.

Prevention of stress ulcers

Gastric and duodenal ulcers develop following injuries and burns that have been complicated by plasma volume deficit and hypovolemic shock. Decreased mucosal blood flow during the period of hypotension increases the permeability of the mucosal cells to the hydrogen ion, which leads to mucosal necrosis and ulcerations that can cause gastric ulcers.

Prevention of stress ulcers and gastric hemorrhage can be accomplished with the use of antacids such as aluminum hydroxide (Amphojel), magnesium trisilicate (Gelusil), and antacids that combine magnesium hydroxide and aluminum hydroxide (Maalox, Mylanta, and Riopan). During the acute stage, the patient is given 15 to 30 ml every hour while awake and during the night when awake. The antacids may be given through a nasogastric tube if necessary.

Following recovery from the acute stage of hypovolemic shock, the patient can be given antacids four times each day, 1 hour after meals and at bedtime. These drugs reduce gastric acidity and prevent the formation of a stress ulcer following massive hemorrhage or burn injuries. The histamine H_2 receptor antagonist cimetidine (Tagamet) can be used to block the release of hydrochloric acid from the parietal cells in the gastric mucosa. This drug is available for oral and intravenous administration. It has gained wide popularity for use in the prevention of stress ulcers. Cimetidine and antacid therapy may both be prescribed.

Emotional support

The nurse should stay with the patient at all times during the initial resuscitation and stabilization phase of therapy. The presence of the nurse will provide reassurance and reduce psychological stress. Communications should be simple, direct, and easy to understand. Lengthy explanations of procedures will only confuse and tire the patient. Fluid supplies and monitoring equipment should be handy to prevent confusion and inefficiency in the delivery of care. An ordered, controlled appearance should be presented to instill confidence in the patient that everything is being managed properly and that he will survive.

INDICATORS OF SUCCESSFUL MANAGEMENT

Evidence that the plasma volume deficit has been corrected and that the shock state has been reversed are obtained by assessment of the patient's response to initial and ongoing therapy.

Clinical signs

Skin and tongue. If the therapy for hypovolemia has been adequate, the skin will be pink and free of excessive moisture except for the axillae and groin, which should always be damp because of sweat gland activity in these areas when the circulating blood volume is adequate. Capillary refill time of the nailbeds and hand vein filling should be brisk. Skin turgor will be normal and the tongue will not be furrowed. In addition, the patient will not be thirsty.

Jugular veins. In the absence of congestive heart failure, changes in neck vein filling provide information about the plasma volume. If the plasma volume is adequate, the neck veins will fill to the anterior border of the sternocleidomastoid muscle when the patient is supine. Collapsed neck veins when the patient is supine would indicate that more fluid infusions are necessary.

Blood pressure and pulse. Blood pressure will return to normal once the plasma volume has been restored. What is considered a normal blood pressure for each patient will depend on his baseline blood pressure before this emergency. Higher blood pressure readings should be anticipated for patients who are known to be hypertensive. The pulse should be below 100.

Level of consciousness. The patient who has been successfully resuscitated from shock should be alert and respond appropriately to the environment. Adequate cerebral perfusion will be evident by a decrease in anxiety, confusion, lethargy, or feelings of impending doom.

Urine output. Hourly urine output is the most sensitive and accurate measure of adequate plasma volume. Following fluid therapy, hourly output from 50 to 100 ml is not unusual and will indicate that resuscitation has been successful. Output should be maintained above 30 ml/hour.

Hematocrit. If the plasma volume deficit is caused by hemorrhage, hemoglobin levels of 12.5 to 14 gm/100 ml will indicate that adequate blood transfusions have been given. Normally, the hematocrit is maintained at 35%. This indicates a moderate hemodilution that reduces blood viscosity to improve small vessel flow to all body tissues.

Hemodynamic values

Although the normal CVP is below 5 cm H_2O, it should be raised to 15 cm H_2O in the shock state to maximally stretch the left ventricular fibers and increase stroke output. Once the hypovolemia has been corrected and the patient's state stabilized, the rate of fluid infusion can be decreased to return the CVP to normal.

The normal PCWP is from 4 to 12 mm Hg. However, as with the CVP, it can be raised to 16 to 20 mm Hg as long as continuous monitoring and nursing observation is available. The rate of fluid infusion can be adjusted to maintain a PCWP of 10 to 12 mm Hg once plasma volume replacement is completed.

When fluid replacement is adequate, the patient's mean arterial pressure will be 80 mm Hg. Careful monitoring of the ulnar pulse distal to the insertion of the arterial catheter is necessary to prevent gangrene and thrombosis when this monitoring technique is used. Continuous heparin infusion of the arterial line prolongs patency of the catheter.

Measurement of the cardiac output by the Swan-Ganz catheter using the thermo-dilution technique will provide quantitative data about the output of the left ventricle and the adequacy of the plasma volume. Measurement of the cardiac output is helpful but not absolutely necessary to provide successful resuscitation from the shock state. Normal cardiac output is 4.5 to 5.5 L/min. Recall from Chapter 1 that the cardiac index is used to correlate the cardiac output to body surface area. The normal cardiac index is approximately 2.8 to 3.2 L/min/m².

SUMMARY

The patient with hypovolemic shock is critically ill, and nursing care is complex. Replacement of the plasma volume remains the first priority of care. Appropriate fluid therapy is started at once, and continuous observation and monitoring are necessary to ensure a successful outcome. Once the critical or acute phase is over and plasma volume has been restored, astute nursing care is necessary to detect delayed complications of hypoperfusion such as cardiogenic shock, adult respiratory distress syndrome, acute tubular necrosis, or disseminated intravascular coagulation. These complications of shock will be discussed in following chapters.

PATIENT VIGNETTE

Hypovolemic shock following traumatic vascular injury

A 26-year-old construction worker was admitted to the emergency room 1 hour following the collapse of a concrete wall, which crushed his right shoulder and upper arm. Continual bright red bleeding was noted on a pressure dressing that had been applied to his upper right arm by the emergency medical technicians. His blood pressure was 90/50, pulse was 120, and respirations were 36. His skin was cold and clammy. He did not realize that he was in the hospital and asked repeatedly for a drink of ice water. Numerous minor abrasions were present on his face, upper back, right arm, and anterior chest. An x-ray film revealed a compound fracture of the upper humerus. The right radial pulse was faint compared to the left radial pulse. Capillary refill of the right nailbeds was sluggish.

Continual monitoring of the vital signs demonstrated continued hypotension and tachycardia. An intravenous infusion of 1000 ml of Ringer's lactate solution was begun with an 18-gauge needle at the rate of 20 ml/min. Blood samples were drawn for determination of baseline arterial blood gases and hematocrit. A catheter was placed in the central venous pool for frequent monitoring of the CVP. A Foley catheter was inserted into the bladder to monitor urine output.

Thirty minutes after the infusion of 600 ml of fluid, the CVP was still below 5 cm H₂O and the hematocrit was reported to be 30% (normal, 42% to 52%). Urine output was 8 ml for the 30-minute period. The patient was increasingly lethargic and confused by his surroundings. Attempts to remove the pressure dressing from his upper right arm resulted in increased hemorrhage. The decision was made to transfer the patient to the operating room for exploration of his vascular injuries and for open reduction of the fractured humerus.

During surgery, 3 units of whole blood and 2000 ml of Ringer's lactate were required to maintain the patient's systolic blood pressure above 100 mm Hg. A laceration of the brachial artery was sutured and internal fixation of the humerus was accomplished. The patient was returned to the surgical intensive care unit with a blood pressure of 112/70, pulse of 84, and respirations of 24. His skin was warm and dry and he was alert. His CVP was 10 cm H_2O and his urine output was 50 ml/hour. The right radial pulse was fully palpable and capillary refill of the nailbeds was immediate. Sensation and movement were present in the right forearm and hand. The patient was discharged from the hospital 14 days later. Follow-up was on an outpatient basis.

Questions

1. What accounts for the initial symptoms of tachycardia and generalized peripheral vasoconstriction in hypovolemic shock?
   a. Fluid overload
   b. Sympathetic response
   c. Endocrine response
   d. Lactic acidosis

2. Why did the CVP remain below 5 cm H_2O following the initial rapid administration of intravenous fluids?
   a. Cardiogenic shock was developing
   b. Normal blood volume was restored
   c. Hypovolemia caused by hemorrhage was present
   d. All of the above

3. What are the symptoms of traumatic vascular injury to an extremity?
   a. Decreased or absent pulses
   b. Pain distal to injury
   c. Altered sensation
   d. All of the above

4. What is the appropriate fluid for volume replacement following hemorrhage?
   a. Whole blood
   b. Ringer's lactate
   c. Normal saline
   d. Packed red cells

5. Which of the following are indicators of successful treatment of hypovolemic shock?
   a. Urine output of 30 ml/hour or greater
   b. Collapsed neck veins
   c. Warm, dry skin
   d. Semiconscious state

Answers

1. b. During hypovolemia the blood volume is reduced and venous return is decreased. When these events occur, the arterial baroreceptors are stretched to a lesser degree and sympathetic outflow to the heart and peripheral vessels is increased. This sympathetic outflow will result in an increased heart rate and myocardial contractility in an effort to maintain the cardiac output at physiological levels. Sympathetic stimulation of the peripheral vessels results in selective vasoconstriction that redistributes the blood flow to favor the heart and brain at the expense of the kidneys, skin, and gastrointestinal organs. The patient will have symptoms such as rapid pulse rate; cool, clammy skin; and decreased urinary output.

2. c. A fluid challenge may be used to test for pump failure and volume capacity during the initial treatment phase of shock. Since expansion of the intravascular volume is the most important therapeutic maneuver in treating shock, fluid used for expansion is infused at a rate of 10 to 20 ml/min for 10 to 15 minutes. If the CVP remains low or normal (5 cm H_2O) during fluid challenge, hypovolemia is the problem, and volume expansion is continued at the same rate. If the CVP is greater than 15 cm H_2O or increases more than 5 cm H_2O over the baseline measurement, pump failure is probably the major component of the shock, and the fluid infusion is stopped. This patient had volume depletion because of the continual loss of blood from a traumatic vascular injury.

3. d. Clinical manifestations of vascular injuries indicate partial or complete obstruction of blood flow caused by the arterial interruption or spasm. Decreased or absent pulses are accompanied by pallor, altered sensation, and severe pain in the distal portion of the extremity. The pain is caused by ischemia and often is more severe than the pain associated with other body injuries. Fractures or dislocations associated with vascular injury or nerve compression should be manipulated promptly to restore pulses and eliminate nerve compression. The principle of initial treatment is to restore vascular and neural integrity to prevent gangrene or severe functional impairment.

4. a. Patients with rapid hemorrhage usually require whole blood transfusions, and patients with slow hemorrhage require transfusion with packed red cells. Each unit of whole blood (500 ml) will raise the hematocrit 2 to 3 points. When hematocrit values are greater than 30%, plasma expanders usually are more useful than whole blood for volume replacement. If high CVP and myocardial failure should limit transfusion therapy, packed cells should be used as needed to maintain the oxygen-carrying capacity of the blood. If the blood loss is less than 1000 ml to 1500 ml, resuscitation with Ringer's lactate solution alone may be adequate. Plasma and plasma protein fraction (Plasmanate) are transfused when the volume deficit is the result of plasma loss instead of hemorrhage.

5. a and c. A urine output of 30 ml/hour or greater is a positive indicator of adequate volume replacement. Hourly urine output is the most sensitive and accurate measure of adequate plasma volume. Warm, dry skin would indicate the absence of excessive vasoconstriction in the skin and indicate adequate perfusion had been restored to the peripheral vessels following treatment for hypovolemia.

The jugular veins provide information about the plasma volume. If the plasma volume is adequate, the neck veins will fill to the anterior border of the sternocleidomastoid muscle when the patient is supine. Collapsed neck veins when the patient is supine would indicate that more fluid infusions are necessary.

The patient who has been successfully resuscitated from shock should be alert and respond appropriately to the environment. Continued demonstrations of confusion, lethargy, or stupor would indicate inadequate cerebral perfusion.

REFERENCES

Baue, A.E.: Metabolic abnormalities of shock, Surgical Clinics of North America **56:**1059-1071, 1976.

Belloni, F.L.: The local control of coronary blood flow, Cardiovascular Research **13:**63-85, 1979.

Berk, J.L., Sampliner, J.E., Artz, J.S., and Vinocur, B.: Handbook of critical care, Boston, 1976, Little, Brown & Co.

Condon, R.E., and Nyhus, L.M., editors: Manual of surgical therapeutics, ed. 4, Boston, 1978, Little, Brown & Co.

Costrini, N.V., and Thomson, W.M., editors: Manual of medical therapeutics, ed. 22, Boston, 1977, Little, Brown & Co.

Demling, R.H., Will, J.A., and Perea, A.: Effect of albumin infusion on pulmonary microvascular fluid and protein transport, Journal of Surgical Research **27:**321-326, 1979.

Foster, W.T.: Principles of acute coronary care, New York, 1976, Appleton-Century-Crofts.

Ganong, W.F.: Review of medical physiology, ed. 8, Los Altos, Calif., 1977, Lange Medical Publications.

Graber, V.M.: Postoperative care and prevention of postoperative complications for the multiple-injured, Journal of the American Association of Nurse Anesthetists **47:**416-423, 1979.

Hardaway, R.M., III: Monitoring of the patient in a state of shock, Surgery, Gynecology and Obstetrics **148:**339-345, 1979.

Hechtman, H.B.: Adequate circulatory responses or cardiovascular failure, Surgical Clinics of North America **56:**929-943, 1976.

Illner, H., and Shires, G.T.: The effect of hemorrhagic shock on potassium transport in skeletal muscle, Surgery, Gynecology and Obstetrics **150:**17-25, 1980.

Jahre, J.A., Grace, W.J., Greenbaum, D.M., and Sarg, M.J.: Medical approach to the hypotensive patient and the patient in shock, Heart & Lung, **4:**577-587, 1975.

Johansen, B.L.: Third space loss, Focus **7:**34-36, 1980.

Liddell, M.J., Daniel, A.M., MacLean, L.D., and Shizgal, H.M.: The role of stress hormones in the catabolic metabolism of shock, Surgery, Gynecology and Obstetrics **149:**822-830, 1979.

Lucas, C.E., et al.: Questionable value of furosemide in preventing renal failure, Surgery **82:**314-320, 1977.

Lucas, C.E., Ledgerwood, A.M., and Higgins, R.F.: Impaired salt and water excretion after albumin resuscitation for hypovolemic shock, Surgery **86:**544-549, 1979.

Lucas, C.E., Bouwman, D.L., Ledgerwood, A.M., and Higgins, R.: Differential serum protein changes following supplemental albumin resuscitation for hypovolemic shock, Journal of Trauma **20:**47-51, 1980.

Machiedo, G.W., and Rush, B.F., Jr.: Comparison of corticosteroids and prostaglandins in treatment of hemorrhagic shock, Annals of Surgery **190:**735-739, 1979.

O'Donnell, T.F., and Belkin, S.C.: The pathophysiology, monitoring, and treatment of shock, Orthopedic Clinics of North America **9:**589-609, 1978.

Ponsky, J.L., Hoffman, M., and Swayngim, D.S.: Saline irrigation in gastric hemorrhage: the effect of temperature, Journal of Surgical Research **28:**204-205, 1980.

Pruitt, B.A.: The effectiveness of fluid resuscitation, Journal of Trauma **19**(Supp. 11):868-870, 1979.

Robinson, W.A.: Fluid therapy in hemorrhagic shock, Critical Care Quarterly **12**(4):1-13, 1980.

Rothenberger, D.A., Fischer, R.P., and Perry, J.F., Jr.: Major vascular injuries secondary to pelvic fractures: an unsolved clinical problem, American Journal of Surgery **136:**660-662, 1978.

Shah, D.M., et al.: Cardiac output and pulmonary wedge pressure: Use for evaluation of fluid replacement in trauma patients, Archives of Surgery **112:**1161-1164, 1977.

Schwartz, S.I.: Supportive therapy in burn care: consensus summary on fluid resuscitation, Journal of Trauma **19**(supp. 11):876-877, 1979.

Weaver, D.W., et al.: Pulmonary effects of albumin resuscitation for severe hypovolemic shock, Archives of Surgery **113:**387-392, 1978.

8 Cardiogenic shock

ANNE GRIFFIN PERRY

Until the advent of hemodynamic monitoring, counterpulsation, and left heart assist devices, cardiogenic shock had a 100% mortality. Simply defined, cardiogenic shock is a state of low cardiac output associated with an inappropriately elevated left ventricular filling pressure. Cardiogenic shock appears as a complication in approximately 15% of acute myocardial infarction patients (da Luz, Weil, and Shubin, 1976). Patients with severe triple vessel disease and distal coronary occlusion are at even greater risk for cardiogenic shock following acute myocardial infarction. As a result of the myocardial ischemia there is impaired contractility resulting in diminished cardiac output.

Historically, treatment for cardiogenic shock centered around the use of catecholamines. Specifically these catecholamines were norepinephrine (Levophed) and isoproterenol (Isuprel). Norepinephrine is an alpha-adrenergic and beta-adrenergic agent that enhances systemic vasoconstriction, thereby improving myocardial perfusion and oxygenation without any significant increase in cardiac output (Goodman and Gilman, 1980). Isoproterenol is a beta-adrenergic agent whose ultimate effect increases cardiac output but at the expense of an increased cardiac workload and myocardial oxygen requirements (Goodman and Gilman, 1980).

This chapter will review the pathophysiology, the clinical picture, and the medical and nursing management of the patient in cardiogenic shock.

PATHOPHYSIOLOGY

Cardiogenic shock, as a complication of acute myocardial infarction, is a state of low cardiac output associated with an inappropriately elevated left ventricular filling pressure (LVFP). Once 40% of the left ventricle becomes infarcted, the risk of cardiogenic shock is increased (Collier, 1979). Following an occlusion of the coronary vessel, blood flow to a region of the myocardium is diminished with a resultant decrease in contractility of the ischemic region. This contractile deficit is the single most important cause of pump failure in the patient with a myocardial infarction, and it initiates the vicious cycle of cardiogenic shock (Fig. 8-1).

The decreased myocardial contractility subsequently causes a decrease in the stroke volume and cardiac index. While these two hemodynamic parameters are declining, the left ventricle is becoming overloaded and there is a rise in the left ventricular end-diastolic pressure (LVEDP). This results in an increased afterload, and the left ventricle must pump against resistance that further compromises stroke volume. In addi-

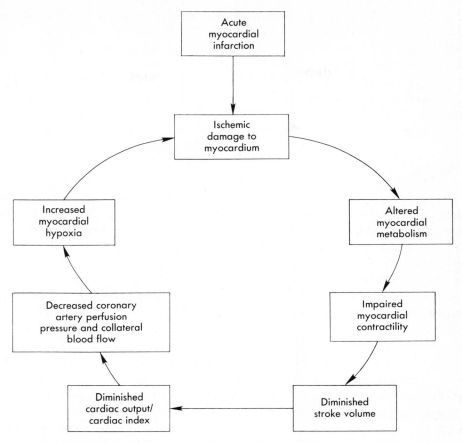

Fig. 8-1. Vicious cycle of pathophysiology in cardiogenic shock.

tion, the increased afterload and decreased contractility of the myocardium allow for an overdistended left ventricle, which occurs at the expense of increased ventricular wall tension and myocardial oxygen consumption and increases the risk of further ischemic injury.

Because of the nature of the circulatory system, the fall in stroke volume and cardiac index results in lower systemic blood pressure. This hypotension decreases coronary artery perfusion and collateral blood flow, causing more myocardial hypoxia with oxygen requirements exceeding the available oxygen supply. As a result there is increased risk for new ischemic episodes to occur.

Eventually pressures in the pulmonary vasculature increase, causing a shift of fluid into the pulmonary interstitial space and the alveoli. Respiratory insufficiency ensues as the surface area available for gaseous diffusion is reduced. This, then, accounts for the pulmonary venous shunting that further compromises oxygen transport (Collier,

1979). Without adequate oxygenation anaerobic metabolism occurs, causing a rise in serum lactate levels producing metabolic acidosis. Blood lactate levels greater than 1.4 mM/L confirm circulatory failure. The severity of shock can be closely correlated to the elevations in serum lactate levels (da Luz, Weil, and Shubin, 1976).

Early recognition and treatment may, however, prevent the onset of the vicious cycle of cardiogenic shock and the loss of the ischemic myocardium. The severity of cardiogenic shock and the prognosis of this syndrome are closely correlated with the percentage of necrotic myocardium. The greater the necrosis, the greater is the risk of mortality.

CLINICAL PICTURE

To decrease the risk of mortality in cardiogenic shock, the nurse must utilize appropriate assessment techniques to ensure early recognition of this syndrome. This syndrome is dominated by hemodynamic alterations of systemic and pulmonary circulation and by neurohumoral mechanisms that result in retention of sodium and water (Giles, 1980). Although cardiogenic shock most commonly follows an acute myocardial infarction, it may also be precipitated by secondary complications of an acute myocardial infarction. These secondary complications include prolonged acidosis, arrhythmias, hypovolemia, hypoxemia, and excessive renal output (Swan, et al., 1972).

Diagnostic criteria

Current literature (Collier, 1979; Mueller, Evans, and Ayers, 1978; Foster and Conty, 1980) is consistent in identifying the diagnostic criteria for cardiogenic shock. Part of the nursing assessment of the patient in cardiogenic shock centers on the evaluation of hemodynamic parameters. The primary parameters include arterial blood pressure, cardiac output and/or cardiac index, and LVFP (Foster and Conty, 1980). The ideal method for monitoring systemic blood pressure is through the use of an intraarterial line. In severely hypotensive patients an indirect cuff measurement is not representative of the central aortic pressure and therefore is not an accurate guide in the assessment of the present or changing status of the patient's blood pressure.

Correct assessment of the patient's cardiac output requires the use of invasive monitoring equipment and a thermodilution catheter. Once the cardiac output is determined, this value can then be converted to the cardiac index (Chapter 1). Noninvasive assessments of decreased mentation, decreased body temperature, rapid thready pulse, arrhythmias, and oliguria are important clinical indices in the evaluation of cardiac output. Although these do not require sophisticated monitoring equipment, one should never minimize their importance in caring for the severely ill patient.

LVFP is measured with the use of the Swan-Ganz catheter and is an indicator of left ventricular functioning; for example, when left ventricular function declines, the filling pressure becomes elevated. The hemodynamic parameters for this measurement are obtained by pulmonary artery diastolic pressure (PAD) and pulmonary artery wedge pressure (PCWP). First, the PCWP is an indirect but reliable means to assess left ventricular preload. Second, this parameter provides continuous evaluation of the capillary

---

Diagnostic criteria for cardiogenic shock

Absent or poor peripheral pulses
Cold, clammy skin
Systolic blood pressure less than 85 mm Hg or, in hypertensive patients, a decrease
    of 80 mm Hg systolic
Urinary output less than 25 ml/hr
Appropriate electrocardiographic and enzyme changes
        ECG: QRS changes, followed by elevated ST segments in leads V_1 to
                V_3 with reciprocal depression in V_4 to V_6. One day after, acute
                myocardial infarction Q waves appear in V_2 to V_4 and ST seg-
                ment elevations and T-wave inversion V_2 to V_6
     Enzyme: Serum glutamic oxaloacetic transaminase (SGOT) elevates 4 to 6
                degrees after infarct
                Lactic dehydrogenase (LDH) elevates 2 to 3 days after infarct
                Creatine-phosphokinase (CPK)-MB elevates 4 to 6 degrees after
                infarct
History consistent with an acute myocardial infarction
Elevated PCWP greater than 18 mm Hg
Cardiac index below 2.2 l/min/m²
Decreased mentation

---

pressures, an important determinant of pulmonary edema (da Luz, Weil, and Shubin, 1976). Clinical studies have identified an increased risk of mortality in patients whose PCWP rose to 20 mm Hg or higher (da Luz, Weil, and Shubin, 1976; Swan et al., 1972; Verdouw et al., 1975). The patient with an elevated PCWP, and consequently an elevated LVFP, is at risk for pulmonary edema. Research has demonstrated that there is an increased risk of pulmonary edema in cardiogenic shock patients whose PCWP exceeds 25 mm Hg (Crexells et al., 1973; Verdouw et al., 1975).

Presently measurements of the plasma colloid osmotic pressure are being utilized to identify the cardiogenic shock patient's risk for pulmonary edema. By relating the PCWP to the plasma colloid osmotic pressure, an oncotic-hydrostatic gradient can be calculated. In 1976 da Luz and associates studied 26 patients and found that there was an absence of pulmonary edema when the gradient was within normal limits and averaged 9.7 ± 1.7 (SEM) mm Hg. They found that the risk of pulmonary edema increased when the gradient was less than 4.0 mm Hg.

Additional signs that may occur with an elevated LVFP are rales, tachycardia, an S_3 heart sound, and ventricular diastolic gallop. Radiographically the heart may be enlarged and demonstrate evidence of pulmonary congestion. The arterial blood gases may be abnormal. Frequently a decreased Pao_2 can precede clinical evidence of pulmonary edema and provide an important indicator of intrapulmonary shunting.

Even though the majority of assessments will focus on increased LVFP and its related clinical changes, it should not be forgotten that right ventricular failure can occur in the patient with cardiogenic shock. The nursing assessment should also evaluate right ventricular function including an elevated CVP, jugular venous distention, hepatomegaly, hepatojugular reflex, and peripheral edema.

MEDICAL AND NURSING MANAGEMENT

The patient in cardiogenic shock requires precise and continuous medical and nursing management because this syndrome can result in rapid physiological deterioration and death. Presently the overall objective in the management of cardiogenic shock is to institute those therapeutic measures that protect the ischemic myocardium. Foster and Conty (1980) stated that the rationale for salvaging the ischemic myocardium is (1) ischemic myocardial tissue has the capability to contract in response to positive inotropic pharmacological agents, (2) the final infarct size is reached over a period of days and is an outcome of factors determining oxygen consumption and coronary perfusion, (3) collateral circulation to the ischemic area is generally present, and (4) animal and human research has demonstrated that well-designed therapeutic measures can control and/or reduce the infarct size.

To adequately meet the overall objective of protecting the damaged myocardium, there are three major goals of treatment for the patient in cardiogenic shock:

Increased oxygen supply to the myocardium

Increased cardiac output

Decreased workload of the left ventricle

The attainment of these goals takes place simultaneously, and they are interdependent.

Increased oxygen supply

Patients in cardiogenic shock must be assessed for adequacy of oxygenation. The patient is experiencing a deficiency in oxygen to the myocardium as well as to the rest of the body. This oxygen need is indicated by restlessness, breathlessness, dyspnea, disorientation, and cardiac arrhythmias. The nurse should note the quality of respiratory functioning as well as the adequacy of blood oxygenation. The best clinical indicators of blood oxygenation are mixed venous arterial blood gases and calculation of P(A − a) gradient. An inspired oxygen concentration of 40% (FI_{O_2} of 0.4) using a venti-mask is sufficient to maintain arterial blood gases within the normal range. When progressive respiratory dysfunction is indicated by hypoxemia (Pao_2 below 70 mm Hg), hypercapnia ($Paco_2$ above 60 mm Hg), and acidemia, it may then become necessary to intubate the patient and institute mechanical ventilation with positive end-expiratory pressure (PEEP). A patient who has the potential for partial or complete ventilatory failure must receive nursing care directed toward maintaining a patent airway, promoting adequate diffusion of oxygen and carbon dioxide, and ensuring complete lung expansion (Rubin, 1977).

Controlling the patient's pain will aid in reducing myocardial oxygen demands. Narcotic analgesics such as morphine sulfate are given intravenously. It is not recom-

---

Assessment parameters for anxiety

Confusion
Dilated pupils
Flushing or pallor
Hyperventilation
Inappropriate laughter or crying
Irritability
Nasal flaring
Tachycardia
Repetitive actions, questions, or statements
Restlessness

---

mended to administer any analgesics intramuscularly because the peripheral blood flow is reduced, and absorption of the drug and subsequent pain relief would be delayed. Analgesics, such as meperidine, that have a hypotensive side effect should be avoided so that an already diminished cardiac output is not further compromised.

Commonly patients entering cardiogenic shock are no longer experiencing chest or referred pain. However, these patients and their families can demonstrate a great deal of anxiety, which can further increase oxygen demands. When assessing the patient in cardiogenic shock the nurse should be sensitive to those signs that indicate various degrees of anxiety. Since some of these signs are also indicative of a declining hemodynamic status, the nurse must then evaluate their presence in relation to the overall physiological condition of the patient. If the signs are truly related to anxiety, the nurse must intervene so that this is reduced. Frequently providing reassurance through the use of touch, eye contract, and information regarding the various procedures and equipment will help to decrease some of the anxiety. Appropriate control of this anxiety will reduce oxygen demands and further myocardial ischemia.

The nurse must also recognize any acid-base disturbances and take appropriate nursing interventions to return the pH concentration to normal levels. Nursing care directed toward the triad of maintaining a patent airway, promoting adequate lung expansion, and adequate diffusion of respiratory gases will assist in acid-base regulation. *Respiratory alkalemia,* which occurs with hyperventilation, can be corrected by various methods. Initially reducing the anxiety can result in a return to normal respiratory rate. If this fails, it may become necessary to sedate the patient, carefully avoiding those drugs that can cause respiratory depression. In some patients who are hyperventilating, instructing them to breathe into a paper bag will restore their pH and bring about a return to a normal respiratory rate. In severe cases, especially in patients with underlying pulmonary disease, it may become necessary to intubate the patient and institute mechanical ventilation. Some degree of *respiratory acidemia* will be present in the patient with cardiogenic shock. This respiratory acidemia will reflect the presence of ventilatory insufficiency in the patient. The greater the failure in ventilation, the greater will be the respiratory acidemia. *Metabolic acidemia,* which results from the shock syndrome itself, reverses once adequate perfusion is restored. da Luz (1976) does not recommend the use of sodium bicarbonate ($NaHco_3$) in the treatment of this acidemia. The rationale for this is twofold. First, excess sodium further potentiates the risk of heart failure by increasing circulating fluid volume and thus increasing cardiac workload. Second, overcorrection may result in a *metabolic alkalemia* that further impairs the unloading of oxygen at the tissue level, shifting the oxygen-hemoglobin dissociation curve to the left.

Controlling oxygen delivery, pain, anxiety, and acid-base balance will assist in increasing the oxygen supply to the myocardium. Although this increased myocardial oxygen supply will not break up the vicious cycle, it will assist in promoting physiological adaptation and preventing further decline in the patient with cardiogenic shock.

Increased cardiac output

The cardiac output of these patients is compromised by the impaired myocardial contractility. There can be further decline in cardiac output because of cardiac arrhythmias, which occur as a result of ischemia, acid-base alterations, or the myocardial infarction itself. Correction of these arrhythmias is essential to prevent continuing circulatory failure.

Bradycardias result in hypotension, which further diminishes cardiac output. This arrhythmia can be controlled with the administration of atropine sulfate intravenously or, if the arrhythmia is prolonged, atrial pacing may be necessary to ensure an adequate heart rate to maintain sufficient cardiac output. Ectopic tachycardias may lead to rapid deterioration of cardiac function as well as an extension of the acute myocardial infarction. Ventricular arrhythmias should be appropriately treated by selected antiarrhythmic agents such as lidocaine (Xylocaine), procainamide, bretylium tosylate, or the newer calcium channel blockers such as verapamil. As the experienced practitioner knows, the life threatening ventricular arrhythmias require prompt treatment with cardioversion and pharmacological agents. Supraventricular arrhythmias are often treated with digoxin (Lanoxin), quinidine sulfate, or cardioversion.

In some patients with cardiogenic shock, hypovolemia may account for continuing hypotension and perfusion failure (da Luz, Weil, and Shubin, 1976). This principle must be remembered because the administration of fluids may result in a reversal of the shock state. Therefore LVFP response to volume loading should be evaluated. The rationale for this is based on Starling's law (Chapter 2). Simply defined this law states that an increase in left ventricular filling pressure should result in an appropriate increase in stroke volume and subsequent cardiac output. However, in the failing heart, volume loading may result in no increase, or even a fall, in the cardiac output (da Luz, Weil, Liu, and Shubin, 1974). It is for this reason that volume loading should be undertaken with caution and in the presence of adequate hemodynamic monitoring equipment. If the LVFP is below 18 mm Hg, volume loading can be initiated (Collier, 1979). Crexells et al. (1973) related the PCWP to the left ventricular stroke index in patients with acute myocardial infarction and found the optimum preload (LVFP) to range between 14 and 18 mm Hg. However, fluid infusion must be abandoned when increases in filling pressure occur without increases in cardiac output. When cardiac output measurements are not available, da Luz, Weil, and Shubin (1976) recommend utilizing the combination of the PCWP and the colloid osmotic pressure. Fluid administration is then continued until the hemodynamic signs of shock are reversed or until colloid osmotic hydrostatic pressure declines to 4 mm Hg or less.

Pharmacological agents have proven beneficial in increasing the cardiac output in these patients. However, research has demonstrated that the sympathomimetic amines have little or no benefit in patients with cardiogenic shock.

Isoproterenol (Isuprel) acts through beta-adrenergic stimulation. The drug improves myocardial contractility and cardiac output; however, studies have shown that there is a resultant rise in myocardial oxygen requirements beyond the available oxygen (Mueller, Evans, and Ayers, 1978). This, then, further increases myocardial oxygen demand and perpetuates the vicious pathophysiological cycle.

Norepinephrine (Levophed) has both alpha-adrenergic and beta-adrenergic action. This drug increases systemic arterial pressure by increasing cardiac output and peripheral vascular resistance. There is an elevation in coronary artery perfusion pressure and oxygen delivery to the myocardium. However, peripheral blood pressure is reduced, especially in the systemic vasculature (Collier, 1979; Mueller, Evans, and Ayers, 1978).

The use of inotropic agents dopamine (Intropin) and dobutamine (Dobutrex) in the patient with cardiogenic shock have been studied. Dopamine occurs naturally as a precursor of norepinephrine. The drug has positive inotropic actions of increased myocardial contractility with increased cardiac output. Dopamine maintains central aortic pressure and enhances renal and splanchnic perfusion through vascular dilation. Recent studies (Mueller, Evans, and Ayers, 1978; Robie, and Goldberg, 1975) have demonstrated that although ventricular performance was increased, this increase occurred at the expense of myocardial oxygen consumption. The study conducted by Mueller, Evans, and Ayers (1978) concluded that an improvement of peripheral circulation is worthless when the myocardial pump itself is deteriorating.

A more recent inotropic agent, dobutamine, acts directly on beta$_1$ (β_1) adrenergic receptors in the myocardium and has positive inotropic and chronotropic actions. The overall physiological result of this drug is an increased cardiac output with a decreased ventricular diastolic pressure and a decreased PCWP (Sonnenblick, Frishman, and LeJemtel, 1979). Perhaps the most beneficial effect of this drug is that it increases cardiac output without increasing myocardial oxygen requirements or a reduction in coronary artery blood flow. The drug is rapid acting and the usual intravenous dosage is 2.5 to 10 μg/kg/min; however, dosages as high as 40 μg/kg/min have been reported in the literature (Sonnenblick, Frishman, and LeJemtel, 1979). Controlling cardiac arrhythmias, assessing and monitoring the status of the circulating blood volume, and proper pharmacological agents will assist in improving the cardiac output of patients in cardiogenic shock.

Effects of vasodilators

Reduced aortic and systemic vascular impedance

Increased left ventricular ejection fraction
Increased effective stroke volume
Reduced left ventricular wall tension
Reduced pulmonary capillary pressure

Reduced pulmonary vascular impedance

Increased right ventricular ejection fraction
Increased effective stroke volume
Arterial hypoxemia

Decreased left ventricular workload

Recent research has proven the efficacy of vasodilators in the treatment of cardiogenic shock. One result of these drugs is improved left ventricular performance without an increased myocardial oxygen consumption. The major physiological effect of vasodilators is the reduction of left ventricular end-diastolic pressure and subsequent increase in stroke volume and improved left ventricular function (Moskowitz, 1975). Although there are multiple effects of vasodilators, the primary goal of these drugs is to reduce the afterload and to facilitate better systolic emptying, which further decreases the preload and myocardial oxygen requirements (Moskowitz, 1975).

Patients with normal LVFP receive no benefit from afterload reduction; therefore the nursing history should include the patient's blood pressure prior to the acute myocardial infarction. This is especially important in patients undergoing treatment for chronic hypertension. While receiving vasodilators, it is essential that these patients have continuous hemodynamic monitoring to evaluate LVFP as well as arterial blood pressure to adequately titrate the rate of drug administration. The infusion of vasodilators should be titrated to maintain LVFP in the range of 15 to 18 mm Hg. Left ventricular function curves tend to flatten or decline when the filling pressures rise above 20 mm Hg.

Prior to the administration of any vasodilator it must be determined that the patient is not hypovolemic. Massive vasodilation will further decrease venous return and result in progressive worsening of the clinical assessment of the hypovolemic patient. Frequently it is wise to fluid challenge the patient prior to the administration of these drugs, unless it has been determined that the patient is indeed normovolemic. Because of the rapid decrease in arterial blood pressure following administration of a vasodilator, there should be vasopressors, such as norepinephrine, available for immediate use in these patients. Postural hypotension is common in patients receiving this medication. If the patient has been horizontal throughout treatment, the nursing care should ensure that the

Table 8-1. Titration schedule for infusion of sodium nitroprusside*

Time (min)	Microdrops/min	μg/min	c.c./min
0	6	10	0.1
5	12	20	0.2
10	18	30	0.3
15	24	40	0.4
20	30	50	0.5
25	36	60	0.6
30	42	70	0.7
35	48	80	0.8
40	60	100	1.0
45	72	120	1.2
50	84	140	1.4
55	96	160	1.6
60	108	180	1.8
65	120	200	2.0

From Ziesche, S. and Franciosa, J.A.: Heart & Lung **6:**99-103, 1977, p. 101.
*50 mg in 500 cc of 5% dextrose and water = 100 μg per cc.

head of the bed remain relatively flat for several hours following discontinuation of the drug.

The common vasodilator drugs utilized are phentolamine and sodium nitroprusside. The action of these drugs is similar, as is the related nursing care. However, when sodium nitroprusside is being used, the nurse must take precautions to prevent exposure of the drug to heat and light. Encasing the intravenous solution and the administration tubing in aluminum foil will avoid exposure to light and the subsequent decreased effectiveness of the drug. For maximum effectiveness, sodium nitroprusside should be titrated to the desired dosage as quickly as possible. Accordingly, the infusion is begun at a rate of 10 μg/min and increased by increments of 10 μg/min every 5 minutes (Table 8-1). This schedule may vary in severely hypertensive patients (Ziesche and Franciosa, 1977). After 4 hours of administration the remaining solution in the intravenous container should be discarded and a new, freshly prepared solution hung in its place.

Intra-aortic balloon pump

The intra-aortic balloom pump (IABP) has proven its effectiveness in the reduction of the left ventricular workload in the patient with cardiogenic shock. Essentially the heart's pumping ability is determined by preload, afterload, and contractility. The level of LVFP is a determinant of cardiac performance, since it affects diastolic ventricular stretch (Crexells et al., 1973). If the left ventricular filling pressure is too low, there is a decline in cardiac output. On the other hand, if this pressure is too high, pulmonary congestion results. Once there is an elevation in LVFP, there is an increased cardiac workload and oxygen demand.

Functional changes in cardiovascular dynamics following ischemia

Decreased contractility
Abnormal ventricular wall motion
Decreased stroke volume
Diminished ejection fraction
Elevated ventricular systolic and end-diastolic volumes
Elevated left ventricular end-diastolic pressure
Altered ventricular wall compliance

From Price, S.A., and Wilson, L.M.: Pathophysiology: clinical concepts of disease processes, New York, 1978, McGraw-Hill Book Co.

Indications for using the intra-aortic balloon pump

Cardiogenic shock secondary to acute myocardial infarction
Other low-output states, i.e., septic shock, burn shock, etc.
Preoperative and postoperative aid to patients requiring open heart surgery
The removal of a refractory patient from total cardiopulmonary bypass
Support for unstable patients undergoing angiography
Intractable left ventricular failure
Intractable angina pectoris
Adjunct in neurosurgery, requiring an increased cerebral blood flow

Data from Bregman, D.: Heart & Lung **3:**916-927, 1974; Durie, M.: Heart & Lung **3:**971-976, 1974.

Ischemia significantly depresses ventricular function by causing the loss of contractility in the necrotic muscle and the surrounding tissue. The functional changes produce the overall decline in hemodynamic parameters and act to delay the decline in cardiac output and perfusion pressure. However, the patient in cardiogenic shock needs measures other than the internal physiological resources to restore adaptation. One of these measures is the IABP.

The present indicators for the IABP are outlined above. Bregman (1974) suggests that dissecting aortic aneurysms, aortic insufficiency, cardiac standstill, abdominal aortic aneurysm, and prior peripheral vascular surgery are either contraindications or reasons for caution in utilizing the IABP. Since the focus of this chapter is on cardiogenic

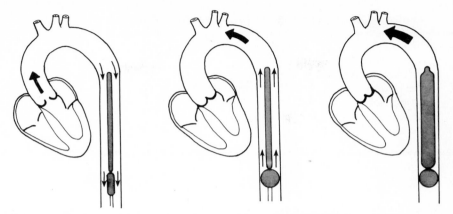

Fig. 8-2. Mechanism of action of dual chambered intraaortic balloon. *1*, Systole: in systole, aortic pressure is increased thus reducing energy expenditure of left ventricle. *2* and *3*, Diastole: during diastole there is an increase in aortic pressure, hence an increase in coronary perfusion pressure and an end result of increased coronary and cerebral blood flow. (From Bregman, D.: Heart & Lung **3:**916-928, 1974.)

shock, the discussion will center on how an increase in coronary perfusion pressure and blood flow and the decrease in left ventricular workload are accomplished with counterpulsation.

The ultimate goals of counterpulsation are to increase cardiac output, increase oxygen supply, and decrease myocardial oxygen consumption. Hemodynamically, the effects of IABP are to break up the vicious cycle of shock; decrease afterload, thereby promoting better ventricular emptying; and reduce preload, which is documented by a decrease in the PCWP (Eckhardt, 1977).

The physiological advantages of the IABP occur as a result of the balloon inflation and deflation cycle (Fig. 8-2). Balloon inflation during the diastolic phase of the cardiac cycle increases aortic diastolic pressure and subsequent coronary artery perfusion pressure. The major coronary blood flow occurs during diastole because the resistance in the coronary vessels is minimal. In the presence of coronary artery disease, coronary artery perfusion pressure is the major determinent of coronary artery blood flow. An increase in the diastolic aortic pressure results in an increase in coronary artery perfusion pressure, coronary and collateral circulation, and myocardial oxygenation. This diastolic augmentation also assists in a more adequate perfusion of the zone of ischemia and the surrounding necrotic region (Durie, 1974).

As mentioned previously, myocardial hypoxia can be directly correlated with serum lactate levels. Studies by Mueller et al. (1971, 1974) have demonstrated that the IABP will result in decreases in serum lactate concentrations, thereby indicating an improved myocardial oxygen metabolism.

Balloon deflation during ventricular systole decreases systolic outflow resistance, which is demonstrated by a decreased systolic aortic pressure (Eckhardt, 1977). For left

---

Factors that affect diastolic pressure augmentation

Position of the intra-aortic balloon
Volume displacement
Occlusivity (ratio of balloon and aortic diameter)
Driving gas
Timing of inflation and deflation cycle

---

ventricular ejection to occur, there must be a build up of intraventricular pressure that exceeds the aortic pressure. This excess in pressure enables the aortic valve to open and blood to flow into the central aorta. This resistance to the left ventricular ejection is referred to as afterload. Therefore as the afterload is elevated, the intraventricular pressure must elevate to a point where it exceeds the pressure in the aorta, which further increases left ventricular workload. Decreases in afterload lead to a decreased ventricular workload and myocardial oxygen consumption. Furthermore, a decreased afterload promotes more efficient emptying of the left ventricle, which in turn increases stroke volume and cardiac output. This decrease in left ventricular workload and myocardial oxygen consumption also assists in salvaging the ischemic myocardium.

Eckhardt (1977) has identified those factors related to the intraaortic balloon that affect the degree of diastolic pressure augmentation and systolic pressure reduction. The intraaortic balloon should be placed immediately distal to the left subclavian artery and descending thoracic aorta, but it should not impinge on the renal arteries (Fig. 8-3). This could result in renal ischemia and renal failure.

As volume displacement and occlusivity increase, further diastolic pressure augmentation and systolic pressure reduction have been observed. It has been recommended that optimal occlusivity should be 90% to 95% to decrease the risk of aortic wall damage and destruction of red blood cells (Weber and Janicki, 1974).

Review of practices has shown that helium and carbon dioxide may be used as the driving gas. The driving gas is the substance that is used to inflate the balloon when it is in proper position. However, carbon dioxide, which may have a delayed filling and emptying time, may be safer to use. In the event of a gas leak, carbon dioxide will readily dissolve in the blood with no ill effects (Eckhardt, 1977).

For optimal hemodynamic effectiveness, exact timing of the balloon inflation during ventricular diastole and deflation during ventricular systole is essential (Fig. 8-4). One method of ensuring this proper timing is by computer control, which automatically adjusts counterpulsation with changes in the heart rate (Eckhardt, 1977).

Studies have demonstrated that demodynamic effects of decreased PCWP, decreased PAD pressure, and increased cardiac index begin within 12 hours after the initiation of IABP, and the peak hemodynamic effect occurs from 24 to 48 hours after

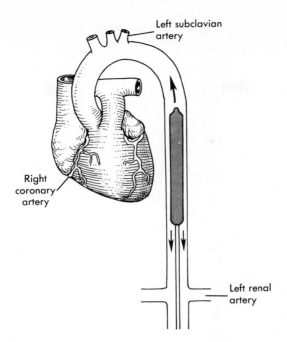

Fig. 8-3. Intraaortic balloon in place, distal to left subclavian artery and proximal to renal arteries. (From Frazee, S., and Nail, L.: Heart & Lung **2:**526-532, 1973.)

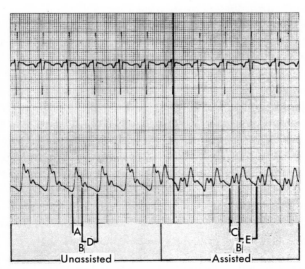

Fig. 8-4. *A,* Period of ventricular systole, and *D,* period of ventricular diastole without intraaortic balloon counterpulsation. *B,* Dicrotic notch. *C,* Balloon deflation decreasing systolic outflow resistance reflected by reduction in systolic pressure. *E,* Balloon inflation augmenting diastolic pressure with intraaortic balloon counterpulsation. (From Eckhardt, E.: Heart & Lung **6:**93-98, 1977.)

initiation (Ehrich, Biddle, Kronenberg, and Yu, 1977; and Bardet et al., 1977). After 48 hours of IABP, there appears to be a decline in left ventricular function and an increased PCWP.

Patients undergoing IABP need expert nursing care to meet their physical and emotional needs. During IABP the patient's mobility is greatly decreased. Because of this immobility virtually every system within the body is at risk for complications. The respiratory system can have multiple risks associated with this syndrome. Frequently these patients are intubated and mechanically ventilated. Once intubation has occurred, there is an increased risk of pulmonary infections from the suction catheter and the ventilator itself. To decrease this risk, strict sterile technique for suctioning should be carried out, as well as appropriate cleansing of the ventilator and related respiratory equipment. Atelectasis is a potential in all of these patients because of the relative immobility imposed by the IABP. Although complete turning and elevation of the head of the bed may be contraindicated, the nurse should encourage the patient to cough and deep breathe to promote as much lung expansion as possible.

In the circulatory system there is the risk of thrombi formation. To avoid this hazard, the patients are heparinized so that their clotting times remain twice the normal baseline value. The nurse should continually assess for signs of impaired circulation such as changes in pulse strength, sensation, and skin color. In addition, passive range of joint motion of the lower extremities decreases the risk of venous stasis.

To correctly monitor fluid balance it is necessary to insert a Foley catheter. This of course predisposes the patient to urinary tract infections. The implementation of correct catheter care can decrease this risk. To determine if the nursing measures are effective in preventing urinary tract infections, frequent urine cultures should be obtained, and appropriate therapeutic measures taken for positive cultures.

The emotional needs of the patients and their families are multiple. The patient who is critically ill suffers from anxiety, but there is also the potential for sensory alterations such as deprivation and/or disorientation. Frequently orienting patients to their surroundings, personnel, and procedures will assist in decreasing some of these sensory problems. It may also be necessary to administer tranquilizers to the patient to assist in controlling anxiety. For patients who are intubated, alternative communication patterns need to be developed. The family may be very effective in the intrepretation of the patient's needs as well as in decreasing the patient's anxiety. Anticipation of the patient's needs will decrease the patient's agitation and frustration over the inability to speak.

The family of the patient in cardiogenic shock also experience anxiety. Their fears are greatly increased with the risk of impending death of their family member. This becomes more increased with the amount of life-support equipment around the bedside. Often clarifying the purpose of the equipment and the reason the patient is using this equipment will decrease the family's concern. Maintaining an open line of communication between the family and the health care team will also assist in decreasing anxiety.

Therapies such as vasodilators and the IABP decrease left ventricular workload. These two therapeutic measures may be used alone, but they are more frequently used in conjunction with one another. Specific nursing therapies are essential in monitoring the patients hemodynamic status and the response to treatment.

PROGNOSIS AND COMPLICATIONS

Through the use of sophisticated hemodynamic monitoring equipment and laboratory analysis, researchers have been able to identify some objective prognostic indicators for the patient in cardiogenic shock. Afifi et al. (1974) found the best prognostic indicators are stroke index, arterial blood lactate levels, and urinary output. Cardiogenic shock patients with a stroke index of 25 ml/beat or greater had a 75% survival. When the serum lactate levels were 2.99 mM/L or less there was an 85% survival. Finally, when the hourly urine output was greater than 56 ml/hour there was a 75% survival. In another study the research showed that cardiogenic shock patients who had a PCWP less than 15 to 20 mm Hg had the greater chance of survival (Verdouw, et al., 1975).

Measurement of the cardiac index may be a more reliable evaluative and prognostic indicator because the cardiac index presents a parameter that controls for variability in body mass. Bleifeld, Hanrath, Mathey, and Merx (1974) correlated the PCWP with the cardiac index and found that patients with pressures greater than 17 mm Hg and cardiac indexes less than $1.81/min/m^2$ had a 70% mortality from cardiogenic shock. In addition, mixed venous oxygen (Pvo_2) saturations are of proven prognostic value. The Pvo_2 saturation is a determination of tissue oxygenation. Cardiogenic shock patients with a Pvo_2 saturation below 55% have a high mortality rate.

Although these patients receive expert nursing and medical care, a high mortality rate and complications are still present. The obvious complication is irreversible pump failure. In this instance the patient is unable to maintain acceptable LVFP, PCWP, cardiac index, Pvo_2 and systemic arterial blood pressure without the presence of therapeutic agents that increase oxygen supply to the myocardium, increase cardiac output, and decrease left ventricular workload.

Because of the diminished cardiac output associated with cardiogenic shock, there can be multiple sytemic organ effects. Cardiogenic shock, a state of low cardiac output, if not identified early, can develop into a vicious cycle that ultimately increases myocardial hypoxia and ischemia, producing a decreased myocardial contractility. The therapeutic goals of increased oxygen supply to the myocardium, increased cardiac output, and decreased left ventricular workload all assist in disrupting the vicious cycle of cardiogenic shock.

PATIENT VIGNETTE

Cardiogenic shock following an acute myocardial infarction

Mr. Kline, a 46-year-old business executive was stricken at his office with crushing substernal chest pain. One hour following the onset of pain he was admitted to the coronary care unit (CCU). Routine blood chemistries including enzymes were drawn in the emergency room. His electrocardiogram (ECG) showed ST segment elevations in leads V_1, V_2, and V_3.

Upon arrival in the CCU his skin was pale, cool, and moist. His vital signs were blood pressure, 160/80; pulse, 96 (regular); and respirations, 16. An ECG rhythm strip displayed multifocal premature ventricular contractions (PVCs). Two 50 mg boluses of lidocaine were administered by intravenous push, and a 4 μg/min lidocaine infusion was piggybacked into the left subclavian intravenous of D_5W. A Venti-mask with 40% oxygen was in place. Admitting arterial blood gases (ABGs) were Pao_2, 86 mm Hg; $Paco_2$, 38 mm Hg; pH, 7.40; percent saturation, 90%. In addition Mr. Kline was catheterized with an indwelling Foley catheter, which immediately drained 150 ml of clear yellow urine.

Mr. Kline's primary nurse completed her baseline nursing assessment, initiated the routine acute myocardial infarction protocols, and oriented Mr. Kline and his family to the procedures and policies of the CCU. Following a brief visit between Mr. Kline and his family, the nurse instructed him to rest and requested that his family return to the waiting room.

During the next 90 minutes Mr. Kline experienced recurrence of chest pain and increased multifocal PVCs, and his skin became cooler, more moist, and a gray putty-like color. He was treated with 8 mg intravenous morphine sulfate, he was given a 50 mg bolus of lidocaine by intravenous push, and the oxygen given by Venti-mask was increased to 70%. The nurse increased the routine assessment from every 2 hours to every 30 to 60 minutes because she thought that Mr. Kline was at risk for developing cardiogenic shock.

Questions

1. What additional significant assessment findings would lead you to suspect impending cardiogenic shock?
   a. Hourly renal output less than 25 ml/hour
   b. Tachycardia
   c. Bounding radial pulse
   d. Agitation
   e. Decreased peripheral pulses

The nursing assessment identified the following significant findings:
   Heart rate, 120 and irregular with multifocal PVCs
   Blood pressure, 80 palpable
   Confused and difficult to arouse
   Urine output less than 15 ml/hr
   Skin cold, clammy, and pale
   Arterial blood gases: pH, 7.35; Pao_2, 60 mm Hg; $Paco_2$, 60 mm Hg; percent saturation, 65%

At this point a Swan-Ganz line was inserted. The initial readings included the following: PCWP, 14 mm Hg; cardiac output, 4.6 L/min; cardiac index, 2.0 L/min/m^2. In addition he was also intubated and eventually placed on 70% O_2 and 6 cm H_2O of PEEP to maintain his Pao_2 at 80 mm Hg, $Paco_2$ at 42 mm Hg, and pH at 7.38.

2. The patient was fluid challenged with two 100 ml boluses of D_5W. What is the rationale for the fluid challenge?

    a. To determine the response of the left ventricle to volume loading
    b. To determine the right ventricular response to volume loading
    c. To assess for any circulating fluid volume deficit

3. The fluid challenge should be abandoned if which of the following changes in hemodynamic values occurs?
    a. Increased PCWP
    b. Decreased PCWP
    c. Increased cardiac output/cardiac index
    d. Decreased cardiac output/cardiac index

It was determined that Mr. Kline was indeed normovolemic and his left ventricular function was declining. The following assessment parameters indicated that Mr. Kline was indeed in cardiogenic shock:

Decreased peripheral pulses
Moist, cool, skin
BP, 80 mm Hg palpable
Urinary output, less than 20 ml/hr
PCWP, 20 mm Hg
Cardiac index 2.0 L/min/m²
Level of consciousness decreased, patient lethargic
CPK, LDH, SGOT, unavailable at the time
ECG: Rate 120/min, greater than 6 multifocal PVCs per minute

4. In patients with cardiogenic shock it is important to decrease left ventricular workload because of:
    a. Increased efficiency of the myocardial contraction
    b. Decreased oxygen consumption
    c. Improved cardiac output/cardiac index
    d. Decreased risk for further ischemic episodes

Mr. Kline was placed on the IABP in order to decrease his left ventricular workload. After 24 hours, weaning from the IABP was begun and hemodynamic values were closely monitored. By the fourth day after the myocardial infarction Mr. Kline was off of the IABP, inotropic agents, and antiarrhythmics. He was carefully monitored for the next 4 days and then discharged to the progressive cardiac unit (PCU).

5. The nursing care for the patient undergoing IABP should include all of the following *except*:
    a. Prevention of the hazards of immobility
    b. Monitoring of arterial blood gases
    c. Assessment of synchronization of the balloon inflation cycle
    d. Monitoring of only the cardiac output/cardiac index
    e. Assessment of renal output
    f. Assessment of pulses in distal extremities
    g. Patient/family education
    h. Monitoring of balloon patency

Answers

1. a, b, d, and e. These are physiological adaptative mechanisms that compensate for diminished cardiac output. In the patient with suspected cardiogenic shock, the cardiac output is diminished because of the impaired contractility. This impairment was initiated by the ischemic episode resulting in a myocardial infarction. If you have difficulty with this concept, the section on pathophysiology and Fig. 8-1 may be of assistance to you.

2. a and b. Persistent hypotension in cardiogenic shock can be secondary to hypovolemia. The fluid challenge is undertaken to determine the response of the left ventricle to volume loading. In the presence of a normal left ventricular filling pressure an appropriate increase in stroke volume and cardiac output should result. This is based on Starling's law of the heart. It is important to evaluate this in the cardiogenic shock patient, rather than blindly administering inotropic agents.

3. a and d. Elevations in PCWP without increases in cardiac output/cardiac index indicate that the persistent hypotension is not caused by hypovolemia. The fluid challenge should then be discontinued so that the workload of the left ventricle is not increased, which would increase the risk for new ischemic episodes.

4. a, b, c, and d. All of these can be affected if the left ventricular workload is increased. Unloading of the left ventricle can improve myocardial contractility, which in turn decreases myocardial oxygen consumption and the risk of new ischemic episodes.

5. d. It is incorrect to monitor only the cardiac output/cardiac index in a patient with cardiogenic shock who is undergoing IABP. The nurse must be aware of the total hemodynamic and oxygenation status of the patient. Since the objective of this treatment modality is to decrease left ventricle afterload, the nurse must assess left ventricular functioning, i.e., pulmonary artery pressures: PAD, PAM, PAS, PCW. If you have difficulty understanding the nursing care for this patient, the section on Intra-aortic balloon pump may be of assistance to you.

REFERENCES

Adams, C.W.: Recognition and evaluation of cardiogenic shock, Heart & Lung **2**:893-895, 1973.

Afifi, A.A., et al.: Prognostic indexes in acute myocardial infarction complicated by shock, American Journal of Cardiology **33**:826-832, 1974.

Bardet, J., et al.: Clinical and hemodynamic results of intraaortic balloon counterpulsation and surgery for cardiogenic shock, American Heart Journal **93**: 280-288, 1977.

Bleifeld, W., Hanrath, P., Mathey, D., and Merx, W.: Acute myocardial infarction V: left and right ventricular haemodynamics in caridogenic shock, British Heart Journal **36**:922-934, 1974.

Bregman, D.: Management of patients undergoing intra-aortic balloon pumping, Heart & Lung **3**:916-927, 1974.

Cohn, J.: Unloading the failing heart. In Fishman, A., editor: Heart failure, New York, 1978, Hemisphere Publishing Corp.

Collier, S.: Cardiogenic shock: principles and management. In Current practice in critical care, vol. 1, St. Louis, 1979, The C.V. Mosby Co.

Crexells, C., et al.: Optimal level of filling pressure in the left side of the heart in acute myocardial infarction, New England Journal of Medicine **289**: 1263-1266, 1973.

da Luz, P.L., et al.: Objective index of hemodynamic status for quantitation of severity and prognosis of shock complicating myocardial infarction. American Journal of Cardiology, **19:**258-263, 1972.

da Luz, P.L., Weil, M.H., Liu, V.Y., and Shubin, H.: Plasma volume prior to and following volume loading during shock complicating acute myocardial infarction, Circulation **49:**98-105, 1974.

da Luz, P.L., Weil, M.H., and Shubin, H.: Current concepts on mechanisms and treatment of cardiogenic shock, American Heart Journal **92:**103-113, 1976.

Durie, M.: Use of an intra-aortic balloon pump following postoperative pump failure and cardiac arrest: case presentation, Heart & Lung **3:**971-976, 1974.

Eckhardt, E.: Intra-aortic balloon counterpulsation in cardiogenic shock, Heart & Lung **6:**93-98, 1977.

Ehrich, D.A., Biddle, T.L., Kronenberg, M.W., and Yu, P.N.: The hemodynamic response to intraaortic balloon counterpulsation in patients with cardiogenic shock complicating acute myocardial infarction, American Heart Journal **93:**274-279, 1977.

Foster, S.B., and Conty, K.A.: Pump failure following myocardial infarction: an overview, Heart & Lung **9:**293-297, 1980.

Frazee, S., and Nail, L.: New challenge in cardiac nursing: the intra-aortic balloon, Heart & Lung **2:**526-532, 1973.

Giles, T.: Principles of vasodilator therapy for left ventricular congestive heart failure, Heart & Lung 1980, **9:**271-276, 1980.

Goodman, L.S., and Gilman, A.: The pharmacological basis of therapeutics, ed. 6, New York, 1980, Macmillan Publishing Co., Inc.

Jackson, G., Cullum, P., Pastellopoulos, A.M., and Jewitt, D.: Intra-aortic balloon assistance in cardiogenic shock after acute myocardial infarction or cardiac surgery, British Heart Journal **39:**598-604, 1977.

Moskowitz, L.: Vasodilator therapy in acute myocardial infarction, Heart & Lung **4:**939-945, 1975.

Mueller, H., Ayers, S.M., and Conklin, E.F.: The effects of intra-aortic counterpulsation on cardiac performance and metabolism in shock associated with acute myocardial infarction, Journal of Clinical Investigation **50:**1885, 1971.

Mueller, H., Giannelli, S., and Ayers, S.M.: Mechanical cardiac assistance in shock following acute myocardial infarction. In Gunnar, G.M., Loeb, M.S., and Rahimroola, S.H., editors: Shock in myocardial infarction, New York, 1974, Grune & Stratton, Inc.

Mueller, H., Evans, R., and Ayers, S.: Effect of dopamine on hemodynamics and myocardial infarction in man, Circulation **57:**361-365, 1978.

O'Rourke, M.: Cardiogenic shock following myocardial infarction, Heart & Lung **3:**252-257, 1974.

Price, S.A., and Wilson, L.M.: Pathophysiology clinical concepts of disease processes, New York, 1978, McGraw-Hill Book Co.

Robie, N.W., and Goldberg, L.I.: Comparative systemic and regional hemodynamic effects of dopamine and dobutamine, American Heart Journal **90:**340-345, 1975.

Rubin, M.B.: Nursing care for the myocardial infarction, St. Louis, 1977, Warren H. Green, Inc.

Russell, R.O., Racklye, C.E., and Pombo, J.: Effects of increasing left ventricular filling pressures in patients with acute myocardial infarction, Journal of Clinical Investigation **49:**1539, 1970.

Sonnenblick, E.H., Frishman, W.H., and LeJemtel, T.H.: Dobutamine: a new synthetic cardioactive sympatheticamine, The New England Journal of Medicine **300:**17-22, 1979.

Swan, H.J.C., et al.: Hemodynamic spectrum of myocardial infarction and cardiogenic shock, Circulation **45:**1097-1110, 1972.

Verdouw, P.D., et al.: Short-term survival after acute myocardial infarction predicted by hemodynamic parameters, Circulation **52:**413-419, 1975.

Weber, K.T., and Janicki, J.S.: Intraaortic balloon counterpulsation: a review of physiological principles, clinical results, and device safety, Annals of Thoracic Surgery **17:**603, 1974.

Whitman, G.: Intra-aortic balloon pumping and cardiac mechanics: a programmed lesson, Heart & Lung **7:**1034-1050, 1978.

Ziesche, S., and Franciosa, J.A.: Clinical application of sodium nitroprusside, Heart & Lung **6:**99-103, 1977.

9 Septic shock

ANGELA SMITH-COLLINS

Septic shock is a series of insults to the cell following circulatory failure and the interaction between an infecting microorganism and the immune system. Patients in the care of most areas of medical and nursing practice may develop septic shock. One percent of all patients admitted to general hospitals develop bacteremia. Septic shock, an outgrowth of bacteremia, has a mortality of 30% to 50% (McCabe, 1973). The frequency and high mortality indicate that further study and research are needed, but in spite of many efforts the progress toward the development of a lifesaving treatment protocol has been slow.

A variety of microorganisms can initiate septic shock. Bacteria, primarily gram-negative but also gram-positive, are the most common. Rare cases of septic shock have been linked to viruses, fungi, and yeast. Bacteremia occurs after a viable microorganism multiplies in the bloodstream. The microorganisms enter the bloodstream from lymphatic drainage or direct involvement of a small blood vessel in an area of local infection. Contaminated instruments or fluids such as intravenous infusions that come in contact with the blood also provide an entry for microorganisms. Approximately 40% of patients with bacteremia develop some degree of circulatory compromise (Eskridge, 1980).

HOST-AGENT RELATIONSHIP

The sequence and severity of septic shock vary. They are dependent on the microorganism and the patient's preexisting disease state. Currently less toxic antimicrobials are more effective in the control of gram-positive than gram-negative bacteria. There are at present no widespread pharmacological therapies to combat viruses. Jackson (1976) reports that the principal determinant of septic shock outcome is the underlying disease. He categorized patients' preexisting disease into three groups: rapidly fatal, ultimately fatal, and nonfatal. The rapidly fatal group included patients with acute leukemia, extensive burns, and aplastic anemia. These patients had a 76% mortality from septic shock. The ultimately fatal group included local neoplasm, renal failure, and systemic lupus erythematosus. These patients had a mortality of 46% from septic shock. The last group included all other conditions and had a mortality of 17%. All of these patient populations had gram-negative septic shock.

Infections that develop into septic shock commonly originate from primary sites within the urinary tract, the respiratory tract, the gastrointestinal tract, and the blood. The urinary tract provides bacteria both a culture medium and access to the highly vascular renal tissue. Organism species most commonly found in the urinary tract are the

172

gram-negative bacteria: *Escherichia coli, Klebsiella-Enterobacter-Serratia* (KES), and *Pseudomonas aeruginosa.* Urinary tract infections are often secondary to urinary catheterization and urinary retention.

A second primary site for infection leading to septic shock is the respiratory tract. The respiratory tract has many of the requirements needed by microorganisms for reproduction. It is a warm, dark, and moist environment. In addition it has the unique property of being the only organ directly exposed to air. Gram-negative organisms commonly causing bacteremia from the respiratory tract are *Escherichia coli* and *Pseudomonas.* Pneumococci are the most common gram-positive bacteria leading to sepsis from the respiratory tract.

The gastrointestinal tract normally contains multiple microorganisms. Surgery, abscesses, or perforations of the gut can provide access for these organisms into the blood. *Bacteroides, Escherichia coli,* KES, and *Salmonella* are the most common organisms from the gastrointestinal tract causing bacteremia (Eskridge, 1980).

The blood can also serve as a primary site for septic shock. The debilitated patient with multiple intravenous or hemodynamic monitoring catheters in place is at risk for sepsis and potential shock. In this case it is perhaps best to institute preventive measures to decrease the risk. Common preventive measures include sterile dressing changes at the catheter insertion site, application of antibiotic ointment over the puncture site, and daily changing of intravenous fluids and tubings.

Populations at risk

There are certain predisposing factors that increase the risk of septic shock. These factors can be grouped into two classifications, those that compromise immunity and those that are caused by invasive procedures. The presence of chronic disease, bone marrow suppression, or stress affects the body's immunological response, therefore increasing the risk for septic shock.

It is important that the nurse be aware of how factors that compromise immunity and invasive procedures increase the risk of septic shock development. This knowledge assists the nurse in early assessment and identification of those patients with the highest risk for septic shock.

There are also particular patient groups in whom bacteremia is more prone to progress into septic shock. Men over 65 are most likely to develop septic shock. Shubin and Weil (1976) believe that the higher incidence in men is related to their tendency to have urinary tract infections when benign prostatic hypertrophy (BPH) is present. Patients with urological disorders are thought to be the patients most at risk to develop septic shock. Neonates and pregnant women also seem more likely to develop septic shock.

Defenses against bacteremia

Transient bacteremia is a common occurrence in daily life. For example, vigorous toothbrushing causes small numbers of microorganisms to enter the bloodstream. These

---

Predisposing factors to septic shock

Compromising immunity

Age (very young or elderly)
Steroids or chemotherapy
Leukopenia
Burns
Chronic diseases (diabetes)
Stress
Nonsteroid anti-inflammatory drugs
Alcoholism
Liver disease
Bone marrow suppression
Dysfunctional spleen

Invasive procedures

Pacemaker insertion
Blood transfusion
Parenteral therapy
Catheters
Tracheostomies
Abortion
Incision and drainage procedures
Drug abuse
Hyperalimentation
Surgery: Gastrointestinal tract, genitourinary tract,
    respiratory tract, reticuloendothelial system

---

bacteria are removed by the efficient work of the reticuloendothelial system (RES). In the RES are fixed macrophages that are lined up along the lymph nodes all over the body. These macrophages remove the bacteria by ingesting them, thus freeing the blood from contamination. This system is so effective that bacteria experimentally administered in high numbers have been removed from the bloodstream in a few hours (Price and Wilson, 1978).

Another protective mechanism against bacteremia from local infection sites is the inflammatory process. The inflammatory process occurs when cells are traumatized by bacterial or other causes. The arterioles supplying the area become dilated, increasing the blood volume in the microcirculation. The increased blood flow delivers the defense components present in the blood to that area. These components, complement, immuno-globins, and white blood cells, work together to remove necrotic tissue and/or infectious

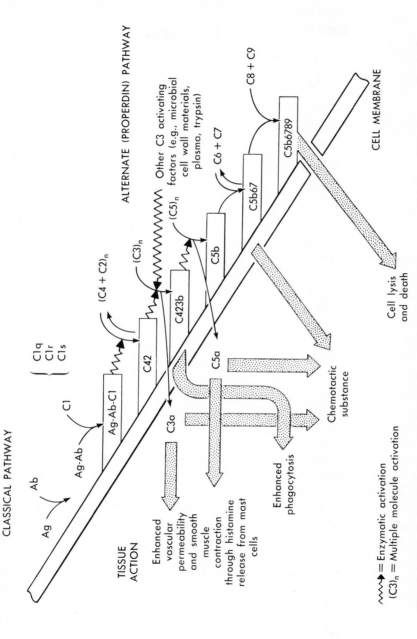

Fig. 9-1. Classical and alternate complement cascade. Sequence of complement activation generates multiple biologically active intermediate molecules, which are active in inflammatory response. (From Phipps, W.J., Long, B.C., and Woods, N.F.: Medical surgical nursing: concepts and clinical practice, St. Louis, 1979, The C.V. Mosby Co.)

agents. Another event at the microcirculatory level in inflammation is that the capillary pores become larger and more permeable to the passage of protein and fluid resulting in edema. This fluid shift dilutes the toxic substances and assists in bringing the defensive components to the inflammation site (Price and Wilson, 1978).

The normal role of complement

Currently 15 complement proteins in the blood have been identified. Complement plays a crucial role in the normal immune response. Complement proteins are inactive until stimulated by a chemical chain of events called the classic pathway of complement stimulation. Another pathway of activation is the alternate, or properdin, pathway. These pathway reactions are also referred to as cascade reactions. A cascade reaction occurs when one activated protein causes the next protein to become active. The pathway proteins are links stimulating the next reaction.

The activation of the complement system can occur in many ways. The most common is the activation of C1 by an antigen-antibody interaction. Other substances that can activate the complement cascade are the Hageman blood clotting factor, plasmin (a clot lysis enzyme), and bacterial endotoxins.

Significant biological activities occur in response to complement activation. The primary response is the selective destruction of cell membranes. Other activities are histamine release, enhanced phagocytosis (white blood cell ingestion of foreign protein), and chemotactic substance formation. Chemotactic substances cause white blood cells to aggregate at an inflammation site (Fig. 9-1).

PATHOPHYSIOLOGY

When bacteremia progresses to septic shock, the body's protective mechanisms are overpowered. This is usually caused by one or more of three factors: immune suppression, overwhelming numbers of microorganisms, or bacteria that are resistant to immune system activity.

Septic shock is characterized by unique pathophysiological features that have their basis in the interaction between the host and the microorganism. However, even though some of the features of septic shock are different, the net result, as with all other types of shock, is decreased tissue perfusion.

Septic shock progresses through three stages. The initial stage is a hyperdynamic cardiovascular and metabolic state frequently termed warm shock. The patient has the following characteristics: high cardiac output, peripheral vasodilation, skin flushing, high renal output, hyperthermia, and respiratory alkalosis. The length of this first stage varies from 30 minutes to 16 hours (Forgacs, 1979). Because the hyperdynamic state or warm shock has an atypical presentation of symptoms, it may remain undiagnosed until signs of deterioration appear.

This clinical deterioration indicates the middle stage of septic shock in which the cardiovascular status changes to a normodynamic pattern (Zschoche, 1981). Although the heart rate remains elevated, blood pressure and cardiac output are reduced. Renal output is reduced and complete renal failure may ensue. Vasodilation persists and the peripheral vascular resistance is below normal. This stage of septic shock has a brief duration and, if the patient is untreated or does not respond to therapy, progression to the final, preterminal stage follows.

This final stage is manifested by a hypodynamic state with diminished cardiac output, vasoconstriction, blood shunting, and poor tissue perfusion. This stage closely resembles other types of shock. If the patient fails to respond to treatment, decompensation continues until death.

The basis for the characteristics of these three stages is the presence of an infectious agent that produces a host-agent relationship. Gram-negative bacterial shock is the most common type of septic shock. It produces a variety of unique effects on the body that are attributed to the effects of endotoxin. Endotoxin is a part of the cell wall of many gram-negative bacteria and is released into the blood when these bacteria are destroyed. It is a lipopolysaccharide-protein complex. Some species have different chemical components in a particular type of endotoxin. Reasons for variations in the degree and severity of the body's reaction to endotoxin are not fully understood.

When the immune system begins to destroy gram-negative bacteria in the microcirculation, high levels of endotoxin result. Endotoxin interferes with the cellular mitochondria and causes the cell to reduce its energy production and decrease its oxygen requirements. The cellular pathways for metabolism are also disrupted. This primary insult to the cell makes the patient's recovery difficult. Indirectly endotoxin can produce cellular hypoxia, which causes an energy deficit that stops the active transport system of the cell. Active transport is used for bringing glucose, amino acids, and fatty acids into the cell and for maintaining the sodium and potassium pump (Gelin et al., 1980).

Endotoxin and the immune system

Inflammation occurs systematically in response to bacterial overgrowth. This is thought to occur because gram-negative bacteria activate the complement system. Complement in turn causes additional bacterial destruction with the release of more endotoxin. The levels of complement drop at the onset of septic shock because they are consumed in the defensive process. The net result of the generalized overstimulation of complement is vasodilation and change in capillary permeability. Complement, specifically C3a and C5a, causes the mast cells of the body to release histamine and bradykinin. These chemical substances result in vasodilation and increased capillary permeability in the microcirculation. The resultant widened capillary pores allow protein and fluid to move from the capillaries to the interstitial space (Fig. 9-2), which causes blood to pool in the microcirculation (Fearon, Ruddy, and Schur, 1975).

Physical findings are related to the systemic responses of the immune system. An elevated temperature, caused by the release of endogenous pyrogens by the neutrophils and macrophages, is often the first sign of septic shock and is accompanied by

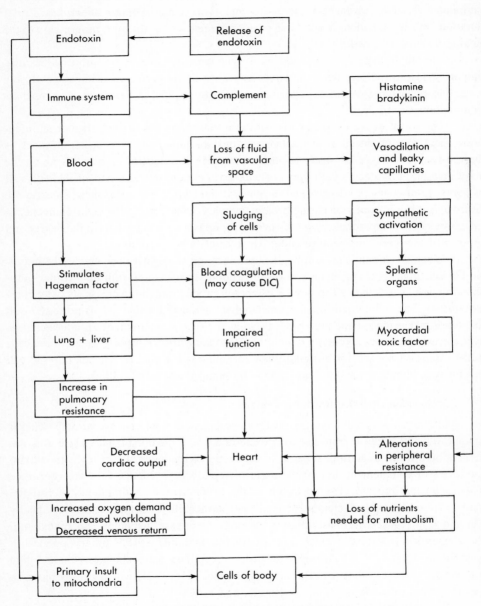

Fig. 9-2. Effects of endotoxin in gram-negative septic shock.

warm and reddened extremities. Endogenous pyrogens communicate to the hypothalamus to increase the body's temperature. Other nonspecific signs and symptoms are malaise, anorexia, weakness, irritability, mental confusion, lethargy, and abdominal cramps. These symptoms are associated with actions of the immune system, although their cause is unknown.

Effects of the blood

Because the fluid elements of the blood are leaving the capillaries, the cellular components are left in a higher concentration in the vessels. The blood has a higher viscosity causing sluggish blood flow and coagulation. Endotoxin also causes endothelial damage by directly activating the Hageman coagulation factor, which can set the stage for the development of disseminated intravascular coagulation (DIC) (Chapter 13). In addition to stimulating the clotting mechanism, the Hageman factor converts kallikreinogen to kallikrein and bradykinin. These substances further increase capillary permeability, thus lowering peripheral vascular resistance.

Effects of endotoxin on the lung, liver and heart

The lung, liver, and heart have alterations caused by endotoxin in septic shock. The lungs become less compliant and more difficult to inflate. The pulmonary vascular resistance is increased, adding additional workload to the right heart. The changes in resistance and compliance have been traced to microembolization of platelets and leukocyte fragments (Gelin et al., 1980). These fragments also trigger the cycle of complement, which stimulates the release of vasoactive substances such as histamine. The resultant change in vascular permeability causes fluid to shift from the capillaries to the alveoli, precipitating ARDS. The respiratory rate increases early in septic shock and usually continues throughout the shock state. This is thought to be a means of compensation not only for metabolic acidosis but also for impaired oxygen diffusion (Gelin et al., 1980).

In septic shock the liver's normal filtering and detoxifying functions are altered. This is partly attributed to white cell microembolism and platelet aggregation. The liver also increases in weight because of fluid accumulation. Liver dysfunction is more pronounced in patients with abdominal infections.

Endotoxin in the initial phase of septic shock indirectly affects cardiac functioning. The increase in cardiac output is caused by beta-adrenergic (sympathetic) stimulation that occurs in response to volume and pressure loss in the vascular bed. This sympathetic activation causes the heart to increase cardiac output within physiological limits. The cardiac output is elevated by increasing the heart rate and force of contraction. Sympathetic stimulation of the heart can precipitate arrhythmias in the diseased heart by increasing myocardial oxygen consumption.

Late in septic shock there is a substance released from the ischemic splanchnic organs called myocardial toxic factor (MTF). This factor is thought to be a byproduct of the enzymes released when the pancreatic cells become necrotic. It is released into the circulation and carried to the heart. MTF is a negative inotropic agent. It profoundly impairs the heart's ability to contract by interfering with calcium ions. this substance directly compromises the ability of the heart to meet the body's oxygen needs (Guyton, 1981).

Endocrine response

Hormone levels are altered in patients experiencing an infectious process. All known hormones are secreted in larger amounts except insulin and thyrotropin (Wilson, 1976b). The response of the body to these hormones is to increase the availability of metabolic fuels. However, in septic shock perfusion is erratic and the message of the hormones may not reach the target organs. On the other hand, higher levels of serum triglycerides and phospholipids are seen in gram-negative septic shock (Gallin, 1969). This is thought to be caused by hormonal stimulation. The lowered insulin level would maintain a higher serum level of glucose, but the insulin-dependent cells would not be able to utilize the glucose. Hormones such as norepinephrine would also provide a vaso-constrictive response, thereby helping the body to maintain blood perfusion.

The net result of the interaction of endotoxin and the body systems is that hemo-dynamics are altered by the change in total peripheral resistance and capillary perme-ability. Fluid is lost into the third space from the vascular bed. Tachypnea and fever also contribute to the fluid loss. Renal, metabolic, myocardial, endocrine, coagulative, hepatic, and pulmonary systems are impaired causing the cell to receive a primary insult to metabolism from endotoxin and a secondary insult related to inadequate oxygenation and nutritional support.

Gram-positive shock

The specific changes seen with endotoxin are not present in gram-positive shock (Weil, Shubin, and Nishijima, 1976). Gram-positive organisms and viral infections are thought to trigger septic shock by effecting the following changes. The interaction be-tween the microorganisms and the inflammatory response causes two responses; vaso-dilation and increased vascular permeability. Generalized vasodilation lowers total peripheral resistance. To compensate for the lowered total peripheral resistance the heart must increase its output. If the heart is unable to do this, the blood pressure drops and the cells become anoxic. The increased vascular permeability causes protein and fluid shift from the capillaries into the interstitial spaces. Because the circulatory volume is sequestered in this space venous return to the heart is reduced, reducing cardiac out-put. Therefore if the body does not compensate, a vicious cycle of fluid and pressure loss occurs (Fig. 9-3). An increased incidence of gram-positive septic shock has been found in children and adults who have a dysfunctional or absent spleen. The spleen is the site of production of some opsonins (Fidler, 1981). Opsonins are chemicals that coat the outer surface of gram-positive bacteria. This coating speeds up phagocytosis of gram-positive bacteria. Therefore persons who have diminished levels of opsonins have difficulty com-

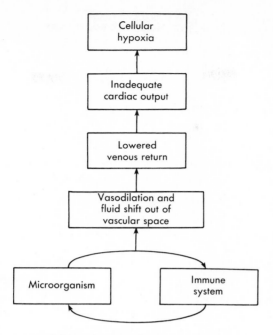

Fig. 9-3. Gram-positive septic shock.

batting this type of microorganism. This is the reason that removal of the spleen, in children particularly, is thought to compromise immune system function.

CLINICAL PICTURE

The clinical presentation of septic shock has no universal pattern of signs and symptoms. This makes septic shock difficult to diagnose because most of the signs and symptoms are nonspecific. However, even if a nonspecific sign such as restlessness appears in a patient at risk, treatment is often started. Unless septic shock can be specifically ruled out there is grave danger in delaying treatment. The signs and symptoms are varied. Any assortment of these cues may signal the onset of septic shock. If septic shock is not diagnosed until overt symptoms of circulatory failure occur, the mortality is greatly increased.

The diagnosis of septic shock is confirmed by microbiological data usually obtained from two sets of blood cultures drawn from different puncture sites as well as cultures of urine, sputum, and vaginal secretions. However, the first reports from cultures are only obtained in 24 hours and treatment must be instituted before that time. Other laboratory tests may include chest x-ray films, arterial gases, and serum electrolytes. All of these tests provide current information about the patient but cannot immediately confirm the presence of septic shock.

Signs and symptoms associated with septic shock

Mental
  Restlessness
  Irritability
  Memory alterations, confusion
  Lethargy
Respiratory
  Tachypnea
  Increased pulmonary resistance
  Greater depth of respirations
Cardiovascular
  Tachycardia
  Altered hemodynamic values
  Decreased preload and arterial
    blood pressure
  Arrhythmias

Renal
  Polyuria*
  Oliguria
Metabolic
  Hypothermia
  Hyperthermia
  Chills
  Malaise
  Respiratory alkalosis*
Gastrointestinal
  Nausea
  Vomiting
  Gastric bleeding
  Distention

*During early stage of septic shock.

MEDICAL THERAPY

The primary goals of the physician in ordering treatment are to eradicate the causative organism and to support vital life functions that are compromised by circulatory failure (Eskridge, 1980). Currently there are three types of intervention directed toward identifying, localizing, and controlling the microorganisms. First, the physician may surgically intervene. Surgery is indicated when sepsis is thought to be secondary to an abscess or retained fetal parts. Incision and drainage promote the resolution of the abscess and a reduction in the number of circulating organisms. In septic abortion the uterus must be scraped to ensure that all fetal and placental parts are removed.

Second, the source of contaminative organisms may be removed. Before invasive lines are removed the health team must consider whether an additional line needs to be inserted with added risk to the patient, the duration of line insertion at this site, and whether the line is the probable site of infection. These considerations are of particular importance with pacemaker wires and hemodynamic monitoring catheters.

Third, antimicrobial drugs are prescribed. This is the most common medical intervention. Treatment is most efficacious if the organism and orginating site are known. In cases of septic shock the route of drug administration is most commonly intravenous.

Antimicrobials

Four clinical variables of presentation are considered when ordering antimicrobials. First, the patient may already be taking some type of antimicrobial agent. In this case the dosage and type of agent will be changed dependent on the microbiology reports and the patient's response to pharmacological therapy (Eskridge, 1980). A second clinical situation may be that the source of the microorganisms is located but the organism is not isolated. In this case the broad-spectrum antibiotics effective against both the gram-negative and gram-positive microorganisms are ordered. Knowing the site is helpful, however, because certain bacteria tend to cause infection in particular sites. For example, since *Escherichia coli* causes most infections from the urinary tract, an agent particularly effective against *Escherichia coli* would be ordered.

The third clinical situation is when the organism is identified. In this case antimicrobial therapy will be chosen on the basis of the sensitivity of the microorganism. This situation is ideal because the pharmacological agent can be ordered specifically for a certain microorganism.

The fourth clinical situation is when both the organism and the site of infection are unknown. In this situation, an infectious disease consultation may be obtained and broad-spectrum antimicrobials will be ordered. Two or three antimicrobials may be utilized together to control the unknown organism (Eskridge, 1980).

Fluid therapy

The medical literature advocates fluid replacement as the most common therapy for supporting vital functions in septic shock. Hypovolemia occurs in septic shock as a result of vasodilation and fluid shift into the third space. Fluids are also lost through increased respiratory rate, fever, sweating, and drainage. In addition, the capillaries are more permeable so that even infused fluids tend to leave the vessels. One of the most prevalent findings in septic shock is a diminished preload as evidenced by low CVP.

Although most sources agree that fluid replacement is needed in septic shock, there is disagreement on which fluid to use. There are primarily two types of fluids, colloids and crystalloids. Colloids are osmotic agents such as human albumin, plasma protein fractions, and dextran. Crystalloid fluids are Ringer's lactate and normal saline (Robinson, 1980). Both types of fluid can help restore intravascular volumes, but crystalloids are more widely utilized because of their lower cost.

Fluid replacement proceeds at a varying rate dependent on the patient's response. The ability of the heart and kidneys to handle the work of increased volume must be assessed. CVP and PCWP are monitored frequently and used as a guide for replacement.

Shubin, Weil, and Carlson (1977), some of the foremost authorities in shock, advocate a 7/3 rule for fluid replacement. They give fluid challenges of 5 to 20 ml/min for 10 minutes. If the PCWP or PAD pressure reading is elevated more than 7 mm Hg above beginning level, the infusion is stopped. However, if the PCWP or PAD pressure rises only to 3 mm Hg above the starting point or decreases, another fluid challenge is given. Because these increments are small, they decrease the risk of fluid overload and further cardiac decompensation.

The physician may order blood components if hemodilution is excessive or if a complication causing blood loss occurs. When whole blood is lost, because of a stress ulcer for example, blood should be replaced. Hemoglobin and hematocrit levels are monitored frequently and serve as a guide. Packed cells are sometimes ordered to improve arterial oxygen transport. Blood that is stored, however, has diminished ability to transport oxygen because of decreased levels of 2,3-DPG. This substance is vital to hemoglobin and oxygen affinity; therefore fresh blood should be used when it is available. DIC or occult bleeding should be suspected when the hematocrit is drastically decreased.

Some institutions use special types of fluid infusions such as glucose, potassium, and insulin (GKI). Because these nutrients are needed intracellularly, their administration should theoretically assist cellular metabolism, but there are no widespread clinical trials of GKI in septic shock at this time. Additional therapies may include specific nutritional support.

Sympathomimetic agents

Vital hemodynamic functions can be impaired by septic shock. To improve the patient's hemodynamic state sympathomimetic agents may be ordered that can improve cardiac output and arterial pressures. There is controversy, however, about the benefit of these agents. Inappropriate use may increase the degree of tissue ischemia. It may also be difficult to determine when such drugs should be used. They may be ordered at the onset of septic shock or only when other therapies fail. Currently there is no conclusive evidence that survival rates are improved by the use of these drugs.

Sympathomimetic drugs work on the alpha-receptors and beta-receptors of the sympathetic nervous system. These drugs magnify the stimulus to certain tissues. Alpha-receptors are located in the smooth muscle of the vascular bed and increase peripheral resistance and venous return. Beta$_1$-receptors are found primarily in the myocardium. Beta$_2$-receptors are located in the muscular lining of the lungs (Plachetka, 1980).

Currently most of the sympathomimetic drugs work by stimulating both alpha sites and beta sites. In theory if the problem in early septic shock is lowered peripheral resistance, a potent alpha agent that causes vasoconstriction would be helpful. The difficulty in using alpha agents is that they would be most effective in early septic shock. The problem is that early septic shock is often not diagnosed in the hyperdynamic (early) stage. Drugs that primarily increase alpha stimulation are less effective in late septic shock. The problem with excessive alpha stimulation in late septic shock is that arterial blood shunting can occur, particularly when the drug is given either at high doses or over a long period of time. This peripheral clamping off of arterioles causes further tissue hypoxia and necrosis. Examples of sympathomimetic alpha agents are methoxamine, phenylephrine, and epinephrine.

The most commonly recommended agents in septic shock are dopamine and dobutamine. Dopamine is a mixed alpha-receptor and beta-receptor stimulator. In therapeutic levels it increases arterial resistance and elevates blood pressure. It also stimulates dopaminergic receptors that increase renal, splanchnic, and mesenteric perfusion. Dopamine can stimulate the body's release of epinephrine, which can further increase cardiac output and peripheral resistance. However, when dopamine is given at high levels or over a prolonged period, it also causes significant tissue ischemia. Again the benefits and potential risks must be weighed.

Dobutamine is used to specifically improve cardiac output, although its use in septic shock is still minimal. Dobutamine acts on the beta-receptors of the sympathetic nervous system. At therapeutic levels it increases the force of contraction of the heart. There is some controversy because it is not known whether dobutamine also increases myocardial oxygen demand (Collins, 1980).

Steroids

There is a diversity of opinion about the use of steroids in septic shock; clinical research studies report conflicting results (Weitzman and Berger, 1974). However, Schumer (1976), in a well controlled human study, showed a decrease in mortality when steroids were used in conjunction with other methods such as fluid replacement and the administration of antimicrobials. Steroids have a variety of actions that may be beneficial in septic shock. Endotoxin causes intracellular hypoglycemia by inhibiting gluconeogenesis. Steroids at high doses seem to prevent this endotoxin action from occurring (Guglielmo, 1980). Steroids also stabilize lysosomal membranes that trigger cellular lysis (Weissmann and Thomas, 1962). Other important actions are reduction of lactic acid concentration and stabilization of the endothelial wall of the pulmonary microcirculation. There is currently a considerable amount of research concerning the use of steroids. Many important questions remain such as dosage, type of preparation, and frequency of administration. There are no definitive answers at present.

Other therapies

Other therapies for septic shock are directed toward the maintenance of vital body functions. For example, a mechanical ventilator may be used to support pulmonary functioning. Any body system can be affected, but systems most frequently compromised are the cardiac, renal, and pulmonary systems.

Future therapies will probably focus on the immune system and new pharmacological agents. Interferon and prostaglandins are agents involved in the immune response that are not fully understood. It is hoped that the more we learn about the immune response, the more we will be able to maximize its effectiveness. Pharmacological agents such as indomethacin, a prostaglandin inhibitor, are being studied (Eskridge, 1980). Nitroglycerin paste is also being used for late septic shock in some clinical settings (Cerra, Hassett, and Siegel, 1975).

NURSING MANAGEMENT

Nursing care of the patient with septic shock requires the utmost skill and competence. The needs of these patients are immense and immediate. The nurse as well as the patient may feel bombarded with the rapidly changing shock state. The high mortality rate also makes caring for the patient more vital and more emotionally draining.

Prevention

The first and one of the most important activities for the nurse is prevention. Septic shock can often be prevented by strict adherence to aseptic principles. This is particularly true of invasive procedures. Aseptic techniques must be utilized when inserting urinary and intravenous catheters and during routine daily care of such invasive catheters. The importance of aseptic techniques cannot be overstated.

Other aspects of prevention are activities that promote the immune response and the correct use of antibiotics. Nurses can promote immune system function by assuring that the patient has adequate nutritional support. Glucose is needed at particular levels for white blood cells to be produced. Nurses should also carefully monitor the progress of an infection. Sensitivity and culture reports should be reviewed when the patient is receiving antibiotics.

Early assessment

Nursing care should be focused on prompt identification of septic shock. Continuous assessment is a learned skill and is based on a knowledge of the multiple signs and symptoms of septic shock. Earlier in this chapter patients at high risk were identified. It is important that these patients be assessed carefully. If signs and symptoms of septic shock are identified early, treatment is much more effective.

Once septic shock is suspected, the nurse has a variety of responsibilities. Before the first dose of antibiotics is given, the nurse or physician will obtain specimens of all suspected sites of infection to be sent for microbiological examination. It is important to carefully label all specimens and to obtain the results as soon as possible. The nurse will also assist with the insertion of hemodynamic lines to improve the accuracy of patient monitoring. Again total system assessment is crucial. A flow sheet of patterns of vital sign measurements and laboratory values is helpful.

Circulatory integrity

Maintenance of circulatory volume and prevention of circulatory failure is a high priority. The nurse must administer the prescribed fluids at the appropriate rate, often titrating the fluid volumes using certain monitoring criteria. For example, the physician may order the fluids to be infused at a rate that will keep the systolic blood pressure at 90 mm Hg. Other clinical criteria observed and used as guides during rapid rate fluid infusion are CVP and/or PCWP, PAD pressure, urinary output, heart rate, blood pressure, respiratory rate, and the presence of pulmonary congestion or rales. Continuous monitoring may be necessary if the circulatory volume is labile. Maintenance of parenteral lines is also a nursing responsibility. A 16 to 18 gauge catheter should be used to accommodate the large amounts of fluids and perhaps whole blood administration.

Peripheral vasodilation occurring early in septic shock mandates the following

---

Points about sympathomimetic drugs

1. Administered by an infusion pump with close nursing supervision.
2. When first starting the infusion, record vital signs every 5 minutes 3 times and then every 30 minutes.
3. Check the compatibility of any medications injected in the parenteral line containing the medication.
4. Monitor the IV site frequently for signs of patency. Infiltration can cause tissue necrosis and may lead to the need for amputation. If infiltration occurs, remove immediately. In case of extravasation ischemia, phentolamine (Regitine), an adrenergic blocker, is often administered locally at the extravasation site. It causes local hyperemia and if given immediately it can overcome tissue anoxia.
5. Check urine output frequently. Some sympathemimetic drugs reduce arterial blood supply to the kidneys.
6. Monitor the therapeutic effects of the agent. Routinely record cardiac output, arterial pressure, level of consciousness, and arterial blood gas values.
7. Assess for signs and symptoms of increasing myocardial oxygen demand, such as chest pain, tachycardia, and arrhythmias.
8. Watch for excessive alpha stimulation of arterioles by assessing peripheral pulses manually and by utilizing a doppler device. This helps the nurse to know when cessation of arterial blood supply has occurred.
9. Assess the adequacy of drug dosage by patient weight, age, and renal and hepatic function. It is also important to note the individual's particular response to the dosage level.

---

interventions. First, swelling of body cavities and extremities is monitored to estimate the amount of third-space loss. Second, the patient's position is changed very carefully from lying to sitting. The effects of postural hypotension can be more pronounced with peripheral vasodilation. Third, the nurse should assess carefully for early signs of peripheral vasoconstriction. The nurse also administers prescribed sympathomimetic agents. These agents are used to improve circulatory pressures and cardiac output. The nurse should administer these agents with caution, using an infusion pump to ensure accurate dosage. Some facts to keep in mind when administering these agents are listed.

Antimicrobial administration

The nurse is responsible for the correct administration of antibiotics. The antimicrobials utilized in septic shock may be toxic and should be administered carefully. The drug groups most commonly utilized are aminoglycosides, penicillins, and cephalosporins (Table 9-1).

Table 9-1. Antimicrobials used in septic shock

Antimicrobial agent	Sensitive microorganisms	Dosage	Nursing implications

Aminoglycosides
Gentamicin
Tobramycin
Kanamycin
Amikacin
	Most gram-negative bacteria
	Pseudomonas aeruginosa
	Klebsiella
	Enterobacter
	Serratia
	Aerobacter
	Acinetobacter
	Escherichia
		Dosage based on ideal weight and
		  creatinine clearance
		Gentamicin and tobramycin,
		  loading dose 1.5 to 2.0 mg/kg;
		kanamycin, 2.0 mg/kg;
		amikacin, 7.5 mg/kg every 12
		  hours
			Aminoglycosides are very ototoxic and
			  nephrotoxic.
			Dosage should be given at precise times.
			Resistant strains are emerging.
			Depending on renal function the drug
			  may be given at 8-, 12-, 16-, or
			  24-hour intervals.
			Nephrotoxicity risk is increased with
			  metabolic acidosis.

Penicillins
Ticarcillin
Carbenicillin
Ampicillin
	Pneumococci used with
	  aminoglycosides for
	  synergistic effect on
	  gram-negative organisms
	Klebsiella synergistic with
	  aminoglycosides
		Ticarcillin, 3 gm every 4 hours
		Carbenicillin, 5 gm every 4
		  hours
		Ampicillin, 2 gm every 4 hours
			Check for history of allergic response
			  to penicillins.
			Check renal function.

Cephalosporins
Cefazolin
		Cephalosporin dosage levels vary
		  depending on type of cephalo-
		  sporin used
			Check that cross-sensitivity from
			  penicillins has been noted.
			Note instability at room temperature

Chloramphenicol Clindamycin	*Bacteroides* Gram-positive *Bacteroides*	100 mg/kg/day in divided doses 600 to 900 mg every 6 hours	Check for depression of bone marrow. Watch for bloody diarrhea associated with colitis

Some key points to consider when administering antibiotics are serum levels, toxicity, and sensitivity patterns. A certain serum level of the drug must be obtained for an antimicrobial to work effectively. The duration of time the drug stays in the body is affected by the function of the kidney and liver. The kidney is the primary means of detoxification and excretion for aminoglycosides. Therefore the amount of drug that stays in the blood has high levels (peaks) when first administered and lower levels (troughs) after renal excretion. This is important because the lower level of antimicrobial should not go below a level that would allow a regrowth of the organism. Also the peak levels should not be at a point where body tissues are damaged by the drug's toxicity. Thus antibiotics should be administered on as precise a schedule as possible. Dosage of antimicrobial agents is dependent on age, renal and hepatic function, weight, and resistance of the organism.

Antimicrobials have a variety of side effects that vary by route of administration. The aminoglycosides cause otoxicity and nephrotoxicity. To assess any early loss of hearing and renal function, laboratory values are helpful. Drug serum levels can be obtained at peak and trough times. If the level is found to be too high, the dosage can be reduced so the likelihood of toxicity is decreased. Another simple means of assessing nephrotoxicity is to watch urine output and creatinine clearance. However, these measures can be altered by other complications of the shock state such as acute tubular necrosis (ATN). The risk of nephrotoxicity is increased when the patient is dehydrated and acidotic (Eskridge, 1980). Cephalosporins can also cause nephrotoxicity. When they are administered with aminoglycosides, the risk of kidney damage may be increased. Clindamycin can produce a severe side effect called pseudomembranous colitis. This occurs because the normal flora of the intestines is suppressed or destroyed and a type of *Clostridium* that also resides in the bowel produces a superinfection. This is evidenced by bloody diarrhea, which serves as an immediate indication to stop the drug. Chloramphenicol has side effects that affect the hemopoietic tissues. A complete blood count should be obtained at regular intervals during the administration of this drug.

Penicillins and cephalosporins are most likely to produce an allergic response in a patient. A history of antimicrobial sensitivities should be elicited from the patient and/or family. Penicillin is currently the major cause of anaphylactic shock.

A final effect of the administration of any antimicrobials is the alteration of normal flora. The normal flora of the intestines produces vitamin K. If the patient does not have normal liver reserves to draw upon, vitamin K should be administered parenterally. This is particularly important to prevent bleeding episodes caused by a lack of clotting factors formed from vitamin K.

Steroid administration

The nurse may administer steroids in septic shock. Steroid administration has a variety of nursing implications. There are only nonspecific indicators by which to monitor the effects of steroids. For example, glucocorticoids stabilize the lysosome membranes, which would decrease cell lysis. Steroids also cause immunosuppression. The resultant decrease in vasodilation and inflammation may be desirable in patients with the endotoxin-immune response. The white blood cell count will decrease over a period of days when the patient has received steroids. As the patient's condition improves, the nurse must remember that administration of steroids suppresses the body's own secretion of corticosteroids. Steroid use must be tapered off so that normal adrenal function can return.

Life support

The nursing care of patients with septic shock will be directed toward vital system support. The nurse should monitor neurological, renal, pulmonary, and cardiac function to assess the onset of decompensation. An example of intervention directed toward support of the systems is the administration of calcium to improve cardiac contractility. Also, the nurse should carefully monitor oxygenation because mechanical ventilation may be necessary. The nurse should assess neurological dysfunction by changes in the level of consciousness and in sympathetic response. In addition, the renal system should be monitored for the onset of acute tubular necrosis. Each decompensation further deepens the shock state and makes recovery more difficult.

Holistic considerations

The physiology of septic shock is complex. However, it is not as complex as meeting the needs of the whole patient. Each patient has many less tangible but no less real spiritual, ethical, moral, and psychological components of nursing care, and no two situations are the same.

There are ethical as well as psychological concerns for the nursing care of the septic shock patient. Many of the people who develop septic shock have an underlying fatal disease. This can cause the team of physicians, nurses, and family to have a number of varying opinions on the appropriateness of expensive and prolonged therapies. The patient may even ask to be allowed to die. There are no easy solutions for this dilemma. The nurse needs to be aware of personal feelings and should seek outside support as necessary.

It is also difficult for the patient and family to adapt to the body changes that occur. If an infected site is draining, it may be purulent and odorous. Families may fear that the person is "rotting." High doses of corticosteroids may also cause facial swelling and distortion. The patient should be bathed and the drainage smells reduced before visiting time to minimize these concerns. It is important to reassure the family that as the patient improves the appearance will also improve.

The physician and nurse need to be able to speak harmoniously about the patient's chance of survival. It is important not to give unrealistic expectations, but on the other hand, not to abolish all hope. The patient's condition is often like walking a tightrope and it is hard to find those "right therapeutic words."

Regardless of what priorities are set for nursing care, the intervention most desired by the patient is human interaction. Reorientation, touch, and simple conversations meet a variety of psychological needs. Detachment is sometimes needed for the nurse to function, but it is important not to detach oneself from the patient's need for humanness.

Nursing management should focus on assisting the person to adapt either to recovery or to death. Perhaps as we understand the dynamics of septic shock more fully, we will be able to improve the outcome. It is also important that nursing research more effective ways for dealing with early recognition of these patients and interventions to promote their comfort. We need to support and educate each other in ways to improve patient care. There is much yet to learn.

PATIENT VIGNETTE
Septic shock following transurethral resection (TUR)

Mr. Bauer, 72, was hospitalized for an admission complaint of pain on urination and difficulty in starting and maintaining a urinary stream. He had been on a 2-week course of trimethoprim and sulfamethoxazole (Bactrim, D.S.) as prescribed by his general practitioner for an *Escherichia coli* infection of the urine. Catheterization for residual urine revealed 250 ml of dark amber urine. Rectal examination found a 4+ prostate enlargement. Other pertinent data from the patient history include a 3-year history of nocturia, intermittent polyuria, and diabetes controlled with an 1800 calorie diet and 16 units of NPH insulin daily. His blood glucose levels have been more labile during the infection. Preoperatively he received four doses of cefazolin (Ancef), 1 gm intramuscularly. The urinalysis preoperatively showed no growth on culture.

Mr. Bauer's obstruction mandated the suprapubic approach TUR. The prostate contained a benign tissue enlargement. At 6:00 PM on the day of surgery his vital signs remained stable at blood pressure, 120/70; pulse 110 (slightly irregular); respirations, 22; and temperature, 98.9 (rectal). His face was flushed and he was disoriented to time, place, and person. His parenteral infusion, D_5W, was infusing at a rate of 75 ml/hour. The 6:00 PM blood glucose was 120 mg/100 ml. Regular insulin was given throughout the afternoon based on his urine sugar, acetone, and serum glucose levels. The continuous bladder irrigation was running well and produced light red drainage.

Questions
1. What factors predispose Mr. Bauer to the development of septic shock?
   a. Diabetes
   b. Age
   c. Surgery
   d. Catheterization

The nurse contacted the urology resident. At 8:00 PM Mr. Bauer's CVP readings ranged between 0 and 3 cm H_2O even when the fluid rates were increased to 180 ml/ hour. Other vital signs were blood pressure, 90 palpation; pulse 160, (irregular); respirations, 28; and temperature, 101.0 (rectal). An electrocardiogram revealed ventricular premature contractions (VPC) at a rate of 5/min. ABG readings were pH, 7.27; Pao_2,

75 mm Hg; Paco$_2$, 35 mm Hg; percent saturation, 80. Oxygen was initiated by Venti-mask at 40% oxygen. A Swan-Ganz line was inserted to monitor hemodynamic data more closely. In addition, multiple cultures were obtained from urine, sputum, and blood. Gentamicin, 80 mg every 12 hours, and cefazolin (Ancef), 1 gm every 6 hours, were given by the intravenous route.

2. What should the nurse assess before giving gentamicin?
   a. Patient weight
   b. BUN and creatinine levels
   c. Allergies
   d. Liver function

3. The blood cultures grew a heavy growth of gram-negative bacteria. What effects of endotoxin might occur?
   a. Increased level of insulin
   b. Increased level of complement
   c. Decreased intravascular volume
   d. Decreased fibrinolytic activity

4. Which laboratory values are important to assess for further physiological compromise?
   a. BUN
   b. CPK
   c. SGOT
   d. Lactic acid

5. Mr. Bauer became severely hypotensive, with a systolic pressure of 60 mm Hg. Dopamine, 400 mg in 500 ml of D$_5$W, was started at 24 drops/min to maintain a systolic pressure of 100 mm Hg. The primary nursing responsibilities are:
   a. Assessment of venous line patency
   b. Assessment of arterial pulses in all extremities
   c. Monitoring of blood pressure every 5 minutes for the first 15 to 30 minutes
   d. Assessment of effects of afterload on the myocardium

Answers

1. a, b, c, and d. All of these factors predispose Mr. Bauer to the development of septic shock (refer to p. 174).

2. a, b, and c. Aminoglycoside antibiotics are excreted through the actions of the kidney. Their dosage is highly dependent upon the patient's age and renal function. History of allergies is vital to the administration of any drug.

3. c. The pathophysiology of septic shock results in a decrease in the level of complement. Because of the nature of this shock the intravascular volume is decreased,

and the clinical picture of septic shock occurs. The section on pathophysiology explains this in detail if you need more information to understand this question.
4. a, b, c, and d. The first three answers are helpful in assessing the function of specific organs. Lactic acid values provide information regarding the level of metabolic acidosis, and they are good predictors for mortality rates in shock.
5. a, b, c, and d. The box on p. 187 provides specific nursing implications in the administration of sympathomimetic agents.

REFERENCES

Cerra, F.B., Hassett, J., and Siegel, J.H.: Vasodilator therapy in clinical sepsis with low output syndrome, Journal of Surgical Research **25:**180-183, 1975.

Collins, A.S.: Dobutamine: a new intropic agent, Nursing '80 **10**(3):62-66, 1980.

Eskridge, R.A.: Septic shock, Critical Care Quarterly **2**(4):55-74, 1980.

Fearon, D.T., Ruddy, S., and Schur, D.H.: Activation of the properdin pathway of complement in patients with gram-negative bacteremia, New England Journal of Medicine **292:**937-940, 1975.

Fidler, M.R.: Maintenance of nonspecific and immunologic defenses. In Kinney, M., Dear, C.B., Packa, D., and Voorman, D., editors: AACN's clinical reference for critical care nursing, New York, 1981, McGraw-Hill Book Co.

Forgacs, P.: Treatment of septic shock, Medical Clinics of North America **63**(2):465-470, 1979.

Gallin, J.I., Kaye, D., and O'Leary, W.M.: Serum lipids in infection, New England Journal of Medicine **281:**1081, 1969.

Gelin, L.E., et al.: Septic shock, Surgical Clinics of North America **60**(1):161-173, 1980.

Guglielmo, J.: Evaluation of the use of corticosteroids, Critical Care Quarterly **2**(4):37-42, 1980.

Guyton, A.C., Textbook of medical physiology, ed. 5, Philadelphia, 1981, W.B. Saunders Co.

Jackson, G.G.: Causative organisms in gram-negative bacteremia and their relation to shock: use of dopamine in shock, McGaw Park, Ill., 1976, American Critical Care Division of American Hospital Supply.

Landesman, S.H., and Gorbach, S.L.: Gram-negative sepsis and shock, Orthopedic Clinics of North America **9**(3):611-623, 1978.

McCabe, W.R.: Gram-negative bacteremia, Disease-A-Month **1:**38, 1973.

Plachetka, J.R.: Sympathomimetic pharmacology, Critical Care Quarterly **2**(4):27-35, 1980.

Price, S.A., and Wilson, L.M.: Pathophysiology: clinical concepts of disease processes. St. Louis, 1978, McGraw-Hill Book Co.

Robinson, W.A.: Fluid therapy in hemorrhagic shock, Critical Care Quarterly **2**(4):1-13, 1980.

Schumer, W.: Steroids in the treatment of clinical septic shock. Annals of Surgery **184:**333-339, 1976.

Shubin, H., Weil, M.H., and Carlson, R.W.: Bacterial shock, American Heart Journal **94:**112-114, 1977.

Shubin, H., and Weil, M.H.: Bacterial shock, Journal of The American Medical Association **235**(4): 421-424, 1976.

Weil, M.H., Shubin, H., and Nishijima, H.: Gram-negative shock: definition diagnosis and mechanisms, Antibiotics & Chemotherapy **21:**178-183, 1976.

Weissmann, G., and Thomas, L.: Studies on lysosomes: the effects of endotoxin, endotoxin tolerance, and cortisone on the release of acid hydrolases from a granular fraction of rabbit liver, Journal of Experimental Medicine **116:**433-450, 1962.

Weitzman, S., and Berger, S.: Clinical trial design in studies of corticosteroids for bacterial infections, Annals of Internal Medicine **284:**1248-1250, 1974.

Wilson, R.F.: The diagnosis and management of severe sepsis and septic shock, Heart & Lung **5**(3): 422-429, 1976a.

Wilson, R.F.: Endocrine changes in sepsis, Heart & Lung **5**(3):411-415, 1976b.

Zschoche, D.A., Mosby's comprehensive review of critical care St. Louis, 1981, The C.V. Mosby Co.

10 Anaphylactic shock

JUDITH L. MYERS

Anaphylaxis is an acute, generalized shock syndrome that results from the interaction of an antigen with antibodies on sensitized body tissues. The antigen reacts with immunoglobulins found on the surface of mast cells in body tissues and basophils in the blood stream. This antigen-antibody reaction causes the release of vasoactive amines, such as histamine, and other biological substances in the body. Release of these pharmacologically active substances produces the clinical manifestations associated with anaphylaxis. This syndrome is life threatening and can be fatal if not recognized and treated early. The nurse in a community setting, emergency room, or hospital division is frequently the first one in contact with the person in anaphylactic shock. Hospitalized patients are often exposed to potentially anaphylactic substances as part of diagnostic procedures or therapeutic interventions. In many instances nurses are responsible for the administration of drugs that can stimulate an anaphylactic reaction. The speed with which anaphylaxis can develop requires that nurses caring for these patients be familiar with assessment criteria and treatment priorities.

Sometimes the term *anaphylaxis* is restricted to an induced, experimental animal model. The human counterpart of anaphylaxis is then referred to as a systemic allergic reaction. Patterson and Schatz (1975) state that "the similarity of the immunologic, cellular and pharmacologic mechanisms in man and in animal models justifies the use of the term anaphylaxis to describe the human systemic allergic reaction."

PATHOPHYSIOLOGY

Anaphylaxis was classified by Coombs and Gell (1963) as a type I hypersensitivity reaction (Table 10-1). The majority of patients who experience anaphylaxis have a true type I reaction. However, anaphylactic reactions can be mediated by type II and type III hypersensitivity states as well as by mechanisms that may activate the alternate pathway of the complement system in the body. For anaphylactic shock to occur the individual must first be exposed to a sensitizing antigen. Following this exposure there is formation of antibodies that attach to tissue mast cells and basophils. The antibodies formed are from the IgE class of immunoglobulins (Table 10-2). This is referred to as the primary immune response. The individual is sensitized to a particular antigen and in some instances to similar antigens. Subsequent contact with the antigen produces a rapid reaction between the tissue bound antibodies and the antigen. The result of this secondary

Table 10-1. Classification of hypersensitivity states

Coombs and Gell (1963)	Mediating mechanism	Examples
Type I: anaphylactic or immediate type	IgE immunoglobulin	Hay fever, extrinsic asthma, anaphylaxis
Type II: cytotoxic type	IgG or IgM immuno-globulins	ABO transfusion reactions, Rh reactions in newborns
Type III: immune com-plex type	Aggregates of immune com-plexes in blood vessel walls or tissue base-ment membranes	Glomerulonephritis, serum sickness, vasculitis
Type IV: delayed type	Sensitized T-lymphocytes	Tissue transplant rejections, rheumatoid arthritis, sys-temic lupus erythematosus, positive TB skin test
Two groups added later		
Type V: stimulatory type	Long-acting thyroid stimu-lator (LATS) on IgG antibody	Thyrotoxicosis
Type VI: miscella-neous type	Alternate pathway of the complement system	Gram-negative endotoxic shock

Table 10-2. Classes of immunoglobulins

Class	Percent of total immunoglobulins	Location	Main function
IgG	75 to 85	Extravascular fluid	Toxin neutralization; viral in-activation; booster im-munity; phagocytosis
IgM	7	Intravascular	Can activate compliment; viral, bacterial inactivation; phagocytosis
IgA	10	Exocrine secretions (saliva, tears, mucin)	Protect mucosal surfaces
IgD	1	?	Unknown
IgE	0.002	Tissue bound to mast cell and basophil	Release histamine in allergic reactions

immune response is a disease state or tissue injury (Fig. 10-1). Not all immune responses are harmful and produce tissue injury. For example, immunizations against childhood diseases represent beneficial primary and secondary immune responses. There are some individuals who have no previous history of contact with an antigen and experience ana-phylaxis as a result of the primary immune response.

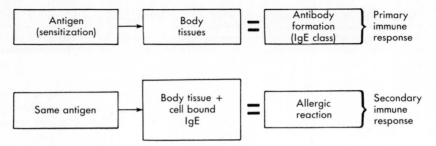

Fig. 10-1. Primary and secondary immune responses.

Classification of antigens

A variety of allergens have been implicated as causes in the development of anaphylaxis. These allergens function as the antigenic stimulus to antibody formation in the immune response. Three main categories of allergens are most frequently identified as causes of anaphylaxis. These categories are classified by the antigen's route of entry into the body and include (1) *injections* of drugs, serum, or contrast media; (2) *ingestion* of food or drugs; and (3) *bites or stings* from venomous animals or insects.

The highest incidence of anaphylactic reactions occurs following injections of antigen substances. There are case reports of anaphylaxis after both subcutaneous and intravenous injections (Goldman, Lewis, and Rose, 1976; Tannenbaum, Ruddy, and Schur, 1975). Routeledge (1976) reports of a previously nonallergic patient who suffered an anaphylactic reaction following a transfusion of blood from a donor with a history of allergy and recent sensitization. Allergic symptoms and systemic anaphylaxis have been reported in up to 2% of radiological studies using contrast media. This accounts for approximately 500 deaths each year in the United States (Gorevic and Kaplan, 1979). Serious allergic reactions in humans are caused by stinging insects from the Hymenoptera class. This group of insects includes bees, wasps, hornets, and yellow jackets. Except for the honeybee, most of these insects can sting repeatedly. The yellow jacket is the most common cause of anaphylaxis from insect stings. Gottlieb (1979) states that 0.4% of the general population experience anaphylactic reactions to stinging insects.

The lack of criteria to predict reactions to allergens causing anaphylaxis has been studied for stinging insects and for contrast media. Settipane, Klein, and Boyd (1978) found that atopic individuals, those with hereditary allergies such as asthma or allergic rhinitis, were not predisposed to acute anaphylaxis. Both the atopic diseases and anaphylaxis are mediated by IgE antibodies. But in the atopic individual the antigen-antibody response occurs primarily at the level of the mucous membranes of the respiratory tract. The presence of this type of sensitivity disorder may have no relationship to an allergic response to an antigen that is primarily encountered by the parenteral route such as bee stings or drugs. However, this same study found that asthmatics who also have bee sting allergy do have a more severe reaction than nonasthmatics. In another

---

Classification of allergens in anaphylaxis

Injections

Drugs: antibiotics (penicillin), analgesics, anesthetics (lidocaine), vaccines, hormones, insulin
Radiological contrast media (iodine based)
Transfusions from a sensitized donor

Ingestions

Drugs: antibiotics
Food: oranges, milk, sesame seeds, mango, soybean, banana, shellfish, nuts, beans, egg whites, and sunflower seed

Bites and stings

Venomous snakes
Insects: bees, wasps, hornets, and yellow jackets

---

report on bee sting reactions, Gottlieb (1979) states that previous reactions are not a good indicator of future responses to insect stings.

In a study of anaphylaxis after injections of radiological contrast media, Epstein (1977) reported that skin testing and intravenous pretesting with small doses of contrast media do not reliably predict adverse reactions to a subsequent diagnostic dose of the same material. Clients with a true fish sensitivity or iodine allergy may be at more risk for allergic reactions to contrast media, iodinated substances, than other individuals.

Since prevention is often the first line of defense in many health care problems, it would be useful if potential victims of anaphylaxis could be identified and exposure to harmful antigens avoided. A complete health history is useful in creating an environment for the client that limits exposure to potential anaphylactic allergens. The assessment data should include a history of allergies, hypersensitivity disorders, and adverse reactions to drugs or diagnostic procedures. In addition to containing information on specific allergens to which the client is sensitized, the assessment should also include the type of reaction that is experienced when the client is exposed to the allergen. However, a history of allergies or a lack of one has not always been a useful aid in identifying those individuals at risk to develop anaphylaxis (Viner and Rhamy, 1975).

Immune reaction

The immune reaction that is responsible for anaphylaxis occurs on the surface membranes of tissue mast cells and basophils in the bloodstream. Mast cells are found in abundance in connective tissue, in the lung and uterus, and around blood vessels. The gastrointestinal tract is another source of mast cells, especially the spleen, liver, and omentum. The kidney, heart, skin, and other organs also contain mast cells. Both mast

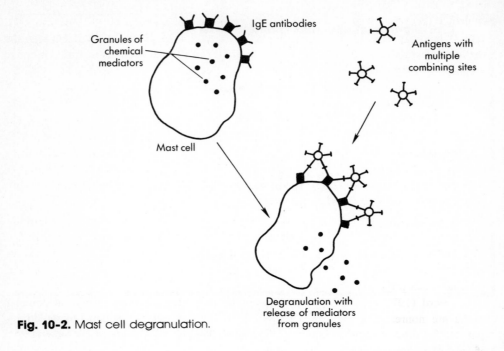

Fig. 10-2. Mast cell degranulation.

cells and basophils are sources of histamine and other chemical mediators responsible for the clinical manifestations associated with anaphylaxis. Reactions between antigens and cell-bound IgE activate a series of enzymes that results in the breakdown of the mast cells and basophils. This cellular breakdown, or degranulation, causes the release of the chemical mediators of anaphylaxis. The histamine and other chemical mediators of anaphylaxis are contained within granules found in the cytoplasm of mast cell or basophil (Fig. 10-2).

Most allergens such as food, drugs, and insect venoms cause anaphylaxis through processes that are reagenically mediated. This means there is an antigen-antibody reaction that causes mast cell degranulation and histamine release. Most of the antigens responsible for inducing anaphylactic shock are multivalent ligands, which have more than one combining site for cell-bound IgE antibodies. In comparison the IgE antibodies have at least two antigen-combining sites. The multivalent ligands are capable of causing aggregation or cross-linking of the cell-bound antibodies. This cross-linking in the antigen-antibody reaction may cause an actual distortion in the cell-bound antibodies that results in degranulation of the mast cell.

Some substances known to cause anaphylaxis function as haptens instead of as true, complete antigens. A hapten is a low molecular weight substance that by itself is unable to stimulate a primary immune response. However, it can combine with a larger "carrier" molecule and produce a primary response. After this initial response is stimulated, the hapten can cause a secondary immune response by itself without a carrier molecule (Bowry, 1977). Penicillin is an example of a substance that functions as a hapten. When an individual is sensitized after an injection of penicillin, it is because the metabolic byproducts of penicillin easily combine with tissue proteins to form complete antigens. This larger molecular complex is now capable of stimulating antibody formation.

There is some controversy about the explanation for anaphylactic reactions to radiological contrast media. Research has yet to identify the mechanisms responsible for anaphylactic reactions. There may be multiple phenomena that produce the responses to the administration of contrast agents. All of the media used for radiological contrast studies contain an iodide that has the ability to cause histamine release. The lung has been considered the target organ in most contrast media reactions. It has the highest concentration of histamine per gram of tissue. Also, since most contrast agents are given intravenously, they must travel through the pulmonary circulation. It has been hypothesized (Epstein, 1977) that some contrast agents may stimulate antibody formation and be classified as reagenic reactions. However, an immunological explanation for contrast media reactions has not been clearly demonstrated since antibodies against contrast media have not been produced experimentally (Viner and Rhamy, 1975).

Ford (1977) has reported that reactions to certain chemicals such as contrast media are nonreagenic processes that seem to involve parasympathetic hyperactivity initiated by patient anxiety or stress. The physical properties and physiological effects of the contrast media may also be responsible for the hypersensitivity reactions experienced by some individuals. The hypertonicity of the contrast media may produce chemotactic effects that cause the crenation and sludging of red blood cells, activation or inhibition of white blood cell enzymes, altered permeability of capillary walls, relaxation of vascular smooth muscle, and changes in nervous function (Gorevic and Kaplan, 1979; Viner and Rhamy, 1975).

The activation of complement pathways (Chapter 9), either classical or alternate, may be another mechanism responsible for anaphylactic reactions to contrast media. Two of the protein fragments formed during complement activation, C3a and C5a, have potent anaphylactic activity. These fragments are called anaphylatoxins because one of their biological activities is to cause the release of histamine from mast cells. C3a and C5a act directly on receptors on mast cells in the absence of antibodies to trigger histamine release. The effect is similar to IgE antibody reactions. These anaphylatoxins can also stimulate type II and type III reactions.

Chemical mediators

The primary chemical mediator of anaphylaxis is histamine. The effects of histamine in the body include the contraction of smooth muscle, the dilation of blood capillaries, an increased capillary permeability, and a fall in blood pressure (Fig. 10-3). There are two known types of histamine receptors in the body, referred to as H_1 and H_2 receptors. Stimulation of H_1 receptors produces vasodilation, increased capillary permeability, and contraction of nonvascular smooth muscle. Stimulation of the H_2 receptors results

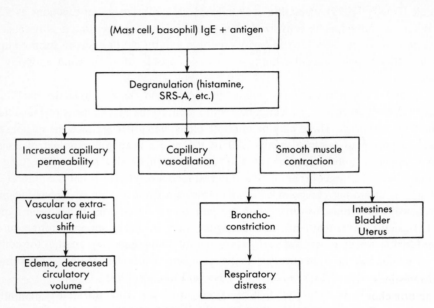

Fig. 10-3. Pathophysiology in anaphylaxis.

Effects of chemical mediators of anaphylaxis

Mediator	Effect
Histamine	Vasodilation (H_1, H_2) Smooth muscle contraction (H_1) (bronchi, intestines) Increased capillary permeability (H_1) Increased gastric acid secretion (H_2)
Serotonin	Increase capillary permeability
Slow-reacting substance of anaphylaxis (SRS-A)	Smooth muscle contraction Enhanced effect of histamine Increased capillary permeability
Prostaglandins	Smooth muscle contraction Increased capillary permeability Potentiation of other mediators
Bradykinin	Smooth muscle contraction Increased capillary permeability

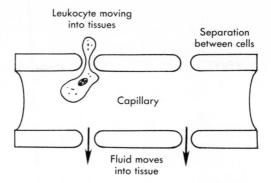

Fig. 10-4. Effect of histamine on capillary.

primarily in increased gastric acid secretion with some minor cardiac stimulation.

Histamine causes contraction of many smooth muscles, such as those in the bronchi and intestines, but powerfully relaxes others, including those in smaller blood vessels. The bronchoconstriction and intestinal contractions are the result of stimulation of the H_1 receptors. The vasodilation, which can produce a fall in blood pressure, is thought to be the combined effect of H_1 and H_2 receptor stimulation.

Capillary dilation is the most characteristic action of histamine. It results from some direct action of histamine on the vessels and is independent of specific innervation. All capillaries are involved, but the effect is most obvious in the face and upper body. These dilator responses are the result of the inhibitory effects of histamine on the smooth muscle of terminal arterioles. The dilation in postcapillary venules, which are devoid of smooth muscle, is mainly passive because of a fall in resistance in terminal arterioles and a rise in pressure in larger veins, which histamine tends to constrict (Goodman and Gilman, 1975).

The effects of histamine on the microcirculation are important not as an isolated event but as an initial step in a process that brings about a shift in fluid balance between the vascular and extravascular fluid compartments. Histamine causes the endothelial cells lining the capillaries to separate at their boundaries and thereby expose the basement membrane, which is freely permeable to plasma proteins and fluid. As a result of this increased capillary permeability there is extravasation of plasma proteins and movement of fluid into the extravascular spaces (Fig. 10-4). Histamine also causes an increased adhesiveness of the endothelial cells. Through capillary dilation and increased blood flow, more leukocytes are delivered to the area. Soon there is diapedesis or ameboid-like movement of leukocytes from the capillaries through the endothelial gaps into tissue spaces. The passage of platelets and injected substances can also occur through the endothelium.

The effects of histamine released from basophils and mast cells are not unique to anaphylaxis. Increased capillary dilation and permeability and increased movement of fluid and cells across the endothelium are part of the normal inflammatory response to tissue injury. The inflammatory response is seen most often as a localized reaction at the site of tissue injury. However, in anaphylaxis the response is magnified to include the entire body and presents a life-threatening situation.

Other chemical substances besides histamines have been identified as mediators of anaphylaxis. These substances include serotonin, bradykinin, slow-reacting substance of anaphylaxis (SRS-A), eosinophil chemotactic factor of anaphylaxis (ECF-A), prostaglandins, and acetylcholine. All of these substances can be released from mast cells. These vasoactive amines are responsible for the manifestations associated with anaphylaxis. The amines cause vasodilation, increased capillary permeability, smooth muscle contraction, and attraction of eosinophils (leukocytes) to the local site of the reaction.

Serotonin, like histamine, causes an increased permeability of pulmonary capillaries. This can produce leakage of plasma into lung air spaces. SRS-A has effects in the body similar to those of histamine. Its chemical composition is unknown, but its name comes from the fact that its effects are slower and more prolonged than histamine. SRS-A is synthesized and released during anaphylaxis rather than being released from a preformed store. Like histamine, SRS-A contracts smooth muscle of the bronchi and may increase the responsiveness of these muscles to the effects of histamine. Increased vascular permeability is also a result of SRS-A activity.

The role of prostaglandins in IgE-mediated reactions is not clearly defined. Their effects are variable based on the type of prostaglandin involved. In general they produce changes in vascular permeability, contraction of smooth muscle, and potentiation of the effects of other vasoactive amines. Bradykinin can produce the contraction of smooth muscles and increased vascular permeability.

In addition to the release of histamine from mast cells during anaphylaxis, heparin is also released. This may account for the reports of clotting abnormalities seen in anaphylaxis. Large numbers of eosinophils may also be present in anaphylaxis. Their main function is to phagocytose the immune complexes and release granular contents that neutralize the vasoactive amines (Bowry, 1977).

NURSING ASSESSMENT

Anaphylaxis has a variety of symptoms involving the eyes, skin, respiratory tract, gastrointestinal tract, and cardiovascular system; hypotension and laryngeal edema are important factors in fatal cases (Bacal, 1978). The fact that the manifestations of anaphylaxis are so variable and involve multiple body systems can make diagnosis a difficult problem. This is especially true if the history of the precipitating event is vague or unknown as might be the case with the emergency room patient or one transferred from another service in the hospital. Ford (1977) identified other disorders for which anaphylaxis may be mistaken, such as vasovagal syndromes, cardiovascular disorders such as myocardial infarction, diabetic coma, pneumothorax, air embolus, and epileptiform seizures. Criteria to be included when a diagnosis of anaphylaxis is made are circulatory failure, wheezing, urticaria, and a past history of allergic-type reactions.

In most cases of anaphylaxis there is a rapid onset of symptoms within minutes after contact with the offending allergen. However, Viner and Rhamy (1975) report cases of anaphylactic reactions to parenteral drugs and contrast media that may not develop symptoms for up to 1 hour after injection. This delay in the onset of anaphylaxis indicates the need for the nurse to carefully observe patients receiving potential anaphylactic drugs for longer than the first few minutes after administration. This is especially true for patients with known drug sensitivities. Patients returning from the x-ray department following contrast media studies should continue to be assessed by the nurse for indications of possible anaphylactic reactions.

Early localized symptoms

The earliest symptoms of anaphylaxis include apprehension or a sense of uneasiness (Fig. 10-5). The patient may complain of lightheadedness and paresthesia. The nurse may observe the appearance of generalized urticaria or hives associated with itching and scratching. Angioedema may develop and is most noticeable in the eyelids, lips, tongue, hands, feet, and genitalia. This swelling is the result of the histamine effect on capillary permeability and the movement of fluid from vascular to extravascular spaces.

Respiratory symptoms

As the anaphylactic reaction progresses, the patient may develop audible respiratory wheezing and dyspnea. There may also be evidence of pulmonary edema developing. These manifestations are produced by the action of histamine on the bronchial smooth muscle, initiating muscle contractions and bronchospasm. The edema occurs because of the shift of fluid from capillaries into tissue spaces. As the patient experiences alterations in respiratory function, the nurse may observe changes in the patient's skin color such as cyanosis or pallor.

As the fluid shift from capillaries to tissue spaces becomes more generalized, the patient develops edema of the uvula and larynx. Because of this upper airway swelling the patient may complain of a choking sensation. This edema can become severe enough to produce an actual respiratory obstruction. Laryngeal edema causes the patient to experience air hunger and impaired phonation. The patient may also have a barking or high-pitched cough.

Smooth muscle contractions

Smooth muscle contractions in the gastrointestinal tract will produce cramping abdominal pain. The patient may even experience diarrhea and vomiting. Contractions of smooth muscles of the bladder will result in urinary incontinence. In women, smooth muscle spasms may affect the uterus and result in vaginal bleeding.

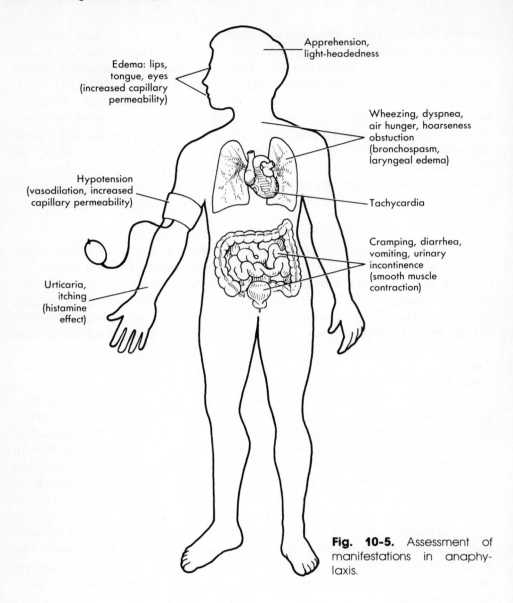

Apprehension, light-headedness

Edema: lips, tongue, eyes (increased capillary permeability)

Wheezing, dyspnea, air hunger, hoarseness obstuction (bronchospasm, laryngeal edema)

Hypotension (vasodilation, increased capillary permeability)

Tachycardia

Cramping, diarrhea, vomiting, urinary incontinence (smooth muscle contraction)

Urticaria, itching (histamine effect)

Fig. 10-5. Assessment of manifestations in anaphylaxis.

Cardiovascular symptoms

The obvious effect of the fluid shift on the circulatory system is a decrease in circulating blood volume. The results are those associated with other types of shock and include hypotension and tachycardia. Anaphylaxis may also be associated with transient changes in the electrocardiogram (Carloss, 1976). The ECG changes are similar to those seen in myocardial injury and may cause confusion in making an accurate diagnosis. In anaphylaxis the ECG may show temporary changes in the ST segment and the T wave that are usually suggestive of coronary insufficiency and ischemia. However, the patient in anaphylactic shock will have normal serum enzymes.

The alterations in ventilation and circulation can eventually cause convulsions and unconsciousness. Death can occur within minutes, unless prompt and appropriate treatment is instituted. Circulatory failure and laryngeal edema are the usual causes of death in anaphylaxis.

Although multiple symptoms usually occur in anaphylaxis, cases have been reported in which hypotension was the only manifestation (Viner and Rhamy, 1975). In these situations vigorous fluid replacement of up to 6 L was required to restore the systolic blood pressure to greater than 100 mm Hg.

MEDICAL AND NURSING MANAGEMENT

The initial goal in treatment of anaphylaxis is to prevent further antigen intro-duction. Additional goals include providing ventilation, restoring adequate circulation, and investigating the precipitating event. Specific treatment protocols show some vari-ations in priorities and the types of drugs used to manage anaphylactic shock. Regardless of the protocol used, the first priority in managing anaphylaxis is preventing further introduction of the causative antigen. In the case of anaphylaxis brought on by intravenous administration of drugs or contrast media the procedure should be stopped immediately. When anaphylaxis is the result of an insect sting, Ford (1977) recommends the application of a tourniquet to the extremity above the site of the sting. Budassi and Barber (1981) recommend removal of the stinger by scraping with a dull object, because a grasping and pulling technique could contract the venom sac and release more toxin into the site.

The establishment and maintenance of a clear and patent airway is another priority that should be considered early in the management of anaphylaxis. Simple oral airways will have little effect on airway patency and will be useless as laryngeal edema progresses. It may be necessary to intubate the patient or perform a tracheostomy to provide adequate ventilatory support.

In conjunction with measures to support ventilation should be the administration of drugs to block or counteract the effects of histamine (Table 10-3). Epinephrine is considered the drug of choice in the treatment of anaphylaxis because it prevents further histamine release and counteracts both circulatory failure and the bronchospasm (Viner and Rhamy, 1975). Since epinephrine is a nonspecific antagonist it is more appropriate as a physiological antagonist in anaphylaxis than other drugs such as the antihistamines (Goodman and Gilman, 1975). In anaphylaxis a number of substances other than hista-mine are released from mast cells. These mediators, such as SRS-A and the kinins, are usually refractory to inhibition by antihistamines. The antihistamines may be useful in controlling localized tissue responses such as edema formation and itching. However, the circulatory failure and bronchoconstriction are not greatly affected by this group of drugs. The antihistamines do not affect the release of histamine from its storage sites.

Management of anaphylaxis

Goal: provide ventilation

Patent airway
  Intubation
  Tracheostomy
Epinephrine
Bronchodilators
Ventilator
Oxygen

Goal: restore adequate circulation

Epinephrine
Intravenous fluids
Vasopressors
Antihistamines
Steroids
Trendelenburg position

Goal: prevent future episodes

Densensitization
Medical identification
Epinephrine kits
Patient education

Table 10-3. Drugs used in anaphylaxis

Drug	Major effects	Implications
Epinephrine	Is sympathomimetic Relieves bronchospasm Increases blood pressure Relieves urticaria, itching, and angioedema	May produce cardiac arrhythmias, especially tachycardias Careful monitoring of cardiovascular status If given by intravenous route, careful regulation of flow rate Temporary effect
Antihistamines	Block histamine receptors on target cells Relieve urticaria, itching, and swelling	Can cause CNS depression Slow acting
Aminophylline	Act as bronchodilator	Can produce cardiac arrhythmias and pulmonary vasodilation
Adrenocortical steroids	Decrease capillary permeability Stabilize basophil membrane to reduce degranulation	

They occupy receptor sites on effector cells to the exclusion of histamine. Another reason antihistamines are not the drugs of choice in anaphylaxis is the fact that they are slower acting than epinephrine.

The powerful bronchodilator action of epinephrine is most evident when bronchial muscle constriction is caused by the effect of substances such as histamine. Other bronchodilators can be given as supportive therapy after the initial use of epinephrine. Aminophylline may be given, but it can worsen the situation by producing pulmonary vasodilation.

Epinephrine can correct some of the circulatory failure by producing a rise in blood pressure. The increase in blood pressure is the result of epinephrine's direct effect on the myocardium to increase the strength of contractions. Epinephrine also produces an increased heart rate and vasoconstriction of precapillary resistance vessels of the skin, mucosa, and kidney.

When epinephrine is administered in anaphylaxis, it is initially given subcutaneously or intramuscularly. The absorption by these routes is usually rapid. The injections of a 1:1000 dilution may be repeated at 10-minute intervals as needed (Epstein, 1977; Ford, 1977). The dosage will depend on the route of administration. For subcutaneous administration a dosage of 0.3 to 0.5 ml is recommended for adults (Epstein, 1977). If the epinephrine is given intramuscularly, the dosage may be increased up to 1 ml for adults (Ford, 1977). If there is no response to the epinephrine given by these routes, a slow intravenous infusion may be tried. The cardiovascular status of the patient receiving epinephrine needs to be monitored carefully. This assessment should include frequent measurement of arterial blood pressure and pulse and continuous monitoring of the ECG. If invasive lines are also available, frequent measurements should be made of CVP and/or PCWP. If the epinephrine is given intravenously, the infusion site needs to be checked at frequent intervals for signs of infiltration that can cause tissue necrosis. The infusion rate should also be monitored closely since slight variations may cause marked fluctuations in the blood pressure.

Epinephrine may not be sufficient to maintain blood pressure in anaphylaxis, since there may be increased peripheral vascular resistance. The use of vasopressor agents in acute anaphylaxis may be of little value and can even make the tissue anoxia worse (Viner and Rhamy, 1975). This implies a third-space loss of fluid caused by the leakage of fluid through damaged capillary walls. To correct this fluid loss and support the hypotension caused by increased capillary permeability, the administration of intravenous fluids is necessary. Hemodynamic studies (Obeid et al., 1975) following acute anaphylaxis to contrast media in the left ventricle showed low filling pressures. The patients responded to volume replacement with normal saline after appropriate drug therapy. The amount of fluid needed to restore water balance and maintain the blood pressure will be variable.

Once the initial therapies of airway maintenance, epinephrine administration, and fluid infusion have been started, additional supportive treatment can be included in the care of the patient. Support of ventilation and cardiac activity should continue as long as the patient seems to require it. Restoration of fluid and electrolyte balance should be a continuous part of treatment. Additional drug therapy can include the administration of adrenocortical steroids and antihistamines.

Adrenocortical steroids in the form of hydrocortisone are given intravenously. Steroids act to stabilize damaged capillary walls and reduce the movement of fluid and plasma proteins into extravascular spaces. Another benefit of steroid administration is their effect on leukocyte membranes. The steroids will stabilize the basophil membrane and reduce the degranulation of the chemical mediators of anaphylaxis.

Antihistamines such as diphenhydramine (Benadryl) can be given parenterally to block further histamine-mediated effects. The patient should be observed closely for signs of central nervous system depression such as changes in the level of consciousness. Other central nervous system depressant drugs such as sedatives, narcotics, and tranquilizers should be avoided.

Once the patient's condition has stabilized, observation should still continue for several hours for any indication of adverse reactions to either the anaphylactic episode or its treatment. The patient should avoid contact with any vasodilators for at least 24 hours after the anaphylactic attack. This includes avoiding the use of any vasodilating drugs, consumption of alcohol, and contact with heat, especially hot showers and baths.

A thorough investigation of the causative agent of the anaphylaxis needs to be done as soon as the patient's status is stable. The patient should be instructed to avoid these substances that are likely to produce future reactions. Desensitization is one method that has been used to decrease the severity of allergic reactions and reduce the risk of anaphylaxis. Desensitization works by introducing small amounts of antigen that gradually exhaust the antibodies bound to mast cells or basophils. In this way the chemical mediators of anaphylaxis are not released in a sufficient amount at any time to bring on shock. In the case of anaphylaxis from bee stings, honeybee venom has been used as immunotherapy to produce IgG antibodies. These IgG antibodies serve to combine with the antigen before the antigen has a chance to react with the IgE antibodies. A study by Busse et al. (1975) using honeybee venom in a desensitization program found a fall in the level of IgE antibodies. This result indicates that the increase in IgG-blocking antibodies during desensitization may depress the development of IgE antibodies.

The nurse should strongly encourage the patient to wear some type of medical identification that lists the allergens to which the patient is sensitive. This identification can be in the form of a bracelet or necklace. In a wallet or purse the patient should carry further medical information about allergic sensitivities. In cases where it is impossible to avoid potential anaphylactic agents such as bee stings, the patient may be given antihistamines and/or sympathomimetic drugs as a preventive measure to reduce the severity of an anaphylactic reaction. Some patients may be instructed in the use of kits that allow self-administration of injections of epinephrine. Family members, neighbors, or co-workers should also be familiar with the use of these kits.

When a patient with known allergies or a history of anaphylactic reactions is admitted to the hospital, all specific allergies should be clearly and noticeably marked in red on the patient's medical records. All requisitions for x-ray films involving the use of contrast media should also indicate the patient's allergic sensitivities. Although anaphylaxis can occur anywhere in a health care institution or outside of one, it is especially important that personnel in the emergency room, in the x-ray department, and on ambulances be thoroughly educated in the recognition and treatment of anaphylaxis. These areas should be adequately stocked with up-to-date drugs and the emergency equipment necessary to treat anaphylaxis.

PATIENT VIGNETTE
Anaphylactic shock following penicillin administration

A 57-year-old woman was admitted to the hospital for treatment of pneumococcal pneumonia. As part of the therapy the patient was to receive aqueous penicillin G, 500,000 units every 6 hours intravenously. In the admission history the patient denied any allergies. Prior to administration of the first dose of penicillin, the nurse questioned the patient about her use of antibiotics. The patient stated she had taken antibiotics before without any trouble, but did not remember the specific names of the drugs. Fifteen minutes after the first dose began infusing, the patient complained of intense itching of her arms and legs and difficulty breathing. The nurse immediately stopped the infusion of penicillin and increased the flow rate of a liter of 5% dextrose in water. The patient became increasingly restless and diaphoretic and had difficulty talking. The blood pressure was 80 mm Hg by palpation and the apical pulse was 124. The cardiac arrest team arrived within 3 minutes. The patient was intubated and received 1 ml of epinephrine intramuscularly and 50 mg of diphenhydramine intramuscularly. A second liter of fluids was given intravenously. Another injection of epinephrine was given 10 minutes after the first dose. Within 30 minutes the patient's blood pressure was 100/68 with a pulse of 100. A third liter of intravenous fluids was infused. Six hours later the endotracheal tube was removed and the patient had no further airway difficulty. Her blood pressure stabilized at 120/70 and the pulse was 80. The remainder of her hospitalization was uneventful.

Questions
1. Which of the following describe the anaphylactic response to penicillin?
   a. An antigen-antibody response involving IgE
   b. A type IV delayed hypersensitivity
   c. An increase in mast cell production
   d. An antigen-antibody response involving IgG

2. In anaphylaxis, what is histamine responsible for?
  a. Increased capillary permeability
  b. Smooth muscle contraction
  c. Mast cell degranulation
  d. All of the above

3. What causes hypotension to occur in anaphylaxis?
  a. A decrease in myocardial pumping activity
  b. A plasma-to-interstitial fluid shift
  c. Peripheral vasodilation
  d. All of the above

4. Why is epinephrine the drug of choice in anaphylaxis?
  a. It blocks histamine receptors in target cells.
  b. It stabilizes capillary membranes.
  c. It acts as a nonspecific antagonist.
  d. It breaks the antigen-antibody bonding.

5. Why was intubation necessary to maintain airway patency?
  a. Increased mucus production
  b. Bronchospasm
  c. Impaired alveolar gas exchange
  d. Laryngeal edema

Answers

1. a. The penicillin served as an antigen to produce an immunological hypersensitivity reaction. Because of the patient's vague past history of antibiotic use, it would be difficult to determine if the anaphylactic shock was a primary or secondary immune response. The intravenous penicillin reacted with IgE antibodies bound to basophils in the blood. This antigen-antibody response stimulated cellular degranulation and the release of histamine.

   IgG immunoglobulins are extravascular and function in response to viral and bacterial infections, as well as toxin neutralization. A type IV delayed hypersensitivity is mediated by sensitized T-lymphocytes. This is an example of cellular immunity.

2. a and b. Histamine is the primary chemical mediator of anaphylaxis. It is released from the mast cells or basophils following the antigen-antibody reaction. The effects of histamine include increased capillary permeability, smooth muscle contraction, and capillary dilation. These actions are the result of histamine binding with both H_1 and H_2 receptors.

3. b and c. The effect of histamine and other chemical mediators of anaphylaxis is capillary vasodilation. This contributes to the hypotension that is characteristic of anaphylaxis. The other factor that contributes to the hypotension in anaphylactic shock is the plasma-to-interstitial fluid shift. The fluid shift is also the result of histamine's effect. Histamine causes the cells lining capillaries to separate at their junctions. The gaps between the cells allow plasma proteins and fluid to move from intravascular to interstitial spaces. The movement of fluid produces a decrease in circulating volume and a decrease in blood pressure.

4. c. Epinephrine is a sympathomimetic drug, and as such it acts as a nonspecific antagonist in anaphylaxis. It acts as a powerful bronchodilator to improve ventilation. Epinephrine improves circulation by vasoconstriction, increased strength of myocardial contraction, and counteracting the systemic effects of histamine and the other chemical mediators.

The antihistamines occupy receptors on target cells to block histamine. These drugs are not effective against other chemical mediators. Although epinephrine has a rapid action, the antihistamines are slower acting in anaphylaxis. Steroids are used in anaphylaxis because of their action in stabilizing capillary membranes.

5. d. Edema of the upper airways and the larynx occur as a result of the fluid shift from capillaries to tissue spaces. This edema can be severe enough to produce respiratory obstruction. Simple oral airways will be useless in maintaining an open airway as the edema progresses.

REFERENCES

Alexander, J.W., and Good, R.A.: Fundamentals of clinical immunology, Philadelphia, 1977, W.B. Saunders Co.

Bacal, E., Patterson, R., and Zeiss, C.R.: Evaluation of severe (anaphylactic) reactions, Clinical Allergy **8:**295-304, 1978.

Bowry, T.R.: Immunology simplified, Oxford, 1977, Oxford University Press.

Budassi, S.A., and Barber, J.M.: Emergency nursing: principles and practice, St. Louis, 1981, The C.V. Mosby Co.

Busse, W.W., and Yunginger, J.W.: The use of the radioallergosorbent test in the diagnosis of Hymenoptera anaphylaxis, Clinical Allergy **8:**471-477, 1978.

Busse, W.W., Reed, C.E., Lichtenstein, L.M., and Risman, R.E.: Immunotherapy in bee-sting anaphylaxis: use of honeybee venom, Journal of the American Medical Association **231:**1154-1156, 1975.

Carloss, H.: Transient electrocardiographic changes in anaphylaxis, Southern Medical Journal **69:**1621-1622, 1976.

Coombs, R.R.A., and Gell, P.G.H.: Clinical aspects of immunology, Philadelphia, 1963, F.A. Davis Co.

Darsee, J.R.: EKG changes and anaphylaxis (letter), Southern Medical Journal **70:**1249, 1977.

Epstein, N.: Acute reactions to urographic contrast media, Annals of Allergy **39:**139-141, 1977.

Ford, R.M.: The management of acute allergic disease including anaphylaxis, The Medical Journal of Australia **1:**222-223, 1977.

Goldman, R.A., Lewis, A.E., and Rose, L.I.: Anaphylactoid reaction to single-component pork insulin, Journal of the American Medical Association **236:**1148-1149, 1976.

Goodman, L.S., and Gilman, A.: The pharmacological basis of therapeutics, ed. 5, New York, 1975, Macmillan Publishing Co., Inc.

Gorevic, P., and Kaplan, A.P.: Contrast agents and anaphylactic-like reactions (editorial), Journal of Allergy and Clinical Immunology **63:**225-227, 1979.

Gottlieb, P.M.: Summary of a consensus development conference on emergency treatment of insect sting allergy, The Journal of Infectious Diseases **139:**250-252, 1979.

Nayes, J.H., Boyd, G.K., and Settipane, G.A.: Anaphylaxis to sunflower seeds, Journal of Allergy and Clinical Immunology **63:**242-244, 1979.

Obeid, A.I., et al.: Fluid therapy in severe systemic reaction to radiopaque dye, Annals of Internal Medicine **83:**317-320, 1975.

Patterson, R., and Schatz, M.: Factitious allergic emergencies: anaphylaxis and laryngeal "edema,"

Journal of Allergy and Clinical Immunology **56:** 152-159, 1975.

Roesel, C.E.: Immunology: a self-instructional approach, New York, 1978, McGraw-Hill Book Co.

Routledge, R.C., DeKretser, D.M.H., and Wadsworth, L.D.: Severe anaphylaxis due to passive sensitization by donor blood, British Medical Journal **1**(6007):434, 1976.

Settipane, G.A., Klein, D.E., and Boyd, G.K.: Relationship of atopy and anaphylactic sensitization: a bee sting allergy model, Clinical Allergy **8:**259-265, 1978.

Tannenbaum, H., Ruddy, S., and Schur, P.H.: Acute anaphylaxis associated with serum complement depletion, Journal of Allergy and Clinical Immunology **56:**226-234, 1975.

Viner, N.A., and Rhamy, R.K.: Anaphylaxis manifested by hypotension alone, The Journal of Urology **113:**108-110, 1975.

Wiener, M.B., Pepper, G.A., Kuhn-Weisman, G., and Romano, J.A.: Clinical pharmacology and therapeutics in nursing. New York, 1979, McGraw-Hill Book Co.

PART THREE

COMPLICATIONS OF SHOCK

11 Introduction to complications of shock

JUDITH L. MYERS

The effects of tissue hypoperfusion associated with shock can produce complications as serious and as life threatening as the original episode of shock. The occurrence of complications can prolong the patient's hospitalization and in some instances contribute to the development of long-term health problems. Early identification of complications prompts treatment measures designed to lessen their severity. However, early detection is not possible in all cases since the early signs of many of these complications can be overshadowed by the shock mechanism. Therefore the tissue injury producing the complications is far advanced before it is recognized. Through continuous assessment of the patient, the nurse assumes a major role in the identification of possible complications.

Assessment of the patient for complications needs to be based on the pathophysiology of the shock and the resultant response of various body systems to reduced cellular perfusion. In addition, the nurse must understand the compensatory adaptive mechanisms of the body in shock. Failure of these mechanisms places the patient at risk for the development of complications. Knowledge of side effects associated with the various treatments of shock should also serve as a guideline for assessment of possible complications.

Are the complications of shock preventable? The key element in answering this question is the duration of shock. The longer a patient is in shock, the longer the body tissues are hypoxic. When tissue hypoxia is prolonged, changes occur in cellular metabolism that can lead to cell death and produce an irreversible stage of shock. Data reported by Shah, Dutton, Newell, and Powers (1977) and Day, Friedman, and Morton (1977) indicate that some changes in peripheral circulation and in cellular electrolytes may not completely recover despite adequate fluid resuscitation of the patient. Delayed recovery in the microcirculation and in cellular metabolism may contribute to the development of many of the complications in shock.

The nursing care given to the patient in shock is important in reducing the risks of complications. Since the major factor in the development of complications is tissue hypoxia, nursing care should focus on measures to decrease hypoxia. Because of the compensatory changes in microcirculation, it may not be feasible to increase the delivery of oxygen to the tissues. However, interventions that decrease the metabolic demands for oxygen may help limit the degree of tissue hypoxia.

Limitation of physical activity obviously decreases oxygen demand. Nursing measures that control infection and reduce the development of fever should be implemented. Infection and fever increase tissue metabolism and further contribute to tissue hypoxia by increasing oxygen demand. Anxiety must be reduced through the use of appropriate analgesics, sedatives, and psychosocial nursing measures. Effective control of anxiety will reduce oxygen demand. Finally it is obvious that any underlying processes that increase metabolic activity, such as hyperthyroidism or pregnancy, must be taken into account when attempting to decrease tissue oxygen demands.

The three chapters in this section will each focus on an organ system and its response to prolonged decreases in cellular perfusion. The adult respiratory distress syndrome (ARDS) will serve as a model for discussion of the lung's response to shock. Changes in blood flow and coagulation that alter normal hemostasis will be examined in the chapter on disseminated intravascular coagulation (DIC). The chapter on acute renal failure will present the effects of decreased renal perfusion. Although prolonged tissue hypoxia affects all body systems and has the potential to produce complications, these three conditions were selected to represent the organizational framework of this text. The frequency with which these complications occur and their potential for producing irreversible damage warrants their discussion in more detail than other complications. The organ failure associated with each of these complications contributes to the irreversible stage of prolonged shock and increases the mortality from shock. In addition to a discussion of the relationship of the particular complication to shock, each chapter will present the necessary nursing assessment. Implications for nursing care will also be included.

SUMMARY OF THE EFFECTS OF SHOCK ON CELLULAR METABOLISM
Anaerobic metabolism

Poor tissue perfusion produces changes in cellular metabolism regardless of the type of shock (Fig. 11-1). A decrease in the delivery of oxygen to the cells changes their metabolism from aerobic to anaerobic pathways. As a result of the changes in metabolism, the patient in shock develops metabolic acidosis. As blood pH levels decrease in acidosis, a compensatory respiratory alkalosis develops leading to a decreased Pco_2. In anaerobic metabolism cells produce very little adenosine triphosphate (ATP) to use for energy. The normal 38 moles of ATP used for energy in aerobic metabolism is reduced to less than 8 moles under anaerobic conditions (Fritz, 1975; Schumer, 1976).

Glucose metabolism

Glucose from glycogen stores is used early in shock to provide fuel for energy metabolism. In normal aerobic pathways the glucose will enter the Krebs cycle and be used to form ATP with carbon dioxide and water byproducts. Any lactic acid that is produced undergoes conversion to pyruvate and follows the usual metabolic route. When oxygen is lacking, as in shock, lactic acid is not converted to pyruvate.

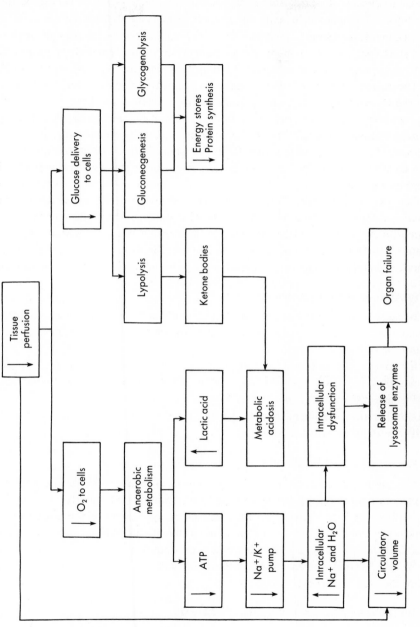

Fig. 11-1. Alterations in cellular metabolism.

Lack of sufficient glucose to support energy production also contributes to the depressed metabolism in shock. A release of catecholamines early in shock stimulates glycogenolysis. The increase in available glucose produces a hyperglycemia to meet the increased demands for energy substrate. Depending on the patient's nutritional status prior to shock, the hyperglycemia will last until glycogen stores are depleted. Schumer (1976) reported that glycogen stores are depleted within 6 hours after the onset of hypovolemic shock. The increased activity of epinephrine in shock inhibits the release of insulin. Without the presence of insulin there is increased glycogenolysis, lipolysis, and release of amino acids from the cell. The use of amino acids for gluconeogenesis has been studied in shock. Alanine, the primary amino acid released from muscles during shock, accounts for most gluconeogenesis (Fritz, 1975; Schumer, 1976). The utilization of alanine is a protective mechanism for the brain. Its use maintains a source of glucose after glycogen stores are depleted.

The increased peripheral uptake of glucose in shock is stimulated by the anoxia and the elevated serum glucose level. This activity is independent of the action of insulin. However, O'Donnell and Belkin (1978) state that the increased extraction of oxygen and substrate fuels by tissues in shock is limited. As blood flow continues to decrease, these mechanisms are no longer compensatory.

Protein and fat metabolism

Because of the impairment of liver function in shock, the conversion of fatty acids and amino acids through gluconeogenesis is also impaired. Decreased blood flow to adipose tissue in shock limits the mobilization of fats for gluconeogenesis. The utilization of fats for energy in this stress situation adds to the acidosis in shock. Ketone bodies, byproducts of fatty acid oxidation, are acid in nature. The liver is normally able to oxidize the ketones. However, poor oxygen perfusion of the liver in shock limits its ability to clear the ketones. Peripheral tissues that normally metabolize ketones are unable to cope with the increased load.

Electrolyte and fluid shifts

The diminished energy supply in the form of ATP alters the function of the sodium-potassium pump on the cell membrane. The ion pump is normally ATP dependent in its function. The result of pump malfunction is the movement of sodium into the cell and a movement of potassium out of the cell. Water moves with the Na^+ into the cell. The fluid shift has two effects. First, it further contributes to the reduction in circulating blood volume. Second, the increased intracellular water causes swelling and more disruption of metabolic activity.

EFFECTS OF SHOCK ON ORGAN SYSTEMS

The effects of tissue hypoxia can be variable, based on the oxygen requirements of each vital organ. The integrity of a specific organ before the onset of shock will also influence that organ's ability to withstand the effects of anoxia. A previously diseased myocardium, lung, or kidney is more prone to permanent injury in shock because of diminished reserve capacity.

Brain

Although compensatory circulatory mechanisms shunt blood to the brain from other areas of the body, disruptions in cerebral function and permanent brain injury can occur in shock. Decreases in cerebral circulation result in cerebral hypoxia. Prolonged shock and brain hypoxia have been implicated as causes of acquired seizure disorders (Norman and Brown, 1981). Brain injury in shock can also develop as a result of cerebral infarction or cerebral thombus formation. Changes in blood flow and coagulation contribute to the occurrence of these problems. Alterations in cellular metabolism throughout the body, accompanied by increasing acidosis and the accumulation of toxic substances, can further depress cerebral function. Even after recovery from shock, the patient may experience permanent alterations in perception and coordination (Jones, Dunbar, and Jivorec, 1978).

In the early stages of shock the patient may experience anxiety and restlessness. As cerebral tissue oxygenation diminishes, the nurse will see decreases in the patient's level of consciousness. Lethargy, stupor, and coma develop as the shock becomes more progressive. In the irreversible stage of shock, cerebral blood flow is decreased to the point of disrupting the normal vasomotor centers in the brain, causing failure of the circulatory compensatory mechanisms. The additional loss of cardiac output further decreases cerebral perfusion pressures, creating a vicious cycle.

Myocardium

The myocardium is more vulnerable to the effects of decreased blood flow because it cannot greatly increase oxygen extraction as can other tissues and organs. The myocardium already extracts more oxygen from the blood than any other body tissues. Decreased

---

Alterations in cerebral function in shock

Contributing factors

Decreased blood flow (cerebral hypoxia infarction)
Metabolic acidosis
Coagulation changes (cerebral thrombosis)

Patient responses

Early: anxiety, restlessness
Later: lethargy, stupor, coma, or seizures
Irreversible: vasomotor center dysfunction

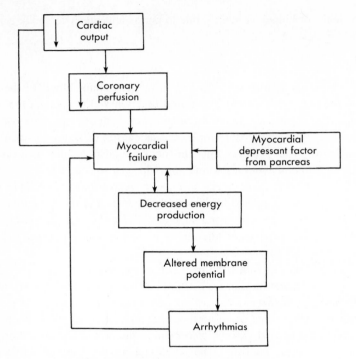

Fig. 11-2. Myocardial failure in shock.

coronary blood flow in shock further contributes to myocardial depression and decreased cardiac output (Fig. 11-2). In shock the coronary arteries are more pressure dependent (Phipps, Long, and Woods, 1979). If the patient already has underlying coronary artery disease, the coronary vessels cannot vasodilate in an autoregulatory way. Another factor that contributes to myocardial failure during shock is the release of myocardial depressant factor (MDF) from the pancreas. The production of MDF is associated with the presence of lysosomal enzymes (Schumer, 1976). The lysosomal enzymes and the depression of myocardial function are implicated in the progression of shock to the irreversible stage. As the heart becomes ischemic, it begins to produce lactate rather than using it for metabolism. Alterations in the ability of the heart to use free fatty acids for metabolism also develop in the ischemic myocardium (Baue, 1976). Disruptions in the normal Na^+/K^+ pump through cell membranes also contribute to complications in the myocardium. Arrhythmias are more likely to develop with alterations in cell membrane potential (O'Donnell and Belkin, 1978). In addition to the occurrence of arrhythmias, other clinical signs of myocardial depression include a continued fall in cardiac output and an increased venous pressure. Baue (1976) states that regardless of the initial cause, when shock is prolonged and severe there may ultimately be depression of the myocardium.

Vascular changes in shock

Vascular component	Early stage	Late stage
Arterial capillary sphincters	Constricted	Open
Venous capillary sphincters	Open	Constricted
Capillary pressures	Low	High
Fluid movement	Extracellular to intravascular	Intravascular to extracellular
Net result	Restoration of circulatory volume	Decreased circulatory volume
		Tissue swelling
		Altered cell metabolism

Peripheral circulation

Shock may impair vascular autoregulatory mechanisms that initially provide compensation for the changes in cardiac output and circulatory volume. The primary mechanisms that support circulatory volume after significant fluid loss are vasoconstriction of capacitance vessels, primarily in the splanchnic bed, and capillary refilling of blood volume from extracellular fluid. In the early stage of shock arterial capillary sphincters remain open. These changes lower capillary intravascular pressure. As a result there is a net movement of extracellular fluid into the intravascular system. The shift in fluid assists in the restoration of plasma volume. When these early compensatory mechanisms fail, circulatory adjustments will occur to maintain blood flow as much as possible in the central circulation of the heart and brain. There will be reduced blood flow to other organs such as the kidney, liver, and skeletal muscle. Secretion of aldosterone and antidiuretic hormone favor retention of sodium and water by the kidney to preserve intravascular volume.

In the late stages of shock the prolonged sympathetic response and vasoconstriction contribute to the development of tissue hypoxia. Kinins from ischemic tissues override sympathetic tone and promote vasodilation. The arterial capillary sphincters dilate, and venous capillary sphincters constrict. These changes in the microcirculation produce an increase in capillary hydrostatic pressure. Fluid movement reverses from that seen during the early stage of shock. Intravascular fluid begins shifting into extravascular spaces. As fluid leaves the intravascular compartment, there is a further decrease in circulatory volume, an additional decrease in arterial pressure, aggravation of tissue hypoxia, and disruption of cellular metabolism.

Gastrointestinal system

As shock progresses and diminished tissue perfusion continues, there is a decrease in the various functions of the hepatic and gastrointestinal systems. Changes in the integrity of the intestines during shock plays an important role in the progression to an irreversible stage. Compensatory vasoconstriction in shock seems to affect the bowel mucosa more significantly than other body systems. Mucosal ischemia and full-thickness gangrene of the bowel wall are manifested as ileus (Silen, 1976). For this reason the assessment of the patient in shock should include auscultation for absence of bowel sounds. Disruption of the bowel wall by necrosis permits the normal bacterial flora of the intestines to enter the circulatory system. Another consequence of the loss of bowel integrity is gastrointestinal bleeding. Changes in coagulation may contribute to the bleeding in the intestines.

Ischemia in the gastric mucosa initiates a superficial erosion that is known as stress ulcers. Silen and Skillman (1976) note that an increase in back diffusion of hydrogen ions in shock may also be important in the pathogenesis of stress ulcers. Bleeding will be the primary manifestation of the presence of ulcers. The prophylactic use of antacids to buffer the contents of the stomach has been successful in preventing the development of stress ulcers.

Hepatic system

Many factors in shock contribute to the depression of the function of the hepatic system. First, there is a decreased blood flow to the liver. The necrotic damage is found primarily in the centrilobular hepatocytes. Vasoconstriction of the splanchnic blood vessels occurs throughout the stages of shock and is aggravated by the administration of vasopressor agents. Changes in the microcirculation result in pooling of blood in the hepatic veins and arteries. Decreased blood flow through the portal circulation also adds to hepatic hypoxia. The portal vein supplies over half the oxygenated blood to the liver. Right-sided heart failure will further compromise hepatic function, resulting in a back flow pressure buildup and pooling of blood in the liver.

This impairment of liver function in shock affects protein, carbohydrate, and fat metabolism. In addition, detoxification of toxic materials, especially those released from bacterial activity, is also diminished. When the reticuloendothelial system (RES) of the liver is lost in shock, there is an increased risk of infection. In this situation septicemia may intensify the problems of the initial shock. Impairment of liver function also contributes to the metabolic acidosis. The liver is no longer able to play a role in lactic acid conversion. Disruption of the liver's ability to manage bilirubin occurs. The uptake, conjugation, and excretion of bilirubin will be altered. Massive transfusions, large hematomas, and hemolysis by bacterial toxins will also contribute to the bilirubin load (Silen and Skillman, 1976; Ledgerwood, 1976).

Jaundice will be an early indication of liver damage associated with shock and may appear as early as 1 to 2 days after the onset of shock. There will also be a rise in serum bilirubin levels and serum enzymes. Without sepsis the bilirubin will usually be less than 4 to 5 mg/100 ml. However, in some cases in which sepsis accompanies the shock, the bilirubin may rise as high as 40 mg/100 ml. Alkaline phosphatase levels will also rise in conjunction with the rise in bilirubin. Even after the patient's recovery,

---

The liver in shock

Factors contributing to damage

Decreased blood flow
Splanchnic vasoconstriction
Vasopressor agents
Pooling of blood in microcirculation
Right heart failure
Bacterial invasion

Changes in liver

Hepatocyte necrosis
Loss of RES
Altered energy metabolism
    Glycogenolysis
    Gluconeogenesis
Decreased lactic acid conversion
Altered bilirubin function

Results of damage

Metabolic acidosis
Jaundice
Decreased glucose availability
Increased infection
Decreased albumin

---

the alkaline phosphatase may remain elevated for several weeks. Elevations of serum glutamic oxaloacetic transaminase (SGOT) and lactic dehydrogenase (LDH) also occur with liver damage. Serum albumin levels will be decreased, and serum globulin levels will be increased. The decreased albumin will affect the transport of substances normally bound to it in the blood; therefore the patient's response to drugs that are normally transported by albumin will be affected in this situation.

• • •

In summary, it is important to remember that in shock the common denominator, regardless of the type of shock, is decreased cellular perfusion. The length of time tissues are hypoxic will be a factor in determining the kind of complications that will occur in shock. The longer hypoxia is present in tissues, the more their ability to compensate for the lack of oxygen diminishes. Changes in cell metabolism and prolonged anoxia lead to cell destruction and organ failure. As shock progresses to an irreversible stage, the patient's chance of recovery without permanent injury decreases.

REFERENCES

Baue, A.E.: Metabolic abnormalities of shock, Surgical Clinics of North America **56:**1059-1071, 1976.

Day, B., Friedman, S.M., and Morton, K.S.: Cell sodium and potassium changes in hemorrhagic shock measured by a lithium substitution method, Surgical Forum **28:**1-2, 1977.

Fritz, S.D.: Energy metabolism in shock, Heart & Lung **4:**615-618, 1975.

Gann, D.S.: Endocrine control of plasma protein and volume, Surgical Clinics of North America **56:** 1135-1145, 1976.

Jones, D.A., Dunbar, C.F., and Jivorec, M.M.: Medical-surgical nursing: a conceptual approach, St. Louis, 1978, McGraw-Hill Book Co.

Ledgerwood, A.: Hepatobiliary complications of sepsis, Heart & Lung **5:**621-623, 1976.

Luckmann, J., and Sorensen, K.C.: Medical-surgical nursing: a psychophysiologic approach, ed. 2, Philadelphia, 1980, W.B. Saunders Co.

Norman, S.E., and Browne, T.R.: Seizure disorders, American Journal of Nursing **81:**984-989, 1981.

O'Donnell, T.F., and Belkin, S.C.: The pathophysiology, monitoring and treatment of shock, Orthopedic Clinics of North America **9:**589-610, 1978.

Phipps, W.J., Long, B.C., and Woods, N.F.: Medical-surgical nursing: concepts and clinical practice, St. Louis, 1979, The C.V. Mosby Co.

Schumer, W.: Metabolism during shock and sepsis, Heart & Lung **5:**416-421, 1976.

Shah, D.M., Dutton, R.E., Newell, J.C., and Powers, S.R., Jr.: Vascular autoregulatory failure following trauma and shock, Surgical Forum 1977, **28:**11-13, 1977.

Silen, W., and Skillman, J.J.: Gastrointestinal responses to injury and infection, Surgical Clinics of North America **56:**945-952, 1976.

12 The adult respiratory distress syndrome

PATRICIA POTTER

The adult respiratory distress syndrome (ARDS) is becoming a familiar term to critical-care nurses. ARDS has become more readily recognized largely because of a developing consensus of its clinical picture. ARDS is a relatively new syndrome that was first recognized near the end of World War II but clearly documented during the Vietnam War. Special circumstances during this time in history allowed physicians to observe the course of ARDS in patients who suffered this unique syndrome. These circumstances included the rapid helicopter evacuation of soldiers with massive trauma and blood loss, who would have died early in previous wars, and the opportunity for these soldiers to obtain medical care at special treatment centers 15 to 20 minutes later. As a result of a greater survival rate the injured soldiers were observed for a longer period of time. A pattern formed in which patients received rapid treatment and recovered from initial shock and trauma. However, they were also noted to develop respiratory failure after a period of 12 to 24 hours. Since the Vietnam War, a similar syndrome has been identified in civilian settings. The term *ARDS* has been used synonymously with many others. Currently it has come to be recognized as a common clinical entity complicating diverse disease states.

As is the case with various terminologies, definitions for ARDS have not often been concise. The syndrome has no common etiology or diagnostic test. For this reason it is often defined descriptively on the basis of clinical findings. It is a clinical and pathological condition characterized by pulmonary edema that occurs in the presence of normal left atrial and pulmonary venous pressures (Burki, 1978). Conditions associated with noncardiogenic pulmonary edema, such as fluid overload and acute bacterial pneumonia, are excluded from the syndrome. The physiological hallmark of ARDS is severe hypoxemia that is unresponsive to high concentrations of inspired oxygen. The syndrome is characterized by respiratory alterations including severe dyspnea and tachypnea. Physiologically ARDS impairs lung function by decreasing compliance and oxygen transport. Because of the nonspecificity of defining characteristics, there are a number of conditions that superficially resemble ARDS:

Cardiac pulmonary edema

Acute hypersensitivity lung disease

Fluid overload

Chronic interstitial fibrosis

Acute exacerbation of chronic lung disease

Common terms that describe the adult respiratory dystress syndrome

Shock lung
White lung
Wet lung
Da Nang lung
Pump lung
Respirator lung
Congestive atelectasis
Progressive pulmonary failure
Adult hyaline membrane disease

Causal factors associated with adult respiratory distress syndrome

Trauma and hemorrhage shock (Chest, abdominal, other)
Aspiration of gastric contents
Septic and nonseptic shock
Disseminated intravascular coagulation
Fat and air embolism
Drug ingestion
Oxygen toxicity
Homologous blood transfusion
Pancreatitis
Viral pneumonia
Uremia
Anaphylaxis
Fluid overload

However, the differences seen in pathophysiology, pathology, and treatment support their exclusion from the syndrome.

It is the purpose of this chapter to discuss ARDS as a complication following shock. It is of interest to note that ARDS may have a multiplicity of causes. Note that any number of these conditions may occur as added complications of shock. As a result the course and prognosis of ARDS are quite variable. The precipitating factors leading to the pathogenesis of ARDS must be identified so that proper management can be attained.

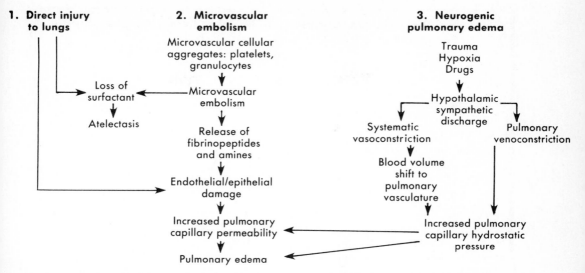

Fig. 12-1. Postulated mechanisms of development of ARDS. (From Burki, N.K.: Southern Medical Journal **71:**1411-1415, 1978.)

PATHOPHYSIOLOGY

The precise pathological mechanism of ARDS is still unclear. Current concepts describing the precipitating events leading to ARDS are summarized in Fig. 12-1. The eventual development of pulmonary edema is believed to result initially from a period of pulmonary hypoperfusion. When ARDS is associated with shock, particularly septic shock, it appears that the primary event is the development of microvascular aggregation of formed blood elements, including white blood cells and platelets. These aggregates create mechanical obstruction to blood flow within the pulmonary microcirculatory bed. Peripheral venous thrombi may develop and embolize into the pulmonary circulation. Coupled with the obstruction to pulmonary blood flow is the release of humoral vasoactive substances. Many of these agents, such as adrenocorticotropic hormone, may simply be released as part of the stress response rather than being responsible for the pathophysiology of ARDS. However, certain of these agents create specific pathological alterations. Serotonin, when released into the pulmonary circulation, causes constriction in the postcapillary venules. Histamine, bradykinin, and catecholamines result in vasoconstriction, bronchoconstriction, and alterations in alveolar-capillary membrane permeability. The fact that the lung becomes vulnerable to the effects of these vasoactive substances is particularly significant. Normally the lungs play a role in regulating the homeostasis of these mediators. A pathological effect on the lung itself by the vasoactive substances implies a prior impairment of metabolic activity of the lung.

The vasoactive agents affect the capillary membrane itself, causing the endothelium to become more permeable. There is initially intense vasoconstriction on the

---

Humoral vasoactive substances believed to have a role in development of ARDS

Adrenocorticotropic hormone (ACTH)
Adrenocortical hormone
Catecholamines
Renin
Serotonin
Kinins (e.g., bradykinin)
Prostaglandins
Histamine
Angiotensin
Complement
Fibrin

---

arterial and venous ends of the pulmonary capillaries. Eventually the precapillary arterial end relaxes, but the postcapillary venous end remains constricted. This increases the hydrostatic pressure within the pulmonary circulation, creating a net force that drives fluid out of the damaged capillary endothelium and into the alveoli. Fluid initially enters the interstitial spaces surrounding alveoli. There can also be perivascular and peribronchial edema and thickening of alveolar septa (Burke, 1978). Eventually protein escapes through the capillary membrane, upsetting the balance of oncotic pressure and pulling more fluid into the alveoli themselves.

The impairment of local pulmonary capillary blood flow creates metabolic alterations including hypoxia and lactic acidosis. The normal physiological response of the pulmonary circulation to local hypoxia is vasoconstriction. This occurs in an effort to shunt blood flow away from underventilated alveoli and toward adequately ventilated alveoli. Vasoconstriction eventually increases PA pressure complicating the pathological picture of ARDS by forcing more fluid into alveoli.

Persistent hypoxemia increases the cellular and mitochondrial hypoxia produced as a result of deficient microcirculatory perfusion. Mitochondria of the alveolar type II cell are believed to produce surfactant. Impaired capillary perfusion seen in ARDS decreases surfactant production by the alveolar type II cell. Atelectasis occurs, decreasing the available surface area for gas exchange and aggravating the hypoxemia. Atelectasis and edema combine to reduce the compliance of the lung, making it extremely stiff. Impairment in the ability of the lung to increase its volume for a given change in pressure results in a reduction in functional residual capacity and vital capacity.

As to the exact cause of hypoxemia there is some controversy whether ventilation-perfusion abnormalities, diffusion impairment, or right to left intrapulmonary shunting are the mechanisms involved. The degree to which ARDS has advanced seems to determine which of these physiological alterations dominates the pathophysiological picture. In the early stages it is doubtful that peribronchial, perivascular, and alveolar interstitial edema significantly interfere with gas exchange. Later as the syndrome progresses, it was found that the hypoxemia is caused by the presence of shunt or units of a very low ratio of ventilation to perfusion (Dantzker et al., 1979).

NURSING ASSESSMENT

Early recognition is the key to the successful management and cure of ARDS. Prompt identification of clinical signs can avoid complications resulting from mismanagement of oxygen, ventilators, fluids, and drugs. However, early clinical signs are often subtle, failing to lead the clinician to early detection of the syndrome. Being alert for the development of clinical signs in patients most at risk can facilitate reaching a diagnosis.

Clinical signs

Dyspnea. Difficulty in breathing is directly related to the increased work of breathing. The stiffness of a noncompliant lung demands a gerater expense of energy for ventilation to occur. In a young, healthy individual dyspnea may not appear early because of the capacity of doubling or tripling minute ventilation during rest.

Restlessness. Restlessness occurs as a result of the developing hypoxemia. Cerebral hypoxia is manifested by behavioral alterations and impaired levels of consciousness.

Cough. The cough of ARDS develops as a result of the presence of edema within the airways.

Grunting respirations with active use of intercostals. The individual who must increase the work of breathing exhibits the active use of the accessory muscles of ventilation. The resultant increased movement of the chest wall works to increase the volume of gas delivered to the airways.

Cyanosis. If arterial oxygen desaturation develops, the color of circulating blood takes on a darkened tint. If the Pao_2 stays above 60 mm Hg, the hemoglobin oxygen saturation is greater than 85% and cyanosis will not appear. Cyanosis is not a reliable index. Identification is influenced by hemoglobin concentration, peripheral perfusion, and the ability of the examiner to perceive color changes.

Pallor. The skin will likely appear pale if peripheral hypoperfusion is present. Vasoconstriction shunts blood flow away from the skin to organs in greater need.

Lung sounds. Continuous assessment of lung sounds may reveal the progressive nature of ARDS. Early in the course of the disease lung sounds remain clear. As ARDS advances, rales may be auscultated as a result of developing edema in the airways. Harsh bronchial sounds can be heard over all lung fields as a late development.

Ventilator inspiratory pressure. If a patient is already on a ventilator as ARDS develops, the first finding may be an increase in the pressure required to deliver a given tidal volume. An increase in the inspiratory pressure is evidence of a drop in pulmonary compliance.

Diagnostic measures

A sensitive test for the early detection of ARDS does not exist. Tests of gas exchange, tests of mechanical function, and roentgenographic analysis are used in evaluating and managing ARDS. Hematological studies of formed blood elements, such as the DIC profile, and of liver and kidney function may assist the clinician to understand the patient more fully or yield clues to the etiology of the syndrome.

Proper interpretation of arterial blood gases is critical. A key finding in ARDS is a lowered Pao_2 that fails to respond to increased oxygen concentrations in the inspired air. Peters (1979) provides some guidelines for the interpretation of the adequacy of alveolar ventilation. If the pH is below 7.35, then the clinician must check whether the Pao_2 is above or below 40 mm Hg. A $Paco_2$ greater than 40 mm Hg indicates inadequate alveolar ventilation. Looking at another situation, if the pH is below 7.35 and the $Paco_2$ is at 40 mm Hg, alveolar ventilation is still inadequate. This is because the patient is unable to increase alveolar ventilation in response to the metabolic acidosis. Likewise if the Pao_2 is below 75 mm Hg and the $Paco_2$ is at 40 mm Hg, alveolar ventilation is unsatisfactory since the patient fails to hyperventilate in response to lowered oxygen levels.

A more precise means to interpret alveolar function is the use of $P(A - a)o_2$. This value assesses the difficulty with which oxygen diffuses from the alveolus across the alveolar capillary membrane and into the arterial blood. The normal $P(A - a)o_2$ value should be less than 15 mm Hg on room air. In ARDS the $P(A - a)o_2$ may reach values of 200 to 500 mm Hg or more. This measurement is more useful than the arterial Po_2 level to indicate what is occurring at the alveolar membrane. Chapter 4 provides a complete discussion of $P(A - a)o_2$.

The shunt fraction may also prove a useful indicator of the progression of ARDS. In a shunt, blood reaches the arterial system without passing through ventilated portions of the lung. The higher the shunt fraction the greater the inadequacy of oxygenation and carbon dioxide removal.

Tests of mechanical function reveal the patient's cardiac and pulmonary status. The cardiac output plays an indirect role with regard to intrapulmonary shunting. When the cardiac output is decreased, the tissues normally extract more oxygen from the blood to meet oxygen demands. As a result oxygen content in venous blood is lowered. In the presence of an intrapulmonary shunt, a decreased venous Po_2 will decrease the arterial oxygen content. In ARDS the lung cannot compensate to increase oxygenation of venous blood. Therefore since venous Po_2 is dependent on cardiac output, the cardiac output indirectly controls the Pao_2 and available oxygen. The cardiac output in ARDS may remain normal or even elevated as a compensatory response to hypoxia. However, as a side effect of the ventilatory support often required in ARDS the cardiac output may drop. Careful monitoring via the Swan-Ganz catheter is vital. It is impossible to differentiate ARDS from left ventricular failure without the use of hemodynamic monitoring. The PCWP as well as PA pressure should be normal in ARDS.

Diagnostic tests used to detect ARDS

Tests of gas exchange
   Arterial blood gases
   Alveolar-arterial oxygen difference
   Shunt fraction
Tests of mechanical function
   Cardiac
      PWCP, PA pressure, cardiac output
   Pulmonary
      Compliance
      Lung volumes
Roentgenographic

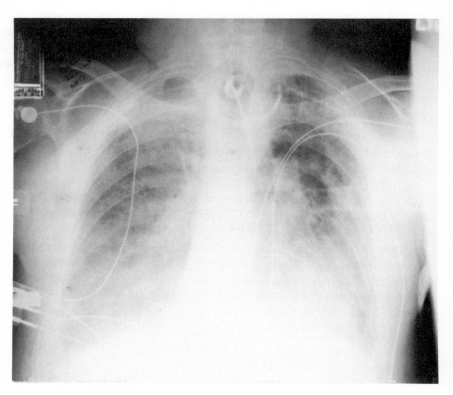

Fig. 12-2. Typical chest film revealing the "white-out" of ARDS.

Tests of mechanical lung function reveal decreases in static and dynamic compliance. The presence of fluid in the lungs prevents their normal ease of expansion under slight changes of intrathoracic pressure. With a noncompliant lung more energy is required to maintain lung expansion and lung volumes are altered. The functional residual capacity (FRC) and vital capacity (VC) are decreased. The ratio of dead space to tidal volume is increased, indicating a reduction in the percentage of air reaching those airways responsible for gas exchange.

The chest x-ray film does not serve as an early indicator of ARDS. It usually appears normal early in the course of the disease. Eventually changes in the radiological picture occur as the result of the movement of fluid out of the pulmonary capillaries and into the interstitium and alveoli. A large increase in lung water is required before the chest x-ray film is seen as abnormal. The "white out" seen on x-ray films is characteristic of ARDS (Fig. 12-2). Heart size should be normal, a finding that discriminates ARDS from left heart failure.

MEDICAL AND NURSING MANAGEMENT

The physician and nurse must work collaboratively in managing the patient with ARDS. The nurse may be the principle source of valuable assessment data used in predicting the occurrence and progression of the syndrome. Prevention is the key to success, but when ARDS does develop clinically, a multisystems management approach must be utilized. The goals of management of ARDS are mutually agreeable among most clinicians. However, controversy exists over the best treatment format. Most debate focuses on the type of pharmacological agents best suited for treating ARDS.

Treatment of underlying condition

Treatment of the underlying or precipitating condition is the first priority of care. The early complete correction of hypovolemia in shock is one of the best modes for preventing ARDS. Lake (1977) reported a general correlation between the severity and

---

Goals for management of ARDS

Treatment of underlying condition
Maintenance of adequate oxygenation
   Improvement of oxygen delivery
   Reduction of oxygen consumption
   Maintenance of oxygen transport
   Maintenance of cardiac output
Maintenance of fluid balance
Prevention of concomitant infection

length of hypotension and the development of ARDS. Collins (1977) reports that there may be an even greater association of ARDS with septic shock than with hypovolemia. In this case measures aimed at preventing pulmonary infection are of paramount importance.

Maintenance of oxygenation

Maintenance of adequate oxygenation becomes a priority concern once the diagnosis of ARDS has been established. This is achieved by way of four therapeutic modalities: (1) improvement in oxygen delivery, (2) reduction in oxygen consumption, (3) maintenance of oxygen transport, and (4) maintenance of cardiac output.

Initial attempts are made at increasing the FIO_2 to keep PaO_2 at or above 60 mm Hg. A PaO_2 above 60 mm Hg assures that the oxygen saturation will be greater than 85%. Below 55 mm Hg the hemoglobin saturation falls precipitously along the oxygen dissociation curve. Unless the FIO_2 is limited to a concentration of less than 50%, alveolar capillary damage, alveolar collapse, and oxygen toxicity may ensue (Bone, 1980; Peters, 1979). Typically advanced ARDS does not respond to conventional means of increasing the arterial oxygen (O_2 Venturi mask, nasal cannula, etc.). If maintenance of the PaO_2 requires an FIO_2 of greater than 50% for more than 24 hours, ventilatory management becomes necessary. The patient will be intubated with a low-pressure, cuffed, endotracheal tube.

Most patients in shock should be intubated and placed on a volume-cycled ventilator. The advantages of mechanical ventilation (Chapter 4) serve to benefit the patient with ARDS. When the patient is first ventilated, 100% oxygen is used to avoid hypoxic complications from a prolonged intubation procedure and/or misplacement of the endotracheal tube. The first arterial blood gas specimens are more acceptable if they show excess oxygenation instead of hypoxemia. Soon the FIO_2 is lowered below 50% to meet the goals of avoiding oxygen toxicity and maintain the PaO_2 at or above 50 mm Hg.

The patient connected to a volume ventilator is typically delivered a volume of 10 to 15 ml/kg body weight, which is nearly twice the normal tidal volume (Bone, 1980).

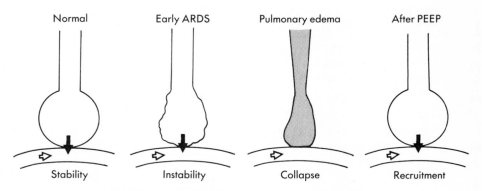

Normal	Early ARDS	Pulmonary edema	After PEEP
Stability	Instability	Collapse	Recruitment

Fig. 12-3. Influence of PEEP on alveoli in ARDS.

The elevation of tidal volumes serves to increase the FRC, maintain optimal compliance, and decrease oxygen consumption. If arterial hypoxemia persists, a common finding in ARDS, more aggressive therapy is warranted.

PEEP and continuous positive airway pressure (CPAP) are the therapies of choice. PEEP is the artificial maintenance of a positive pressure at the end of expiration. CPAP is the maintenance of above-atmospheric pressure throughout the respiratory cycle. The patient on CPAP is spontaneously breathing and may not be on a ventilator, whereas with PEEP the patient is ventilator dependent. Both PEEP and CPAP serve to increase the FRC, keep marginal alveoli from collapsing, and open collapsed alveoli. Dantzker et al. (1979) have evidence that PEEP increases the Pao_2 by decreasing the perfusion of unventilated lung units. The mechanism for this remains unclear.

The literature speaks to the use of PEEP more frequently in the management of ARDS. Research has demonstrated that the early use of PEEP significantly reduces the incidence of ARDS as well as the incidence of deaths and pulmonary morbidity (Weigelt, Mitchell, and Snyder, 1979). Knowledge of the patient's past medical history is crucial if PEEP is employed. Use of positive-pressure ventilation is contraindicated when the patient has a history of chronic obstructive pulmonary disease. Extremes in pressure can cause the rupture of already fragile alveoli and lung tissue.

PEEP is usually started at 3 to 5 cm H_2O and increased by increments of 3 to 5 cm H_2O until oxygenation is improved (Bone, 1980). Some clinicians prefer to set the level of PEEP on the basis of compliance curve measurements. In this situation the optimal amount of PEEP is believed to be the pressure at which tidal ventilation takes place on the point of maximum compliance. However, if the Pao_2 is adequately achieved at lower levels of PEEP, complications are less likely to occur.

PEEP can cause serious side effects including (1) increased work of breathing, (2) barotrauma to the lung (pneumothorax), and (3) depression of cardiac output. During PEEP, alveolar pressure must drop below atmosphere to initiate inhalation. Negative alveolar pressure during the inspiratory cycle is normal, but the degree to which it must become negative can dramatically increase the work of breathing. Rapid fatigue may develop, a factor that further places demands on the patient's depleted oxygen reserves.

High PEEP levels and/or tidal volumes may cause alveolar rupture leading to the collapse of all or part of the lung. In addition, PEEP has the potential for lowering cardiac output since an increase in airway pressure will increase the mean intrathoracic pressure and thus decrease venous return. However, since the lungs in ARDS are extremely stiff, the elevated airway pressure may not cause a significant increase in intrathoracic pressure. PEEP also increases the alveolar pressure of ventilated alveoli. The increased alveolar pressure compresses the pulmonary capillaries and reduces blood flow. Cardiac output may be lowered as a result of the increased vascular resistance. Simultaneously blood flow is redirected to collapsed alveoli, aggravating the degree of pulmonary shunt and the resultant hypoxemia.

Monitoring the patient on PEEP is critical. The nurse must be alert to signs of developing complications as well as signs of improved ventilation. Arterial blood gases must be measured to observe the response of arterial oxygen levels. The nurse responsible for drawing blood for arterial blood gases should recognize that any nursing or patient activity that temporarily alters oxygen delivery or demands should be avoided at least 15 minutes before the blood is obtained. Skelley, Deeren, and Powaser (1980) found that endotracheal suctioning without preoxygenation produced a fall in PaO_2 30 seconds after suctioning. Changing ventilator tubing or prolonged episodes of coughing may likewise significantly lower arterial oxygen values.

The nurse can also assist in the early recognition of pneumothorax. The ventilator's peak inspiratory pressure should be closely monitored. An acute increase in this pressure reading suggests a pneumothorax has developed. Collapse of all or part of a lung may also be assessed by the sudden absence or decrease in lung sounds over the involved lobes. It is wise for the nurse to auscultate lung sounds hourly. Tracheal deviation toward the uninvolved side is a sign of a developing tension pneumothorax. Palpation of the trachea's position will indicate if a dangerous mediastinal shift is developing.

Evidence of a lowering in cardiac output can quickly be detected by the use of the Swan-Ganz catheter through the thermodilution technique. Measurement of the PCWP as an adjunct source of information may be misleading. If the alveolar pressure under PEEP is greater than the pulmonary venous pressure, the PCWP reading will reflect alveolar pressure and not left atrial pressure (Peters, 1979). When the Swan-Ganz monitoring is not utilized, clinical signs of a decrease in cardiac output resemble those of shock: pallor, tachycardia, diaphoresis, and a decrease in hourly urine output. Since the patient in ARDS may also be suffering shock, the nurse must be alert for sudden changes in the patient's condition. Change may be the key to identifying complications of PEEP. If signs suggest a drop in cardiac output as the result of PEEP, ventilator adjustments will probably be required.

The patient's survival may not allow the physician to regulate PEEP levels when a lowering of cardiac output occurs. If the PaO_2 should fall when the PEEP levels are lowered, the dangerously high PEEP levels may be necessary for the patient's survival. In this case fluids and inotropic agents may be required to maintain the cardiac output, although care must be taken to avoid fluid overload.

The patient on the ventilator will of course require vigorous pulmonary hygiene. A buildup of secretions may cause the patient's respiratory rate and work of breathing to increase. The airway manometer reading on a volume ventilator will rise, accompanied often by the ventilator's pressure alarm. On a pressure ventilator the manometer reading will remain the same, but the delivered tidal volume will likely fall.

The nurse should not allow suctioning to be ruled by a ''numbers routine.'' In other words, suctioning every 1 or 2 hours may be insufficient. Copious secretions may develop quickly, requiring suctioning several times within the hour. The nurse must also consider whether or not suctioning is being performed too often. Hemorrhage from the tracheal mucosa and bronchospasm are just two complications resulting from excessive catheter insertion. Observation of the character and volume of sputum as well as frequent auscultation of lung sounds provide criteria to determine the need for suctioning.

It is also wise before suctioning to assess the patient's mental status, cardiac rate, and rhythm to determine suctioning tolerance.

Intrapulmonary secretions may be removed more readily by instillation of 3 to 5 ml of normal saline via the endotracheal tube (Kirilloff and Maszkiewicz, 1979). The saline should be introduced during inspiration to improve disbursement. Many clinicians ventilate the patient briefly with an Ambu bag to further spread the saline. Benefit of the saline is derived from the vigorous cough it elicits. Some clinicians think it may temporarily aid in liquefaction of mucus. The procedure is absolutely safe as long as the nurse stands by with the necessary suction equipment.

Turning and postural drainage with percussion and vibration are routine pulmonary hygiene measures applicable to the needs of the ARDS patient. It is prudent on the nurse's part to remain aware of x-ray findings that localize areas of mucus consolidation. This information will guide the nurse to correctly position the patient so that affected lobes of the lung may drain effectively.

When the patient with ARDS shows signs of stabilization, PEEP must not be suddenly discontinued. The use of PEEP should be maintained until the alveoli are sufficiently stable to stay open alone. Premature discontinuance of PEEP can result in rapid atelectasis. Weaning from the ventilator is initiated when a Pao_2 of 60 mm Hg or more is reached consistently (Glover and Glover, 1978). When the patient is on high PEEP and Fio_2 levels, the Fio_2 is first reduced to a safe level (40%). Fio_2 and PEEP should not be lowered simultaneously (Glover and Glover, 1978). After the Fio_2 is reduced, the PEEP is lowered a few centimeters at a time. Throughout the weaning process arterial blood gases and cardiovascular dynamics are monitored closely. Once PEEP has been discontinued, final weaning from the ventilator has become safer with the use of intermittent mandatory ventilation, which allows the patient to breathe a humidified gas mixture spontaneously at the patient's own chosen rate. The use of intermittent mandatory ventilation is particularly beneficial in patients with wasting of respiratory motor mechanisms.

There are other methods of improving oxygen delivery to the patient in ARDS without intubation and mechanical ventilation. Although some techniques are still somewhat experimental, they hold promise for effective therapy without the risk of lethal side effects. One technique is the use of continuous negative chest wall pressure. In a report by Sanyal, Bernal, Hughes, and Feldman (1976) continuous negative chest wall pressure was used to treat progressively severe hypoxemia in a spontaneously breathing adult with diffuse alveolar disease. A modified tank respirator was attached to a 5 hp vacuum pump, which applied a continuous negative pressure of −1 to −18 cm H_2O around the chest wall and lower body. Within 24 hours of this therapy the patient's respiratory rate lowered, intrapulmonary shunt decreased, and Pao_2 increased. There were no adverse effects on blood pressure or heart rate. Although this technique has been more commonly used with children, it holds promise for the treatment of adult clients.

The other method involves the use of alterations in posture to improve oxygenation. Standard care of patients requiring mechanical ventilation is most commonly carried out with the patient in a supine position. Periodic turning from side to side is usually performed as part of the patient's pulmonary hygiene and skin integrity maintenance. However, these positions do little to promote ventilation in the dorsal aspect of the lungs. In a study with six patients in acute respiratory failure, subjects were positioned with the aid of a CircOlectric bed from supine to prone positions (Douglas et al., 1977). The upper thorax and pelvis were supported on specially constructed pads allowing the abdomen to protrude. The head was supported in a fashion to avoid pressure on the eyes. It is critical that the abdomen does not bear the weight of the torso or intra-abdominal pressure will increase. Increased intra-abdominal pressure may compress the vena cava, causing hypotension, or it can impede the diaphragm's descent.

As a result of the prone positioning the arterial Po_2 increased by a mean of 69 mm Hg at the same tidal volume, same FIO_2, and same level of PEEP (Douglas et al., 1977). In four of the five patients on mechanical ventilators the maneuver made it possible to reduce the FIO_2. Likewise it led to deferring intubation in the one patient who breathed spontaneously. Although this technique required meticulous nursing care, it holds promise for a simple but highly effective means of improving oxygen delivery.

Reducing oxygen consumption

Oxygenation can be further improved in the ARDS patient by reducing oxygen consumption. This is achieved through the prevention of fever, chills, and restlessness. Fever causes a shift of the oxyhemoglobin dissociation curve to the right (Chapter 4). As a result, the red blood cells tend to freely give up oxygen to the tissues at a particular Pao_2. Although more oxygen is made available to the tissues, it increases the demand for more oxygen delivery. In the case of ARDS this demand will likely go unmet.

Frequent monitoring of body temperature is of course vital. In addition to the administration of antipyretics, environmental controls aid in lowering body temperature. Reducing the amount of linen covering the patient, using tepid water for bathing, and controlling room temperature are simple measures that may prove helpful. All must be conducted in a manner that prevents the onset of chills. Shivering and the accompanying muscular work increase metabolic heat. As much as 50% of the increased heat production caused by shivering can be retained in the body (Mountcastle, 1980). The advent of chills can cause the body temperature to rise, further increasing oxygen demands for the body's metabolism.

Any increase in patient activity, as in the case of restlessness, will increase oxygen consumption. The presence of the ventilator and monitoring equipment may evoke anxiety in the patient who is alert enough to recognize his plight. Care must be taken to avoid depersonalization of this acutely ill patient. All procedures, from measuring cardiac output to instituting oral hygiene, should be explained clearly and concisely. Alternative means of patient communication by note pad, magic slate, word cards, or sign language should be instituted.

Comfort becomes the goal of the nurse who strives to reduce the patient's restlessness. Instituting comfort measures through frequent correct positioning, suctioning of the hypopharynx around the endotracheal tube, avoiding movement of endotracheal or ventilator tubing, and keeping the patient off wires and tubing may be enough to relieve restlessness. Although it is often difficult in an intensive care setting, the nurse should take care not to "overnurse." This is to say that caution should be taken to use all time spent with the patient purposefully. The nurse, concerned with the critical nature of the patient and confronted with the highly stressful intensive care environment, may initiate excessive and unnecessary contacts with the patient. Sensory bombardment can cause the patient to become disoriented, confused, and even more restless. Judgment therefore should be used to appropriately space nursing activities, allowing for the patient's rest. If the patient is stable, taking vital signs every 15 minutes may not be required.

The nurse must be cautious in seeking pharmacological means to reduce restlessness. Restlessness can be an indicator of hypoxia, acidosis, or hypercapnia. Sedation should be avoided if possible. If there is concern that restlessness and resultant movement by the patient will cause airway trauma from the endotracheal tube, small doses of diazepam (initial dose, 5 mg intravenously) may be given (Bone, 1980). There are some physicians who prefer using morphine to reduce restlessness, since adverse cardiorespiratory effects can be reversed with naloxone hydrochloride (initial dose, 0.4 mg intravenously) (Bone, 1980).

Maintenance of oxygen transport

Maintenance of oxygen transport is achieved through careful monitoring of the patient's complete blood count. The oxygen content of blood is dependent on the hemoglobin concentration. If the patient's hematocrit falls, the resultant drop in hemoglobin makes less oxygen available to the tissues. The treatment of choice for anemia in this case is usually the administration of packed cells.

Maintenance of cardiac output

The final mode of treatment used in maintaining oxygenation is the maintenance of an adequate cardiac output. It is essential to maximize available oxygen delivered to the tissues. The available oxygen is equal to the product of cardiac output and arterial oxygen content. As was previously discussed, if there is a lowering of cardiac output, venous Po_2 and eventually the arterial Po_2 will decline. Because the cardiac output has this indirect effect on available oxygen, its status in ARDS must be closely monitored. Inotropic agents will be employed if cardiac output lowers as a direct effect of the syndrome itself or from PEEP therapy.

Maintenance of fluid balance

Since pulmonary edema is a dominant pathological factor in ARDS, the maintenance of fluid balance is clearly a priority of treatment. Overexpansion of interstitial water will lead to an exacerbation of the edema. The clinician is faced with two concerns in treating the shock patient with ARDS: (1) the possible leakage of excess fluid through the damaged alveolar capillary membrane and (2) the risk of volume depletion aggravating the hypotension of shock. Controversy exists as to the volume of fluids to administer and the type of fluids that will serve to benefit the patient most.

No agreement can be found as to the exact volume of fluid used in management. Agreement does exist as to the avoidance of using saline solutions in intravenous fluid therapy. Obviously careful hemodynamic monitoring is required to determine therapy suitable to the individualized needs of patients.

Albumin infusion has become a popular mode of therapy in the fluid management of ARDS. Its use is aimed at restoring hemodynamics and tissue perfusion through plasma volume expansion without fluid volume overload by pulling fluid out of interstitial compartments. This would lessen the likelihood of pulmonary edema developing. The frequent objection to the use of albumin is that it "leaks" into the peripheral and pulmonary interstitial spaces, pulling fluid with it and thus aggravating pulmonary edema.

A closer look at the physiology of albumin is necessary. The "leaking" of albumin may be confused with the normal equilibration of the body's albumin supply as well as with albumin metabolism. Albumin is normally manufactured by the liver and secreted into the plasma to exert oncotic pressure vital to fluid balance. It then equilibrates in the interstitial space where 55% to 60% of the albumin pool resides (Shoemaker and Hauser, 1979). A majority of the albumin in the interstitial space is tissue bound and thus fails to exert oncotic pressure.

With the insult of shock the catabolic result is an increase in albumin metabolism and a reduction in its synthesis. Therefore the "leakage" of albumin from plasma to interstitial spaces may be simply rapid equilibration or increased tissue demand instead of true leakage (Shoemaker and Hauser, 1979). If such is the case, the patient should be able to satisfactorily handle infusions of albumin. It then seems appropriate to correct low plasma albumin concentrations and plasma oncotic pressures with required amounts of 25% albumin. However, current research continues to reveal conflicting findings. There is evidence, as reported by Collins (1977), that administration of albumin to patients with increased capillary permeability to other materials of like size was ineffective. These patients suffered a greater risk of pulmonary flooding.

Physicians concerned over postoperative patients retaining salt water keep postoperative ARDS patients dry by fluid restriction and diuretics. The goal again is to avert pulmonary edema. Diuretics are used especially if the PCWP is elevated. However, if hypovolemia results and third-space fluid stays expanded, a worsening of circulatory shock and ARDS may ensue. Therapy must keep the interstitial spaces dry and not the intravascular space. For this reason albumin seems to hold greater therapeutic qualities since it maintains plasma volume by drawing fluid out of interstitial spaces.

In a study reported by Shoemaker and Hauser (1979), albumin and crystalloid therapy using Ringer's lactate were compared. Critically ill surgical patients with early ARDS were treated in two groups, one with 1 L Ringer's lactate and the other with 25 gm of 25% albumin. The albumin increased plasma volume significantly by shifting fluid from the interstitial space to intravascular water; Ringer's lactate only temporarily increased plasma volume and then leaked back into the interstitial space. As a result of using albumin the patient's cardiac index, mean arterial pressure, ventricular stroke work, oxygen delivery, and oxygen consumption improved. The result in the case of ARDS was improved oxygen delivery and consumption. Ringer's lactate caused cardiopulmonary indexes to decline. If there were any temporary changes in circulatory status following Ringer's lactate infusion, it was attributed to a central reflex response affecting cardiac contractility. No long-term hemodynamic benefit was derived from crystalloids.

Because of the disagreement existing over the best means for fluid management in ARDS, the nurse should be prepared to see numerous combinations of therapy. No one therapy for decreasing pulmonary edema has been widely accepted. Corticosteroids have been used in ARDS. Theoretically their purpose is to reduce capillary inflammation and thereby reduce capillary permeability. Studies on the effects of steroids in ARDS are still somewhat conflicting. Schumer (1976) reported that corticosteroids improve survival in sepsis and seem to be beneficial in fat embolism. Both sepsis and fat embolism may cause ARDS.

To summarize, most resources acknowledge the need to maintain the ARDS patient's volume status on the "dry" side. This can be achieved through a combination of fluid restriction and/or diuretics. Yet if hypovolemia becomes a concern, volume expansion may be attained more safely through colloid administration and not crystalloid therapy.

Rigorous attention must be made to monitoring the patient's fluid volume status. The strict recording of intake and output and daily weights is crucial for determining gross changes in fluid balance. Pflaum (1979) investigated the accuracy of nursing practice in using intake and output records to determine body fluid balance. Her study of 30 adult patients revealed a mean error in intake and output figures of 799.5 ml per day when compared with weight calculations. The nursing literature has often argued the accuracy of intake and output measurements. Daily weights are further argued to be more sensitive indicators of fluid gain or loss. Pflaum (1979) suggests that intake and output records should continue to be collected and compared with daily weights to alert practitioners to insensible losses, fluid shifts, or calculation inaccuracies. To ensure accuracy of daily weights patients should be weighed at the same time, with the same scale, and with the same weight of clothing.

Arterial blood pressure and PCWP reflect more subtle changes in the patient's intravascular fluid volume. Inspecting for peripheral edema and auscultating lung sounds will give clues as to the site and nature of fluid buildup. The alert nurse will correlate observations with knowledge of the pathological course of ARDS to reach relevant nursing judgments.

Prevention of concomitant infection

The lungs lie in a vulnerable position. They are one of three large "external" surfaces of the body, the others being the skin and intestine, which are directly exposed to bacteria. Of these three surfaces only the lower airway must remain sterile to function properly. The lungs are equipped with specialized defense mechanisms to guard against bacteremic assault. However, the ability of the lungs to clear and kill inhaled bacteria is impaired by serious injury, hemorrhage, aspiration, hypoxia, oxygen toxicity, and other causes (Collins, 1977). Furthermore the risk of infection is increased by factors such as intubation and retained secretions.

Care must be given to the use of antimicrobial therapy in ARDS. Use of prophylactic antibiotics is worthless and may give rise to superinfection by highly resistant gram-negative organisms such as *Pseudomonas*. *Pseudomonas* is particularly difficult to eradicate once it is found in the lower airway (Collins, 1977). Diagnosis of gram-negative pneumonia can be extremely difficult in an already critically ill patient. Fever, leukocytosis, pulmonary infiltrates, and hypoxemia can be indicative of other conditions and be masked by ARDS, but when they occur in the presence of purulent sputum, the clinician should be alerted. Evidence of specific pathogens from tracheal cultures is needed before antibiotic therapy is instituted.

Infection is prevented by the nurse's rigid use of sterile technique during suctioning, endotracheal tube care, and ventilator tubing management. The intensive care setting often demands quick action but should not negate the need for diligent technique. Another means of prevention lies in meticulous oral hygiene. Studies have demonstrated a phenomenon in which oropharyngeal flora of sick, hospitalized patients are converted to predominantly gram-negative bacteria (Collins, 1977). Removal of retained oropharyngeal secretions in the intubated patient is essential to prevent aspiration from around the endotracheal tube. Positioning the less responsive patient on his side to allow secretions to drain forward out of the mouth can also be helpful. Oral hygiene itself should not be limited to the occasional use of glycerin swabs. Although they may afford lubrication to dry mucous membranes, there is no bacteriostatic benefit. A solution of diluted peroxide and normal saline (half and half) can be used to loosen debris between teeth and to remove coating on the tongue. As an oxidizing agent hydrogen peroxide does have antiseptic qualities. Care must be taken to dilute peroxide to avoid burns to the mouth. The peroxide solution should be rinsed thoroughly with saline or a commercially prepared mouthwash if available. The nurse should be sure that any liquids used for oral hygiene are not aspirated by the patient. Oral hygiene should be administered frequently enough to avoid excess debris and mucus accumulation.

PROGNOSIS: IMPLICATIONS FOR NURSING

The prognosis of ARDS is largely dependent on early recognition, competent management, and the availability of sophisticated treatment facilities. Survival from the acute episode of ARDS varied from 50% to 70% as reported by Burki (1978). However, the fact that the syndrome is becoming more recognizable may improve these statistics. Among those patients who do survive, a mild residual restrictive lung defect with a slight decrease in gas transfer is common (Burki, 1978).

The nurse has been shown to play a critical role in the management of the ARDS patient. Despite the overwhelming pathogenicity of the disease process, its course can be controlled to avoid permanent severe pulmonary crippling. Likewise, recognition of the multiple causes related to ARDS can lead the nurse in these situations to initiate aggressive pulmonary hygiene, infection preventive measures, and fluid regulation restraints. ARDS can present an exciting challenge to the nurse who acknowledges that knowledge of pathophysiology, current treatment modalities, and skilled nursing care go hand in hand.

PATIENT VIGNETTE
ARDS following multiple trauma

A 55-year-old man was admitted to the surgical intensive care unit following an automobile accident. The patient was in mild respiratory distress with respirations 30 and labored. Blood pressure was 90/50, pulse, 118 and thready. The abdomen was distended and dull to percussion. A paracentesis revealed sanguinous fluid return. Two intravenous infusions of Ringer's lactate were started and the patient's blood was typed and crossmatched for 6 units of whole blood. During emergency surgery a splenectomy was performed. The patient was estimated to have lost 4 units of blood as a result of the injury.

Postoperatively the patient was placed on 40% oxygen with a high-humidity mask. A nasogastric tube had been inserted for abdominal decompression and was to be irrigated every 2 hours. Twenty-four hours postoperatively the arterial blood gases revealed the following measurements: pH, 7.38; $Paco_2$, 40; Pao_2, 85. The evening of his second postoperative day the patient complained of nausea. The nurse checking the nasogastric tube found that it was not draining effectively. During her attempt to irrigate the nasogastric tube, the patient began vomiting. Despite placing the patient on his side, there was concern he had aspirated stomach contents. One hour after nasotracheal suctioning, arterial blood gases revealed measurements of pH, 7.35; $Paco_2$, 40; and Pao_2, 75. Over the next 24 hours the patient began to develop dyspnea and signs of restlessness. Despite aggressive pulmonary hygiene and institution of a 40% oxygen face mask, arterial blood gases worsened. New arterial blood gases showed pH, 7.32; $Paco_2$, 42; Pao_2, 60. A chest film showed the white-out pattern of ARDS. The patient was intubated and placed on a volume ventilator with 5 cm PEEP. One month later after successful ventilatory management the patient was discharged.

Questions

1. What is the common precipitating factor leading to ARDS believed to be?
  a. Hyperinflation of alveoli
  b. Transfusion of crystalloids following traumatic injury
  c. Pulmonary hypoperfusion
  d. Bronchial inflammation

2. What is the main factor in arterial blood gas interpretation that can indicate the development of ARDS?
  a. Lowered Pao_2 that fails to respond to increased oxygen concentrations in the air

b. A rise in the level of arterial carbon dioxide tension
c. Lowering of arterial pH accompanied by an increase in $Paco_2$
d. Failure of arterial carbon dioxide tension to lower in response to increased oxygen concentrations in the inspired air

3. What is the purpose of PEEP in managing ARDS?
a. To increase airway pressure during inspiration so as to expand collapsed alveoli
b. To increase the functional residual capacity and open collapsed alveoli by maintaining positive pressure at end of expiration
c. To maintain above-atmospheric pressure throughout the respiratory cycle to prevent atelectasis
d. To lower the inspiratory force needed to expand collapsed alveoli

4. What do the most common complications resulting from the use of PEEP include?
a. Increased cardiac output
b. Pneumothorax
c. Bronchospasm
d. Oxygen toxicity

5. Treating fluid balance alterations in ARDS involves all of the principles *except* which of the following?
a. Avoid volume depletion
b. Promote plasma volume expansion
c. Increase pulmonary interstitial oncotic pressure
d. Reduce pulmonary capillary permeability

Answers

1. c. The initial development of pulmonary edema associated with ARDS is believed to result from pulmonary hypoperfusion. Development of microvascular aggregation of blood elements creates a mechanical obstruction to blood flow. Coupled with hypoperfusion is the development of increased pulmonary capillary permeability. Leakage of fluid into the pulmonary interstitium creates pulmonary edema.

2. a. The hypoxemia of ARDS does not improve as a result of exposure to increased inspired oxygen concentrations. Indeed the patient will likely be acidotic with an elevated Pco_2. However, these findings alone are not solely indicative of ARDS. In the progressive stages of ARDS the hypoxemia is believed to result from shunting in areas where the ratio of ventilation to perfusion is low.

3. b. Positive end expiratory pressure is as the name implies. An artificial pressure is maintained via a mechanical ventilator during the end of expiration. When positive pressure is exerted at the end of expiration, fewer of the smaller airways collapse. Likewise the functional residual capacity, or volume of air remaining in the lung at the end of expiration, is increased. PEEP works to keep atelectatic alveoli open and increases the available surface area for gas exchange.

4. b. Pneumothorax is particularly a risk when high PEEP levels are used. PEEP can cause alveoli to rupture, leading to the development of a pneumothorax. A lowering of cardiac output is also a potential side effect resulting from PEEP because of lowered venous return and increased pulmonary vascular resistance.

5. c. Increasing pulmonary interstitial oncotic pressure would be a treatment principle devastating to the ARDS patient. Pulmonary edema would naturally worsen and likely become fatal. In treating ARDS a major goal is to maintain the plasma volume intravascularly to avoid escape of fluid into the pulmonary interstitium. Many physicians desire to keep the patient relatively dry intravascularly to avoid further pulmonary edema. However, if volume depletion occurs, circulatory shock may ensue. The use of steroids by some physicians is designed to minimize pulmonary capillary permeability.

REFERENCES

Anderson, R.R., et al.: Documentation of pulmonary capillary permeability in the adult respiratory distress syndrome accompanying human sepsis, American Review of Respiratory Disease **119:** 869-877, 1979.

Ayres, S., et al.: The lung in shock, American Journal of Cardiology **26:**588-594, 1979.

Bone, R.C.: Treatment of severe hypoxemia due to the adult respiratory distress syndrome, Archives of Internal Medicine **140:**85-89, 1980.

Burki, N.K.: Adult respiratory distress syndrome, Southern Medical Journal **71:**1412-1415, 1423, 1978.

Collins, J.A.: The acute respiratory distress syndrome, Advances in Surgery **11:**171-225, 1977.

Dantzker, D.R., et al.: Ventilation-perfusion distributions in the adult respiratory distress syndrome, American Review of Respiratory Disease **120:** 1039-1052, 1979.

Douglas, W.W., et al.: Improved oxygenation in patients with acute respiratory failure: the prone position, American Review of Respiratory Disease **115:**559-565, 1977.

Glover, D.W., and Glover, M.M.: Respiratory therapy: basics for nursing and allied health professions, St. Louis, 1978, The C.V. Mosby Co.

Greenfield, L.J.: Adult respiratory distress syndrome, American Surgeon **44:**133-136, 1978.

Kirilloff, L.H., and Maszkiewicz, R.C.: Guide to respiratory care in critically ill adults, American Journal of Nursing **79:**2005-2012, 1979.

Lake, K.B.: The adult respiratory distress syndrome ("shock lung"). In Burton, G.G., Gee, G.N., and Hodgkin, J.E., editors: Respiratory care, a guide to clinical practice, Philadelphia, 1977, J.B. Lippincott Co.

Mountcastle, V.B.: Medical physiology, vol. 2, St. Louis, 1980, The C.V. Mosby Co.

Peters, R.M.: Lifesaving measures in acute respiratory distress syndrome, American Journal of Surgery **138:**368-373, 1979.

Pflaum, S.: Investigation of intake-output as a means of assessing body fluid balance, Heart & Lung **8:** 495-498, 1979.

Sanyal, S.K., Bernal, R., Hughes, W., and Feldman, S.: Continuous negative chest-wall pressure: successful use for severe respiratory distress in an adult, Journal of the American Medical Association **236:**1727-1728, 1976.

Schumer, W.: Steroids in the treatment of clinical septic shock, Annals of Surgery **184:**333-340, 1976.

Shoemaker, W.C., and Hauser, C.J.: Critique of crystalloid versus colloid therapy in shock and shock lung, Critical Care Medicine **7:**117-124, 1979.

Skelley, B.F., Deeren, S.M., and Powaser, M.: The effectiveness of two preoxygenation methods to prevent endotracheal suction-induced hypoxemia, Heart & Lung **9:**316-323, 1980.

Weigelt, J.A., Mitchell, R.A., and Snyder, W.H.: Early positive end-expiratory pressure in the adult respiratory distress syndrome, Archives of Surgery **114:**497-501, 1979.

13 Disseminated intravascular coagulation

ANGELA SMITH-COLLINS

For the last 20 years, a syndrome of profuse bleeding has been associated with a variety of clinical conditions. This syndrome has been called consumption coagulopathy, hypofibrinogenemia, temporary hemophilia, and defibrination syndrome. The name most commonly used at present is *disseminated intravascular coagulation* (DIC).

DIC is a complication of shock and many other clinical conditions. It never appears alone but always as a sequelae to some other disorder. DIC is characterized by what seems to be a contradiction: the patient has widespread coagulation in the capillaries but is hemorrhaging elsewhere. Thus DIC reduces the blood's ability to support cells that have already been damaged by the primary condition.

DIC is a clinically complex syndrome; the nurse is often the one who first notices its symptoms in the patient. The physician and nurse also monitor the laboratory reports that give indication of the progress of DIC and administer prescribed treatments. Nursing management of DIC is based on knowledge of coagulation and fibrinolytic systems, trigger states for thrombohemorrhagic disorders, clinical presentation, and therapeutic management.

NORMAL DYNAMIC STATE OF BLOOD

The blood exists in the vascular bed as a fluid comprised of cells, water, and dissolved components. Blood maintains the metabolic balance of every cell in the body by providing the nutrients necessary for aerobic metabolism and by removing the cells' waste products. Blood also serves as a systemic transport system for the body's chemical messengers, such as hormones.

Perhaps the most unique property of the blood is its ability to change from a fluid to a solid plug. Under normal conditions, blood is a fluid because (1) the normal vascular system is lined with endothelial cells whose surface is such that it is difficult for platelets and fibrin to attach to their walls, (2) the blood travels at a speed that prevents the damage of platelets or the promotion of stasis, and (3) the blood's coagulation system is protected by a system of checks and balances (Price and Wilson, 1978). These factors usually protect the body from inappropriate clot formation (Fig. 13-1).

Hemostasis

Hemostasis is the cessation of blood flow caused by a partial or traumatic defect in the blood vessel wall (Mason and Saba, 1978). The process is dependent on the

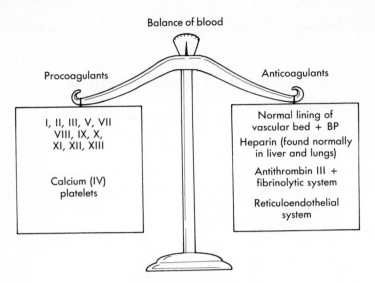

Fig. 13-1. Balance of blood.

presence of adequate numbers of functioning platelets, the adequate function of vessel endothelium, normal support structures for blood vessels, and adequate numbers of properly functioning clotting factors.

Platelets are the "glue" of the blood. In normal blood, they are present in concentrations of 150,000 to 400,000/mm³. When platelets come into contact with damaged tissue, they stick to the exposed collagen forming a physical barrier to blood flow. The platelets then degranulate and exude tissue thromboplastin (factor III), serotonin, epinephrine, and ADP. All of these substances cause platelets to gather together and clump into a platelet "plug." Platelets are the activators of the intrinsic pathway of blood coagulation.

The endothelial lining of blood vessels contains substances that promote or deter coagulation. This can either activate or inhibit plasminogen, which is the trigger for the fibrinolytic (clot-destroying) pathway. The endothelium can also produce certain prostaglandins; their function is not well understood, but they appear to interact with platelets to promote aggregation.

Supporting structures around the blood vessel help the vessel to constrict and further stimulate coagulation. Trauma to the vessel activates the sympathetic nervous system, causing a reflex of vasoconstriction along the vessel for several centimeters in the vicinity of the trauma. Vasoconstriction causes a decrease in the diameter of the lumen of the vessel so that a smaller plug is needed. The supporting structures also constrict, which further contains the blood volume. When supporting structures are exposed, their

Table 13-1. Clotting factors

Factor	Name	Source	Pathway
I	Fibrinogen	Liver	Intrinsic and extrinsic
II	Prothrombin	Liver (vitamin K dependent)	Intrinsic and extrinsic
III	Tissue thromboplastin	Present in most tissues	Extrinsic
IV	Calcium	Dietary intake and parathyroid secretion	Intrinsic and extrinsic
V	Labile factor	Liver	Intrinsic and extrinsic
VII	Stable factor	Liver (vitamin K dependent)	Extrinsic
VIII	Antihemophilic factor	Reticuloendothelial system	Intrinsic
IX	Christmas factor	Liver (vitamin K dependent)	Intrinsic
X	Stuart-Prower factor	Liver (vitamin K dependent)	Intrinsic
XI	Plasma thromboplastin antecedent		Intrinsic
XII	Hageman factor		Intrinsic
XIII	Fibrin stabilizing factor		Intrinsic and extrinsic

exposed collagen fragments attract the platelets and further stimulate hemostasis.

The clotting factors include eleven known plasma proteins and calcium (Ca^{++}) ions (Table 13-1). The protein clotting factors are made in the liver; hence abnormal liver function can result in a coagulation disorder depending on the degree of hepatic failure. Dietary intake and absorption of protein, vitamin K, and calcium are needed to maintain a normal level of clotting factors. Vitamin K is needed by the liver for formation of factors II, VII, IX, and X.

Clotting factors circulate in the blood in an inactive form and are believed to react in a cascade manner. This means that stimulation of one factor serves as the enzyme activator for the next step in the sequence. The activation of clotting factors occurs when there is a disruption of the vasculature of trauma to the blood. There are two cascade pathways leading to clot formation: the extrinsic pathway and the intrinsic pathway. The extrinsic pathway requires the release of thromboplastin by damaged endothelial cells or other tissues. The extrinsic pathway, which is activated by thromboplastin, causes factors I, II, V, and X to react. The intrinsic pathway is stimulated by platelets and platelet factor release. The intrinsic pathway causes factors I, II, VIII, IX, X, and XI to interact.

Both pathways unite to stimulate the same end pathway of coagulation. As can be seen in Fig. 13-2, both the extrinsic and intrinsic pathways activate factor X. Factor X in turn stimulates factor II to change to thrombin. The sequence of cascade reactions caused by factor X is called the common pathway of coagulation (Moses, 1981).

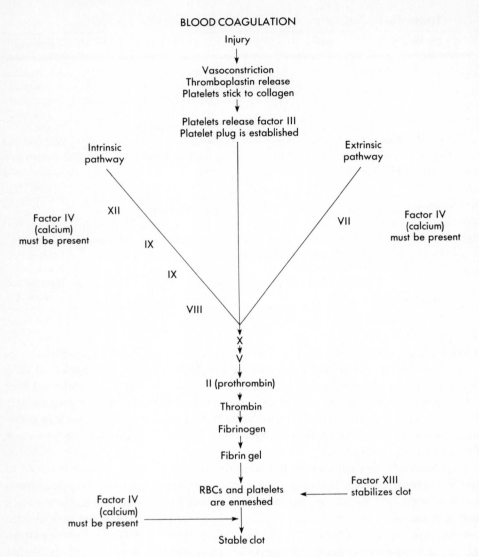

Fig. 13-2. Pathway of coagulation.

Thrombogenesis

The interaction between the four components in hemostasis is complimentary. The platelets, endothelium lining, supporting structures, and clotting factors all contribute to the end product, the blood clot. Appreciation of the intricate nature of the clotting mechanism will help the nurse to recognize how the absence of any one component can cause hemorrhagic effects.

Hemostasis begins at the site of tissue and/or vascular injury. Vasoconstriction occurs in response to a release of epinephrine. Platelets stick to collagen fragments and release factor III and ADP, establishing a weak platelet plug that slows down bleeding. Tissue thromboplastin (factor III) activates the intrinsic system, beginning a cascade of chemical reactions involving factors XII, XI, IX, and VIII. Simultaneously the extrinsic system is activated by thromboplastin from the endothelium lining. The extrinsic pathway stimulates factor VII. Both the intrinsic and extrinsic pathways can only react in the presence of calcium (factor IV). The two pathways then unite and stimulate the reactions of factors X, V, and II. This is the common pathway of the coagulation cascade. Prothrombin (factor II) is converted to thrombin. Thrombin is a potent coagulant because it stimulates the conversion of fibrinogen to fibrin. Fibrin is a threadlike protein that forms a netlike plug, which entangles platelets and blood cells. Calcium and fibrin stabilizing factor (factor XIII) stabilize the clot structure, completing hemostasis. This takes about 3 to 6 minutes. Within an hour, the clot is retracted, meaning that the serum is squeezed out of the clot and either fibrinolysis or inflammatory repair of the defect occurs.

Fibrinolytic system

Hemostasis stops blood flow temporarily, but as the trauma heals, a method of removing the clot is necessary. This is accomplished by the fibrinolytic system, which functions as a counterbalance of hemostasis. The key to this system is a protein called plasminogen, which circulates in the blood in an inactive form. It is thought to be manufactured in the kidneys and in granulocytes (Mason and Saba, 1978).

When trauma stimulates clotting, clotting stimulates the body's immune and fibrinolytic systems (Fig. 13-3). Fibrinolysis is activated by the kallikrein cycle. Kallikrein's nature is unknown, but it is a multipurpose substance that causes the conversion of kinase. Kallikrein is formed in the initial stage of clotting in response to the activation of factor XII. This process is linked to the immune system's complement activation. Complement stimulates the conversion of prekallikrein, which then becomes kininogen. Kininogen becomes kinin, the direct activator of plasminogen. Kinin is a specific type of kinase that changes (catalyzes) plasminogen into plasmin. Plasmin is an enzyme that degrades fibrin into fibrin split products. Plasmin also inactivates factors V and VII (Mason and Saba, 1978).

Other kinases have been found that convert plasminogen to plasmin. Some researchers think that these kinases are made by the endothelial lining of the blood vessel. Urokinase, found in the urine, is also a potent stimulus of this conversion. Streptokinase, used in hypercoagulable states, is a pharmacological agent that will cause fibrinolysis.

Antithrombins function as a check against excessive clotting. Antithrombins are not known to dissolve a stable clot, but they can prevent expansion of the clot and formation of new clots by acting directly against thrombin. The most currently researched is antithrombin III, which chemically binds with thrombin and thereby inactivates it (Cham-

FIBRINOLYTIC SYSTEM

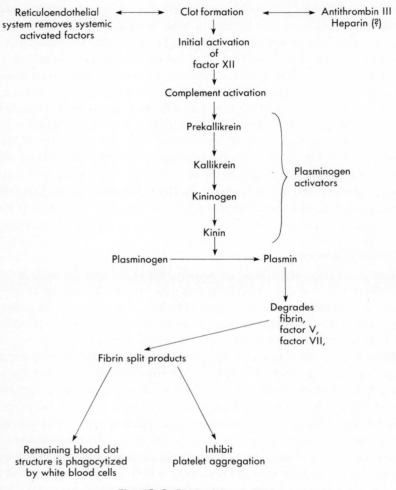

Fig. 13-3. Fibrinolytic system.

berlain, 1980). Heparin is also a type of antithrombin that is normally secreted in small amounts by liver cells and mast cells in the lung (Guyton, 1981). The actions of heparin primarily work on the common pathway of blood coagulation. However, because of its small concentration in the healthy body, these effects are not normally pronounced.

Fibrin split products inhibit coagulation in three ways: coating platelets to reduce their tendency to aggregate, inhibiting thrombin, and preventing fibrinogen from assuming a stable chemical state (Jennings, 1979).

The reticuloendothelial system is also a check against excessive clotting. This sys-

Actions of heparin
Inhibits thrombin-mediated conversion of fibrinogen to fibrin Potentiates the action of antithrombin III Inhibits the activation of factor IX Neutralizes activated factor X
Modified from Weiner, M.A., Pepper, G.A., Kuhn-Weisman, G., and Romano, J.A.: Clinical pharmacology and therapeutics in nursing, New York, 1979, McGraw-Hill Book Co.

tem includes the liver, spleen, and lymph nodes. If activated clotting factors leave the area of localized trauma, the reticuloendothelial system removes them from the bloodstream. Patients with spleen or liver damage can be expected to have impaired functional capacity in this system. Patients receiving steroids can also expect to have difficulties since steroids depress this system.

PATHOPHYSIOLOGY

There are a large number of different conditions that can trigger DIC, but they all have one thing in common: they disrupt the checks and balances of the coagulation system. The causative agent or agents of DIC are not known. DIC is always found to be a secondary state in response to some other condition. It is not known why some people with triggering states develop the disease and others do not. There is no consensus on a common pathophysiological pattern for DIC. It is possible that each trigger state interacts with the coagulation system differently (Fig. 13-4).

The trigger states fall into four groups of clinical conditions. The first group activates procoagulant activity and includes transfusions of incompatible blood, obstetric catastrophe, and heat stroke. The second group triggers DIC by endothelial injury, which can be caused by septic reactions, toxic shock syndrome, and metastatic malignant disease. The third group is one that includes insult to the reticuloendothelial system such as splenectomy and hepatic disease. The fourth group includes conditions that promote vascular stasis. Pulmonary embolism and polycythemia are examples of this group (Gralnick, 1977).

DIC may be either acute or chronic. The chronic states are usually associated with cancer. The pace of this type of DIC is such that sometimes the bone marrow and liver are able to compensate. Many cases go undetected because of the lack of overt signs and symptoms.

Any type of shock can trigger DIC. Five aspects of shock are conducive to its development: sluggish blood flow caused by poor perfusion and capillary shunting, metabolic acidosis, the release of ADP and phospholipids from traumatized cells, hypoxemia

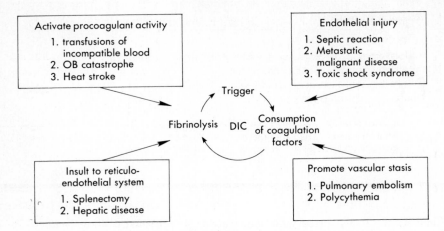

Fig. 13-4. Triggers of DIC.

POSSIBLE TRIGGER OF DIC IN SEPTIC SHOCK

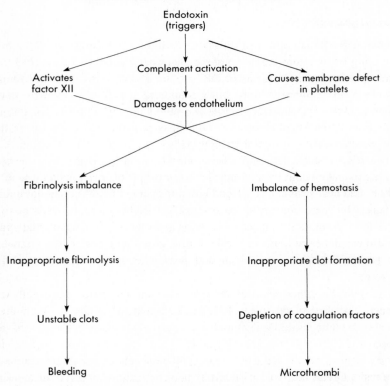

Fig. 13-5. Possible trigger of DIC in septic shock.

of cells, and endothelium damage. The pathophysiology will be illustrated by the example of gram-negative septic shock, which is thought to trigger DIC by acting on all of these aspects (Fig. 13-5).

Endotoxin is released into the bloodstream as the immune system destroys the cell walls of the bacteria. Endotoxin affects the body's clotting, fibrinolytic, and kinin systems and directly stimulates the initial factor in the intrinsic pathway (Factor VII) to start the inappropriate clot formation. The Hageman factor (Factor XII), when activated, stimulates the immune system's complement response. Complement, in turn, starts the kinin cycle, which stimulates fibrinolysis. Endotoxin may damage the endothelium, which could magnify the stimulus to the coagulation pathway and fibrinolytic system.

Other checks and balances of the blood are disturbed by septic shock. Blood is shunted away from the reticuloendothelial system to more vital organs. Poor capillary oxygen and nutrient exchange occurs, resulting in lysis and cellular death. This releases ADP and stimulates platelet aggregation. Metabolic acidosis alters the pH of the blood, which changes the rate of the body's chemical reactions.

Therefore septic shock does not simply disrupt the blood's checks and balances at only one point, it makes multiple assaults. This is why it is impossible to pinpoint one aspect of septic shock that is the trigger for DIC.

CLINICAL PICTURE

The cause of DIC is elusive and may be associated with a wide variety of triggering conditions, but a similar clinical picture is seen in most cases. The basic problem is that clots form in capillary beds where they are not needed, which depletes clotting factors so that clots cannot form at trauma sites where they are needed. The fibrin network in the capillaries causes erythrocytes to be damaged or destroyed during passage through the capillaries. The formation of the microthrombi causes excessive activation of the fibrinolytic mechanism so that even stable clots will dissolve, resulting in bleeding. The hemostatic mechanism and fibrinolytic system are no longer balanced. Thus even a slight trauma can produce excessive bleeding because stable clots cannot be formed.

The clinical indications of DIC reflect the condition's thrombohemorrhagic nature. Hemorrhagic events are usually the presenting signs of DIC. Overt bleeding is seen from puncture sites, body orifices, drainage tubes, and suture lines. Other frequent sites of bleeding are cutaneous purpura and petechiae. The onset of covert bleeding may appear as a change in mental status, a fluctuation of vital signs, or a progressive increase in abdominal girth.

Thrombotic events manifest themselves in many ways. Acral cyanosis is cyanosis of the toes, fingers, or extremities. It is distinctive because specific landmarks of circulatory borders are seen on the skin (Fig. 13-6). This is secondary to microthrombi occluding blood flow to a specific body region (Dressler, 1980). Other thrombotic events, secondary to microemboli, induce cerebrovascular events, pulmonary thrombosis, and tissue necrosis. Organ necrosis, particularly acute tubular necrosis, is also secondary to the microthrombi.

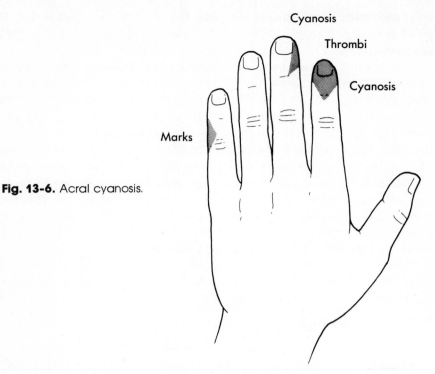

Cyanosis

Thrombi

Cyanosis

Marks

Fig. 13-6. Acral cyanosis.

Abnormal hemostasis is primarily monitored by laboratory tests. Laboratory values in DIC should be monitored as closely as the blood pressure. An arterial or CVP line may be needed for obtaining multiple blood specimens. This avoids the need for multiple puncture sites that will result in additional bleeding.

The basic screening battery of laboratory tests consists of prothrombin time, fibrinogen, platelet count, and fibrin split products. The prothrombin time (PT) and partial thromboplastin time (PTT) are lengthened in DIC because of the consumption of clotting factors. Fibrinogen levels are low because of the fibrinolytic action of DIC. The platelet count is low because of the aggregation and lysis of platelets in the microcirculation. Fibrin split products are elevated because of excessive fibrinolysis (Table 13-2).

Different medical centers may have preferences for other laboratory tests. Other measurements may include the protamine sulfate test, factor assays, and examination for schistocytes and monomer products. The protamine sulfate test is strongly positive in DIC. Factor assays will help to determine percentages of the depletion of specific clotting factors such as factors II, V, and VII. Schistocytes are erythrocytes that have been trapped by intravascular fibrin. The erythrocyte walls are damaged by passage through fibrin nets. Monomer products are not usually found in large concentrations in the bloodstream in healthy individuals, but they are found during DIC. Fibrin monomers occur because plasmin breaks fibrin into four degradation products.

Table 13-2. Laboratory tests utilized in DIC

Tests and assays	Normal values*	DIC
Hemostasis		
Prothrombin time	12 to 17 seconds	Increased
Activated partial thromboplastin time	Under 35 seconds	Increased
Thrombin time	Less than 15 seconds	Increased
Factor analysis	50% or more	Variable
Coagulation time (Lee-White method)	6 to 8 minutes	Increased
Bleeding time (Duke method)	3 to 6 minutes	Increased
Cellular		
Platelet count	150,000 to 450,000/mm³	Decreased
Erythrocytes	4.5 to 5.5 million/mm³	Decreased, schistocytes are present
Hemoglobin	14 to 17 gm (male)	Dependent on degree of blood loss
Hematocrit	42 to 52 gm (male)	Dependent on degree of blood loss
Fibrinolytic system		
Fibrin split products (monomers)	0 to 10 μg/ml	Increased
Fibrinogen	70 to 410 mg/100 ml	Decreased
Euglobulin lysis test	12 to 15 minutes	Shortened

*Normal values are dependent on the manner in which the test is run. Normals therefore are variable from institution to institution.

Blood coagulation and monitoring tests

Component	Measurement
Platelets	Platelet count, clot retraction, tourniquet test, prothrombin consumption time
Factors VII, IX, X, XI, XII, Ca⁺⁺	Prothrombin time, partial thromboplastin time
Prothrombin, thrombin, factors V, VII, X	Prothrombin time, partial thromboplastin time
Fibrinogen, fibrin, factor XIII	Venous clotting time, plasma fibrinogen, protamine sulfate test, clot lysis

Modified from Tilkian, S.M., Conover, M.B., and Tilkian, A.G.: Clinical implications of laboratory tests, ed. 2, St. Louis, 1979, The C.V. Mosby Co., p. 190.

MEDICAL MANAGEMENT

There is no complete agreement on the medical management of DIC. Some medical protocols include life-support functions, combating the trigger states, the use of anticoagulants and/or fibrinolytic agents, and blood component therapy. Usually the physician will choose one, two, or more of these therapies for a specific patient.

The most prevalent recommendation is to treat the triggering condition. Successful resolution of the underlying condition usually decreases the severity of DIC (Sharp, 1977). Because shock is often the triggering state, medical efforts are directed toward the stabilization of body systems. Management priorities are the control of acidosis, hypotension, hypoxemia, and electrolyte imbalances. It is theorized that these alterations potentiate the DIC syndrome (Dressler, 1980).

Medical therapy also includes the vital functions compromised by DIC. The pulmonary and renal capillaries can be occluded by microthrombi, compromising the organs' adaptive capacities. Often during the acute phase, the patient may require mechanical ventilation and dialysis assistance. Mechanical ventilation allows the physical manipulation of oxygen delivery and thus some control of acid-base balance. Dialysis can help remove toxic wastes and assist in restoring normal acid-base balance. Some physicians think that peritoneal dialysis is contraindicated in DIC because the insertion procedure may increase further bleeding. Hemodialysis can be used but is still hazardous for the bleeding patient. The hazards can be minimized by modification of the amount of heparin used and the volume of blood in the system.

Physicians do not agree on the use of anticoagulants during DIC; however, heparin is the most commonly prescribed drug. There is literature supporting low-dose heparin of 5000 units every 12 hours (Gurewich and Lipinski, 1977). There are also advocates of therapeutic heparin usage at 500 to 3000 units per hour (Colman, Minna, and Robboy, 1974). There is evidence that heparin works more effectively in DIC states triggered by specific conditions. Sharp (1977) reports that heparin therapy decreases the severity of renal disease DIC when it is caused by incompatible blood transfusions. Early in heat stroke, heparin may prevent further stimulation of the DIC process. Some research indicates that heparin therapy may decrease platelet dysfunction in septic shock (Sharp, 1977). However, heparin is not recommended in DIC secondary to snakebite (Warrel, Pope, and Prentice, 1976).

Medical management of blood therapy is dependent on the needs of the specific patient. If the patient is hypovolemic, packed cells or whole blood may be indicated. Whether blood is prescribed is also dependent on the functioning of the patient's immune, cardiac, and renal systems. If clotting factors or platelets are almost totally consumed, fresh frozen plasma (containing clotting factors) or platelet units may be ordered. However, there are some authorities who think that blood component replacement activates further DIC. The theory is that the transfused components serve as more ''fuel added to the fire.'' In other words, any added hemostatic agents will be consumed as well (Dressler, 1980).

In some research centers other medical management is used. Some experiments are underway with epsilon and aminocaproic acid (Amicar) to control the fibrinolysis of DIC. Other centers use a combination of anticoagulants such as dipyridamole (Persantine), sulfinpyrazone (Anturane), and aspirin (acetylsalicylic acid). Future therapies may include the use of antithrombin compounds and new pharmacological agents.

NURSING MANAGEMENT

Nursing care of the patient with DIC demands knowledge, organization, coordination, and communication. The patient with acute DIC is critically ill and has a high mortality risk. Because of this, the demands of care pose stress for the family as well as the nurse.

Bleeding observation checklist

Head and neck
  Change in affect (restlessness, lethargy)
  Change in neuromuscular response (stroke)
  Aphasia
  Headache
  Disorientation
  Blurred or impaired vision
  Retinal hemorrhages
  Malaise
  Nose bleeds
  Gingival bleeding
  Posterior nasopharynx, swallowing of blood
Skin
  Visual inspection of mucous membranes
  Presence of pallor, purpura, petechiae
Internal
  Change in CVP or Swan-Ganz readings, indicating decrease in preload
  Change in girth of cavity (abdominal bleeding)
  Pain
  Tachycardia
  Falling hematocrit
Gastrointestinal
  Guaiac-positive stool or emesis
Renal
  Low urine output (oliguria)
  Hematuria
  Increased BUN
  Increased creatinine
  Backache

Identification of DIC

Initial nursing care is based on prompt identification of DIC. An assessment checklist for subtle signs and symptoms of bleeding can be used for patients who have disorders that trigger DIC. The more quickly the DIC is noted, the better the probability of appropriate management. It is important that the assessment data be reported and charted. Testing of all drainage for occult bleeding is recommended.

Prevention of bleeding

Prevention of bleeding is also an important priority. Preventive measures include informing the health care team about the DIC so that unnecessary procedures are not performed. For example, a respiratory therapist should not be allowed to do vigorous postural drainage. Other preventive measures are directed toward maintaining the integrity of body linings. Simple interventions are increasing the humidity on respiratory equipment and decreasing the amount of vacuum power used in suctioning. The skin should be protected from trauma with sheepskins, bed cradles, and flotation devices and siderails should be padded if the patient is confused or having seizures. Thermometers and nasogastric tubes must be well lubricated before insertion. Trauma can be further avoided by using gentle mouth care and electric razors for hygiene measures. The administration of medications by subcutaneous or intramuscular routes should be avoided, as hematomas will develop (Jennings, 1979). If a puncture is necessary, the nurse should use the smallest needle gauge possible and apply local pressure. In addition, if the clot at the trauma site seems unstable, it should not be removed. An intermittent pressure such as that caused by a blood pressure cuff can cause superficial bleeding. Arterial lines are recommended for blood pressure monitoring and for obtaining blood specimens. It takes additional effort to prevent bleeding, but without prevention the results can be catastrophic.

Many interventions are directed toward the control and measurement of bleeding. When the patient begins to ooze blood, local pressure, nasal packs, cold application, and topical clotting agents (such as thrombin powder) may be used. A laboratory flow sheet is helpful in monitoring the progressive bleeding and clot lysis. During periods of acute bleeding, traumatic procedures such as turning or suctioning should be kept at a minimum. Blood loss found in linens, dressings, and drainage equipment must be accurately measured so replacement is exact. Careful observation of bleeding is needed because hematocrit values often lag behind true values. Blood specimens should also be counted as blood loss.

Nursing care also includes measures to help the patient compensate for the anemia and acid-base imbalances caused by blood loss. The anemia occurs because of the loss of erythrocytes that transport oxygen. The nursing goal with this imbalance is to decrease oxygen debt. Administering oxygen, providing opportunities for rest, and decreasing temperature can be helpful to minimize oxygen needs. If the volume of blood loss is at a level where the blood pressure is unstable, the nurse should move the patient slowly to minimize orthostatic changes (Jennings, 1979). Acid-base balance is disrupted by blood loss because blood buffers acids. Blood gases should be checked carefully for acidosis. Any acidosis requires prompt intervention because it is thought to increase the severity of DIC.

Anticoagulant administration requires careful monitoring and technique. Heparin doses and infusions should be carefully noted for time and concentration. The intravenous site should be checked frequently for inflammation and oozing. It is advisable to check the compatibility of any other medications before infusing them through the same line. Blood for the coagulation panel should not be drawn from this line because the concentration of heparin would be higher at the venous infusion site, thereby giving inaccurate values. Heparin's effects will be more difficult to monitor in DIC because the PTT is already altered. These effects may be seen as a decrease in bleeding episodes and an improvement of hemostatic balance. The nurse must be aware that heparin can cause immune-mediated thrombocytopenia (Rhodes, Dixon, and Silvers, 1977). Platelet monitoring is essential. The nurse should take the same precautions against bleeding that would be taken with any anticoagulant.

Pain relief

Pain relief also demands the nurse's attention. The pain of DIC is primarily caused by tissue ischemia because of occluded or sluggish blood flow. Ischemic pain is thought to be caused by neural stimulation from localized acidosis, hypoxia, and necrosis of cells. The pain varies in intensity and may be diffuse or localized. It is important to frequently assess the pain and give analgesics as needed. Intravenous morphine is often the drug of choice. However, respirations and blood pressure must be stable enough to withstand the analgesic depression. Vasoactive drugs, if already in use, can be titrated to maintain the desired blood pressure by counteracting the vasodepressive aspects of analgesics. If a ventilator is being used, the respiratory depression of analgesics can be overcome. The analgesic should not contain aspirin or any other drug that has anticoagulant properties.

Aspirin (Ascriptin, Empirin)

Propoxyphene (Darvon compound, Darvon compound-65)

Pentazocine (Talwin compound)

Some patients are reported to have joint and muscle pain. Passive range of motion and repositioning during nonbleeding periods can reduce the pain. Backrubs may promote capillary bleeding and vigorous skin massage is contraindicated. Other measures to reduce pain are touch, reassurance, and visits by family or close friends.

Blood administration

Another commonly prescribed treatment is blood component administration. Nurses are responsible for the proper checking and administration of blood, the monitoring of tranfusions, and the prevention of transfusion complications. Checking the blood unit for the patient's name and blood type is routine, but its importance cannot be overstated. The use of blood administration tubing and filters is also important. Before starting a blood transfusion, the nurse should make sure the line is patent and the needle gauge is wide enough to accommodate the volume and/or blood cell size. Blood should never

---

Complications caused by blood administration

Hemolytic reaction
  Results from antibody reactions on red blood cells
  Severity is measured by:
    The number of cells involved
    The type of red cell antigen involved
    The immunoglobin class of the antibody
    The degree to which incompatible cells are sensitized (the number of anti-
      body molecules per cell) (McLeod, 1980)
Febrile reaction
  Results from incompatible leukocytes and platelet antigens
Urticarial reaction
  Results from incompatible plasma protein antigens
  Washed packed cells can decrease incidence
Anaphylactic reaction
  Results from IgA plasma and other immune-mediated sensitivities
Pathogen contamination
  Results from viral or bacterial contamination caused by improper handling
    of the blood

---

be given through a Swan-Ganz line. The CVP port on a standard Swan-Ganz line is a 23-gauge opening, which may damage erythrocytes and some proteins. If a pressure bag is used for rapid infusion, it should not be inflated above 200 mm Hg. If more pressure than that is needed, there is probably some occlusion of the line.

Blood component infusion can cause a variety of complications. Hypersensitivity to the transfusion can occur at any time during the administration. Usually it occurs in the first 30 minutes of administration. The patient should be monitored for fever, chills, hives, itching, or backache. Measurement of vital signs is needed before the transfusion, 15 minutes after beginning the transfusion, and hourly during the transfusion. Monitoring vital signs may be time consuming, but it is also life saving. The risk of hypersensitivity reactions increases during the administration of whole blood and fresh frozen plasma. McCleod (1980) has an excellent discussion of factors to consider when giving a blood transfusion.

If multiple transfusions are given, the nurse must be aware of additional complications. Fluid overload may occur if too much blood is given rapidly to a patient with poor cardiac function or poor renal status. Hypothermia can be secondary to administering blood that is not properly warmed beforehand. Hyperkalemia can occur when whole blood or packed cells are given because of erythrocyte damage during drawing and storing procedures. When a red blood cell is destroyed, potassium is released in the serum; therefore the unit has a higher potassium level. Citrate intoxication poses a particular threat in DIC. Citrate is added to blood units to keep them from clotting.

Citrate binds ionized calcium, which is essential for hemostasis. Therefore the nurse must monitor the calcium levels and be alert for signs of hypocalcemia, such as tetany, muscle cramps, convulsions, and serum calcium levels below 4.5 mEq/L (Metheny and Snively, 1979).

The transfusion of platelet units requires particular nursing care. Platelet infusions contain plasma and random leukocytes as well as platelets. A febrile reaction is the most common hypersensitivity caused by this type of infusion. Platelets are usually given 8 to 10 units at a time with a special filter. Each set of infused platelets should increase the platelet count by 5000. The nurse should be certain all the fluid is administered because platelets are fragile and expensive.

Nutrition

If the patient's course of recovery from DIC is a prolonged one, a catabolic state will occur. For the patient to recover, nutritional needs must be met. The patient's nutritional needs are magnified because protein and vitamins are needed to replace lost blood components. Since many of the clotting factors are dependent on vitamin K, it may be administered parenterally. Energy or caloric requirements often double in a patient with such a depleting illness. Protein is needed for iron replacement and the manufacturing of new red blood cells. The outcome of a functional recovery after the acute episode of DIC is often linked to adequate nutrition.

Hyperalimentation (total parenteral nutrition) is indicated if absorption from the gastrointestinal tract is altered. A hyperalimentation line must be carefully monitored and sterile technique must be vigilant. The patient is already immunosuppressed if malnourishment has existed for a period of time. Hyperalimentation is only used if the patient cannot meet nutritional needs in any other way.

Tube feedings and soft foods are usually the first choices to meet nutritional needs. The nurse must make sure that the foods do not traumatize the lining of the gut, promoting further bleeding. Constipation should be avoided because straining during bowel movement can cause intracranial bleeding. Bowel sounds must be carefully assessed and nasogastric systems must be aspirated before any additional intake is given. All stools should be checked for blood.

Psychological support

The patient with DIC, if conscious, may verbalize a variety of feelings. Anger is common and may be an expression of helplessness because of one's condition. Families may also be angry for a number of reasons, not the least of which would be the high cost of treatment and the uncertainty of the outcome. Also, because DIC is secondary to a primary state, some patients and families may feel that improper medical treatment caused the DIC. Acceptance of the patient and family and their anger is critical. Explanations of procedures and the problems of DIC should be given by both the physician and the nurse. Often the anger may be a result of the pain. If so, pain control can lessen the problem. Also allowing the family their visiting time may help them feel more in control of the situation.

Fear and isolation are also feelings that the patient may have. The bleeding of DIC is often profuse and visible, thus increasing the feeling of fear and weakness. The supportive equipment may make the patient feel pinned down and unable to communicate. Endotracheal tubes destroy the ability to talk, thereby isolating the patient from others. Magic slates and picture boards are helpful but not easy to use, especially if fatigue is a problem. Human touch and simple conversation often are vital links for the patient. When a patient looks up from the bed, lines, tubes, buzzers, and machines are immense, tangled webs of confinement. The nurse needs to see the patient who longs for human kindness behind the familiar monitors.

Sensory overload and sleep deprivation are also problems that nurses can reduce. Frequent orientation to time and place are helpful in minimizing disorientation. The nurse should try to reduce the personnel traffic near the patient's area and decrease environmental stimuli (Lidenmuth, Breu, and Malooley, 1980). Sleep periods and rest are essential. It takes extra planning, but research continues to indicate the high priority of rest for recovery. The nurse should try to plan at least 30 minutes of rest for the patient after exhausting or lengthy procedures. The nurse is the primary person who can help alleviate the constant stimulation of the patient.

The patient and family need to be aware of the possibility of death from DIC or the underlying condition. Death spawns a variety of feelings. The nurse can intervene in many ways. Empathetic listening is a powerful skill, though draining to the caregiver. The nurse needs to recognize personal feelings about the patient's death. If the nurse is unable to assist the family, another support person should be located for the family. Spiritual rituals and visits by religious counselors may be requested by the patient and/or family. The nursing management of the patient with DIC is full of challenges. It is the responsibility of the nurse to intervene in the best manner for the patient.

PATIENT VIGNETTE

DIC following gastrointestinal hemorrhage

Mr. Lemberg is in the medical intensive care unit on the fourth day following a massive gastrointestinal bleed that progressed to hypovolemic shock. He received 6 units of whole blood, 10 units of packed cells, 10,000 ml of normal saline, and 7 bottles of 12.5 gm of albumin. His hemoglobin is 12.0 gm/100 ml and the hematocrit is 38. His arterial pressure stabilized at 120/70 with the pulmonary artery diastolic pressure at 12 to 15. Gastric aspirate from the nasogastric tube is lightly guaiac positive. He is oozing small amounts of black tarry stools at frequent intervals.

Mr. Lemberg's medical history reveals alcohol abuse and decreased liver function. His bleeding was located by gastroscopy and found to be gastric in origin. Vitamin K, 5 mg intramuscularly, has been administered daily. Other medications are cimetidine (Tagamet), 300 mg intravenous piggyback every 6 hours, and magnesium aluminum hydroxide (Maalox), 30 ml by nasogastric tube every 2 hours.

At 3 PM Mr. Lemberg appears to be resting, but the nurse notes an increase in swallowing by the patient. The nurse conducts a further assessment.

Questions

1. Which of the following factors predispose Mr. Lemberg to the development of DIC?
   a. Blood transfusions
   b. Liver alterations
   c. Kidney alterations
   d. Shock
   e. Hypovolemia

2. Which of the following data are useful in the assessment of bleeding?
   a. Capillary wedge pressure
   b. Frequent swallowing
   c. Level of consciousness
   d. Pupil reactivity
   e. Urine output

Mr. Lemberg starts oozing blood from his Swan-Ganz catheter site, and bright red blood can be aspirated from the nasogastric tube. A panel of coagulation tests is done. The physician orders normal saline at 175 ml/hour or at a rate necessary to maintain the systolic pressure at 90 mm.

3. Which of the following is (are) reason(s) for ordering normal saline?
   a. Decreased liver congestion
   b. Cause fibrin to dislodge from capillaries
   c. Increase intravascular volume
   d. Decrease activation of fibrinolytic system

4. A stat dose of vitamin K 100 mg is given intramuscularly. What does this nutrient help to do?
   a. Prevent the activity of the reticuloendothelial system
   b. Promote the synthesis of clotting factors by the liver
   c. Prevent the action of heparin
   d. Promote the neutralization of gastric secretions

Low-dose heparin was ordered because his renal system started to show signs of microthrombi.

5. How would you monitor the patient's response to heparin?
   a. By checking the partial thromboplastin time
   b. By checking for acral cyanosis

c. By checking the prothrombin time

d. By noting a reduction in bleeding

6. What nursing interventions are relevant to caring for Mr. Lemberg?

a. Frequent suctioning and turning to decrease pulmonary complications

b. Padding of siderails and use of bed cradle

c. Removing loose clots

d. Administering oxygen with increased humidity

Answers

1. a, b, d, and e (Fig. 13-4). Blood transfusions are in the group of disorders that are believed to trigger DIC by procoagulant activity. Liver alterations are triggers of DIC because the liver is part of the reticuloendothelial system. Kidney alterations are not known to be triggers of disseminated intravascular coagulation at this time. Shock is often the trigger of DIC. The text of this chapter discusses the five aspects that are conducive to development of DIC. Hypovolemia would not *directly* trigger DIC. Hypovolemia in Mr. Lemberg's case led to hypovolemic shock, therefore it is *indirectly* associated with DIC.

2. a, b, c, d, and e. For an explanation of this answer, see the bleeding observation checklist, p. 257.

3. c. (a) Normal saline could not decrease the congestion in the liver. Liver congestion could be caused by cirrhosis or microthrombi. (b) Fibrin deposits would not be dislodged by increasing intravascular volume. Fibrin must be broken down by the fibrinolytic system. (c) Normal saline helps to increase intravascular volume lost because of bleeding. (d) Normal saline does not decrease the activity of the fibrinolytic system.

4. b. (a) The reticuloendothelial system functions to remove activated clotting factors from the blood. Vitamin K does not interfere with this function. (b) Vitamin K is stored and is needed by the liver to manufacture clotting factors. The liver is part of the reticuloendothelial system, but vitamin K assists the liver in performing its vital functions. (c) Vitamin K is the antidote for excessive Warfarin sodium (Coumadin) dosage. Warfarin sodium is an anticoagulant not used in DIC. Heparin's action is not prevented by the administration of vitamin K. Heparin works in another portion of the coagulation cycle. (d) Vitamin K is a fat-soluble vitamin. When administered intramuscularly, it has no contact with gastrointestinal secretions.

5. d. (a) Partial thromboplastin time is a good indicator of heparin function in all conditions except DIC. (b) Acral cyanosis is a sign that is associated with microthrombi. (c) Prothrombin time is a good indicator of vitamin K–dependent blood clotting functions.

6. b and d. (a) These procedures would cause additional bleeding. Nursing judgment, however, must be used to balance prevention of bleeding with pulmonary compromise. (c) Removing loose clots will cause additional bleeding. Even an inadequate plug is better than no sealing in the vascular defect.

REFERENCES

Chamberlain, S.L.: Low-dose heparin therapy, American Journal of Nursing **80:**1115-1117, 1980.

Colman, R.W., Minna, J.N., and Robboy, S.J.: Disseminated intravascular coagulation: a problem in critical care medicine, Heart & Lung **5:**789-796, 1974.

Deykin, D.: The clinical challenge of disseminated intravascular coagulation, The New England Journal of Medicine **283:**636-644, 1970.

Dressler, D.: Disseminated intravascular coagulation I and II, Proceedings of the seventh annual 1980 National Teaching Institute, Irvine, Calif., American Association of Critical Care Nurses, 1980.

Eskridge, R.A.: Septic shock, Critical Care Quarterly **2**(4):55-74, 1980.

Franco, L.A.: Acute disseminated intravascular coagulation, Cardiovascular Nursing **15**(5):22-26, 1979.

Gralnick, H.R.: Intravascular coagulation, Postgraduate Medicine **62**(5):68-75, 1977.

Gurewich, V., and Lipinski, B.: Case report: low dose intravenous heparin in the treatment of disseminated intravascular coagulation, American Journal of the Medical Sciences **274:**83-86, 1977.

Guyton, A.C.: Textbook of medical physiology, ed. 5, Philadelphia, 1981, W.B. Saunders Co.

Jennings, B.M.: Improving your management of DIC, Nursing '79 **9:**60-67, 1979.

Lindenmuth, J.E., Breu, C.S., and Malooley, J.A.: Sensory overload, American Journal of Nursing **80:**1456-1458, 1980.

Mason, R.G., and Saba, H.I.: Normal and abnormal hemostasis: an integrated view, American Journal of Pathology **92**(3):775-803, 1978.

McCleod, B.C.: Immunologic factors in reaction to blood transfusion, Heart & Lung **9:**675-681, 1980.

Metheny, N.M., and Snively, W.D.: Nurses' handbook of fluid balance, ed. 3, Philadelphia, 1979, J.B. Lippincott Co.

Moses, G.D.: The hemopoietic system. In Kinney, M.R., Dear, C.B., Packa, D.R., and Voorman, D.M., editors: AACN's clinical reference for critical care nursing, New York, 1981, McGraw-Hill Book Co.

O'Brien, B.S., and Woods, S.: The paradox of DIC, American Journal of Nursing **78:**1978-1980, 1978.

Palmer, R.L.: Intravascular coagulation and fibrinolysis, Postgraduate Medicine **62:**181-187, 1977.

Price, S.A., and Wilson, L.M.: Pathophysiology: clinical concepts of disease processes, New York, 1978, McGraw-Hill Book Co.

Rhodes, G.R., Dixon, R.H., and Silver, D.: Heparin induced thrombocytopenia, Annals of Surgery **186:**752-758, 1977.

Sharp, A.A.: Diagnosis and management of disseminated intravascular coagulation, British Medical Bulletin, **33**(3):265-272, 1977.

Tilkian, S.M., Conover, M.R., and Tilkian, A.R.: Clinical implications of laboratory tests, St. Louis, 1979, The C.V. Mosby Co.

Warrell, D.A., Pope, H.M., and Prentice, C.R.M.: Heparin use in snake bite, British Journal of Hematology, **33:**335-342, 1976.

Weiner, M.A., Pepper, G.A., Kuhn-Weisman, G., and Romano, J.A.: Clinical pharmacology and therapeutics in nursing, New York, 1979, McGraw-Hill Book Co.

14 Acute renal failure

JUDITH L. MYERS

The ability of the kidney to filter waste products from the blood is directly dependent on the perfusion pressures maintained by the heart and circulatory system. The normal glomerular filtration rate (GFR) averages 125 ml/min (180 L/day) as measured by renal clearance of inulin or creatinine. The volume of protein-free plasma filtrate remains constant if renal perfusion pressures are maintained. Significant changes in cardiac function or decreases in effective circulatory volume produce inadequate renal perfusion. This change in renal perfusion is the most common cause of oliguria in the critically ill patient (Lucas, 1976). Acute renal failure occurs as a result of severe and prolonged shock. It is also seen in situations producing severe fluid volume deficit and endotoxemia. The incidence of acute renal failure in patients who are in shock is difficult to determine since the clinical features of acute renal failure may be overshadowed by manifestations of the initiating process. Suppression of urine output may not be present; the patient may continue to excrete a normal urinary volume (Freedman and Smith, 1975). The greatest incidence of acute renal failure is seen in patients following major trauma, extensive burns, aortic surgery, massive blood loss, severe myocardial infarctions with or without arrhythmias, sepsis, and DIC.

The nurse should carefully monitor the patient in shock for early evidence of decreases in renal function. Cardiovascular and pulmonary failure can be readily diagnosed in their early stages and treated aggressively. However, significant renal dysfunction may go unnoticed until impairment is quite severe (Wilson and Soullier, 1980). When the causes of suppressed renal function are identified early, specific treatment can be started and the renal failure is more easily reversible.

PATHOPHYSIOLOGY

The kidney responds to injury (shock) by maintaining circulating plasma volume at the expense of its own perfusion. Seriously injured, hypovolemic, and septic patients enter into a fluid sequestration phase during which significant amounts of salt and water move from the vascular space into extravascular spaces (Lucas et al., 1977). After 36 to 72 hours (the point of maximum weight gain), this fluid is mobilized and excreted. In studies of anesthetized dogs (Ferguson and Schenk, 1977), hemorrhage significantly altered renal hemodynamics. There was a marked fall in renal vascular resistance and an increase in the renal distribution of the cardiac output. Lucas (1976) found that the high ratio of renal blood flow to kidney weight allows the kidney to effectively preserve blood volume and maintain function after injury or hemorrhage.

Changes in renal blood flow and glomerular filtration rate

Renal vasoconstriction at the postglomerular level permits an increase in renal vascular resistance with a decrease in renal blood flow and yet maintains a normal GFR. When renal vasoconstriction occurs at both the afferent and efferent arterioles, the renal blood flow drops to 500 ml/min without danger of the development of acute renal failure. This allows about 700 ml/min of blood flow to be redirected to core organs. The GFR falls to 50 to 80 ml/min. Autoregulatory mechanisms allow the GFR to be maintained and renal blood flow is decreased to 70% of normal. The renal prostaglandins may play a role in the renal autoregulation of blood flow.

Mortality associated with acute renal failure approaches 40%. However, this rate includes those severely ill persons in whom renal failure is a complication of an extensive underlying illness. The number of deaths from acute renal failure has decreased because of the treatment of hyperkalemia, fluid overload, and acidosis with dialysis.

In the patient in shock, acute renal failure can develop as a complication when the systemic blood pressure drops below 70 mm Hg (Lucas, 1976). At this level the GFR ceases and all renal blood flow is returned to the systemic circulation. The renal tubules begin to increase conservation of salt and water as a result of the decreased GFR, increased ADH secretion, and renin release. The kidney compensates for the drop in systemic pressure by sacrificing its own blood perfusion. This allows more blood to be made available for the perfusion of the heart and brain. On the average, renal blood flow is 40% to 50% of normal following anuria after shock (Reubi and Varburger, 1976). Cortical blood flow in the kidney seems to be reduced more than total renal blood flow.

Several theories have been proposed to explain the mechanisms responsible for the development of acute renal failure. Cronin and Schrier (1976) summarize four theories that explain acute renal failure. The vascular theory states that increased preglomerular vascular resistance reduces effective filtration pressure and causes the cessation of glomerular filtration. The obstruction theory states that cellular debris obstructs the renal tubules and raises intratubular pressure that opposes glomerular filtration. In the backleak theory it is postulated that normally filtered urine leaks back into peritubular capillaries through damaged and abnormally permeable tubules. The theory of altered glomerular permeability states that chemical or morphological alterations in the glomerular capillary basement membrane result in a decreased glomerular filtration. It is possible that factors from each of these theories contribute to the development of acute renal failure. Experimental animal models have been developed to support each of the theories. However, the actual pathogenesis of acute renal failure in humans has yet to be determined (Leaf and Cotran, 1980).

Development of renal tubular ischemia

Freedman and Smith (1975) suggest that a unified concept to explain the development of acute renal failure might be more accurate. One such unified theory is offered by Kashgarian et al. (1976). A situation such as shock produces renal tubular ischemia (Fig. 14-1). This tubular damage leads to an alteration in the reabsorption of sodium and

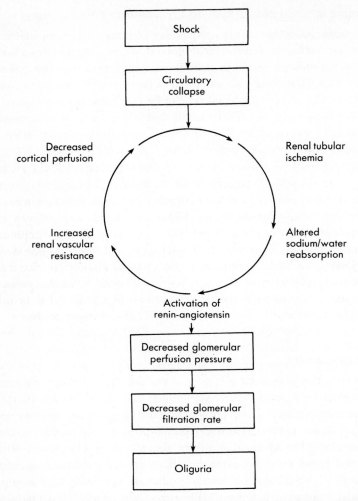

Fig. 14-1. Development of renal tubular ischemia: theoretical model.

water. Ischemia to the tubular cells of the loop of Henle in the juxtaglomerular nephrons impedes sodium reabsorption against a gradient, thus preventing medullary hypertonicity, concentration of the filtrate, and preservation of salt and water. As a result of this alteration, the renin-angiotensin system in the juxtaglomerular apparatus is activated. Lucas (1976) found that increased renin activity may be occurring in the kidney where it is present in greater concentration in the outer cortex compared to the medulla. Locally activated renin-angiotensin leads to the constriction of renin-secreting smooth muscle cells in the arterioles of the damaged tubules. The increased levels of angiotensin alter glomerular and cortical hemodynamics by increasing vascular resistance. The vasoconstriction causes a diminished total renal blood flow. There is a decrease in glomerular perfusion pressure and a decrease in glomerular filtration. The lower GFR leads to a decreased tubular flow and oliguria. The cortical vascular resistance causes a redistribution of cortical blood flow. The cause for decreased cortical flow may be related to increased catecholamine release, increased sympathetic tone, or increased angiotensin II activity (Lucas, 1976). There is a fall in cortical perfusion and a potentiation of tubular damage through hypoperfusion and ischemia.

The cycle of ischemia, tubular damage, decreased glomerular filtration, and increased renal vascular resistance can lead to progressive ischemic damage of the tubular epithelium and basement membrane. Acute tubular necrosis (ATN) is associated with ischemic renal injuries. The development of ATN in ischemia is variable. There may be patchy or widespread necrosis of the tubular epithelium and basement membrane. The degree of involvement depends on the extent of decreased renal blood flow and the length of time ischemia exists. When the basement membrane is disrupted, epithelial regeneration occurs at random, frequently leading to obstruction of the nephron at the site of necrosis. Even after blood flow to the kidney is established, persistent swelling of cells in the corticomedullary margin and an accumulation of cell debris provide evidence of continued tubular obstruction (Frega, De Bona, Guertler, and Leaf, 1976). This cellular swelling and collection of necrotic debris can also contribute to the renal vascular obstruction and potentiates renal ischemia.

CLASSIFICATION

Acute renal failure can be classified in a variety of ways. One method is to divide cases into two major categories, oliguric and nonoliguric, based on urine output volumes. Acute oliguric renal failure can be further categorized according to the causes of the kidney damage. These three categories are prerenal; intrinsic, or renal; and postrenal. Prerenal oliguria occurs from circulatory collapse as in hemorrhage with a consequent decrease in renal blood flow and GFR. If prerenal oliguria is treated early, there is no damage to the renal parenchyma. If the prerenal cause persists, it can progress to acute tubular necrosis. The causes of intrinsic failure are those associated with damage to the renal parenchyma. These include diseases and nephrotoxic substances such as antibiotics. Postrenal causes of oliguria can occur anywhere in the urinary system from the tubules to the meatus.

Acute oliguric renal failure

Acute oliguric renal failure is divided into two main phases based on urine output volumes and serum urea nitrogen (BUN) levels (Table 14-1). The oliguric phase usually begins within 24 to 48 hours after the initial renal injury. The major problems associated with the oliguric phase of acute renal failure include potassium excess, fluid volume excess, metabolic acidosis, and uremia. Other problems can inlcude calcium deficit, sodium deficit, and anemia (Metheny and Snively, 1979). Death is usually the result of cardiac arrest from hyperkalemia or pulmonary edema from volume excess. The oliguric

Causes of acute oliguric renal failure

Prerenal
Circulatory collapse (hemorrhage, pump failure)
Severe dehydration
Renal artery disorders (thrombosis, stenosis)

Renal (intrinsic)
Nephrotoxins (drugs, metals, organic compounds)
Severe infections
Acute glomerulonephritis
Vasculitis

Postrenal
Obstruction (clots, calculi, tumors, strictures, prostate)

Table 14-1. Phases of acute oliguric renal failure

	Oliguric phase	Diuretic phase
Onset	24 to 48 hours after injury	2 to 6 weeks
Duration	1 to 3 weeks	1 week (average)
Urine output	< 400 ml/24 hr	> 1000 ml/24 hr
BUN	Progressive elevation	Elevated early, then returns to normal
Associated problems	Hyperkalemia	Hypokalemia
	Fluid-volume excess	Hyponatremia
	Metabolic acidosis	Hypovolemia

Table 14-2. A comparison of oliguric and nonoliguric acute renal failure

	Oliguric	Nonoliguric
Urine output	< 400 ml/24 hours	Up to 6 L/24 hours
GFR	Decreased	Decreased
Urine osmolality	High (urine concentrated)	Low (urine dilute)
Serum creatinine	Elevated	Elevated
Causes	Refer to box above	Volume depletion
		Hypotension
		Surgical stress
		Nephrotoxins

phase can last from 1 to 3 weeks followed by the diuretic phase. The diuretic phase begins from 2 to 6 weeks after the onset of acute renal failure. Its onset signals the beginning of renal recovery. Early in the diuretic phase, the urine is hypotonic and the BUN and serum creatinine levels may continue to rise. The ability of the kidney to concentrate urine is the last renal function to return (Freedman and Smith, 1975).

Because of the inability of the kidney to concentrate urine, hypovolemia can occur during the diuretic phase. The hypovolemia can lead to further renal ischemia as a result of severe dehydration (Lucas, 1976). The final pathway of acute oliguric renal failure development is a prolonged, progressive decrease in outer cortical flow leading to ischemia.

Acute nonoliguric renal failure

Acute nonoliguric renal failure is increasingly recognized as a clinical form of acute renal failure (Table 14-2). It may be a separate entity or may represent the diuretic phase of acute renal failure when the oliguric phase is short or unrecognized (Lucas, 1976). Some consider it to be a variant form of oliguric ATN (Danovitch, Carvounis, Weinstein, and Levinson, 1979). According to Meyers, Roxe, and Hano (1977), nonoliguric renal failure represents about one third of all renal failure cases. The causes of this type of renal failure include volume depletion, hypotension, surgical stress, and the use of nephrotoxic antibiotics. The primary manifestation is an increased serum creatinine level in the presence of adequate urine production. There is no clear explanation for the differences in urine volumes between the oliguric and nonoliguric forms of renal failure. Danovitch, Carvounis, Weinstein, and Levinson (1979) report the major difference to be the amount of induced renal damage. Renal blood flow and GFR are reduced in nonoliguric failure (Lucas, 1976), but urine output may be as high as 6 L in 24 hours. The urine is dilute and iso-osmolar. These characteristics may represent a diffuse ischemia to both cortical and juxtamedullary nephrons. According to Popovtzer (1979), nonoliguric failure is associated with lower mortality than acute oliguric failure.

MEDICAL AND NURSING MANAGEMENT
Nursing assessment

The manifestations associated with acute renal failure in the patient in shock may be difficult to detect since symptoms of shock can overshadow those of acute renal failure. It is important to measure the patient's urine output frequently. Even after the patient's circulatory status is stabilized, renal ischemia may persist and lead to the development of acute renal failure. A decrease in urine volume to less than 400 ml in 24 hours is an indication of the oliguric phase of renal failure. Kidney functioning may be challenged with either mannitol or furosemide to determine if there is prerenal oliguria or true ATN. In prerenal oliguria, the urine output will increase, and in ATN the urine output will not increase in response to diuretics (Phipps, Long, and Woods, 1979).

Measurement of the fluid balance of the patient is of critical importance during acute renal failure. According to Johnson, Kowalski, Brungardt, and Cotton (1975),

**Assessment of fluid balance in acute renal failure
(oliguric phase)**

Assessment criteria	Expected changes
Urine output	< 400 ml/24 hrs
Body weight	Increased
Pulse	Rapid, pounding
Blood pressure	Increased
Breath sounds	Moist rales
Fluid volume status	Edema (dependent and nondependent), distended neck veins

Table 14-3. Assessment of GFR in acute renal failure

Test	Expected changes	Considerations
BUN	Elevated (normal: 8 to 25 mg/100 ml)	Can be increased by: Increased protein intake Fever Tissue catabolism Gastrointestinal bleeding Liver function changes
Creatinine, serum	Elevated (normal: 0.6 to 1.2 mg/100 ml)	
Creatinine clearance	Low (normal: 115 ± 20 ml/min)	Correct timing of plasma and urine samples 2-hour test as valuable as 24-hour collection

the most valid means of determining a patient's fluid status is the accurate measurement of body weight. Daily weighings with the same clothes and at the same time of day will provide the most accurate indications of changes in body weight. As the oliguric phase progresses, the patient's weight will increase since the kidney is unable to excrete body fluids. Daily blood chemistries and frequent measurement of pulse and blood pressure will also aid in monitoring fluid balance. An increase in the pulse and blood pressure will occur as the circulating blood volume increases. The nurse should also assess dependent areas of the body for indication of edema. As the fluid overload progresses, the patient will have puffy eyelids and distended neck veins. Assessment of breath sounds may reveal moist rales and the patient may experience shortness of breath.

The urinalysis in acute renal failure will reflect changes in the kidney's function. Protein will be present in the urine because albumin is lost through the damaged nephrons.

The urine may also contain casts, red and white blood cells, and other cellular debris from the injured kidney (Brundage, 1980).

An elevated BUN level will occur as the GFR drops below 50 ml/min. However, other factors can cause an elevated BUN level. Increased protein intake, fever, or increased tissue catabolism will markedly increase the rate of urea production and contribute to an elevated BUN level. Changes in liver function and gastrointestinal bleeding can also cause a rise in the BUN level.

Because of the variability of the BUN as a measure of glomerular filtration, clearance tests are a more reliable estimate of the GFR (Table 14-3). A creatinine clearance test will give a more accurate indication of changes in glomerular filtration, since creatinine is excreted during filtration and not reabsorbed or secreted in the tubules. As the GFR drops in acute renal failure, the serum creatinine level will rise above its normal range of 0.6 to 1.3 mg/100 ml and the 24-hour creatinine clearance will be less than its normal range of 115 ± 20 ml/min.

Even though creatinine clearance is a more sensitive and accurate measure of renal function, a 24-hour collection can be difficult and cumbersome in a critical care setting. Accurate collection of urine and storage of the specimen is time consuming and delays the diagnosis of renal failure. Wilson and Soullier (1980) report that 2-hour creatinine clearance tests provide a rapid measure of GFR, and results closely resemble those of 24-hour clearance. Sequential assessments of clearance by the kidney in the critically ill patient can be useful in the early detection of renal impairment (Brown et al., 1980). When creatinine clearance tests are done, the nurse should assume responsibility for the accurate timing of the collection of blood and urine specimens. The usefulness of the results will be limited if specimens are not collected at correct time intervals according to laboratory procedure.

The kidney's excretory functions are decreased in acute renal failure. When the urinary excretion of the acid end products of metabolism is impaired, metabolic acidosis develops. The arterial pH will be low or normal. There will be a low serum bicarbonate level and a low CO_2 combining power. The patient will usually be asymptomatic until the CO_2 combining power drops below 12 mEq/L (Johnson et al., 1975). At this time, Kussmaul's breathing develops as a respiratory compensation for the metabolic acidosis.

The kidney's ability to excrete potassium is also reduced in acute renal failure. This is reflected in a rise of serum potassium levels. Other factors that can contribute to a rise in potassium in renal failure include increased tissue catabolism (fever, steroids, and trauma), hemolysis, and infection. Metabolic acidosis also adds to the increased serum potassium because cells take up hydrogen ions to balance the drop in pH and release potassium ions to balance electrolytes. If no protein or potassium is ingested and sufficient calories in the form of carbohydrates and fats are consumed to prevent tissue catabolism, a potassium excess can be avoided for several days to weeks in the oliguric phase (Metheny and Snively, 1979).

Manifestations of increased potassium levels include muscle weakness, anxiety, restlessness, and changes in the electrocardiogram. The muscle weakness can progress to a flaccid paralysis and a decrease in deep tendon reflexes. When the respiratory muscles

---

Acid-base changes in acute renal failure

Criteria	Expected changes
pH, arterial	Low to normal
Bicarbonate, serum	Low
CO_2-combining power	Low
Respirations	Kussmaul's breathing

Hyperkalemia in acute renal failure

Causes

Reduced renal excretion
Increased tissue catabolism
Hemolysis
Infection
Metabolic acidosis

Manifestations

Muscle weakness, flaccid paralysis, decreased deep tendon reflexes, respiratory difficulty
Anxiety, restlessness
Electrocardiogram changes:
   Potassium 6.5 to 6.0 mEq/L (low amplitude P waves, prolonged PR interval, prolonged QT interval, widened QRS, depressed ST segment, and tall, tented T waves).
   Potassium > 8.0 mEq/L (arrhythmias, arrest, and myocardial standstill in diastole).

---

are involved in this weakness, the patient will have increasing breathing problems. When the potassium levels are between 6.5 and 8.0 mEq/L, the electrocardiogram will show low amplitude P waves, a prolonged PR interval, a prolonged QT interval with a widened QRS complex, depressed ST segments, and tall, tented T waves. These changes will be seen best in leads V_2 and V_4. As the potassium level increases above 8.0 mEq/L, cardiac arrhythmias become more frequent. Cardiac arrest or standstill occurs with the myocardium in diastole (Johnson, Kowalski, Brungardt, and Cotton, 1975; Metheny and Snively, 1979).

The effect of acute renal failure on renal tubular function is seen in the increased concentration of the urine. Tests that measure the ability of the kidney to dilute and concentrate urine are valuable in renal failure since this is one of the first functions to be

Table 14-4. Assessment of renal tubular function

Test	Expected changes	Considerations
Urinalysis	Proteinuria Casts RBC, WBC Debris	Reflects damage in nephrons
Specific gravity	> 0.020 to 1.030 (prerenal) < 1.012 (ATN)	Accuracy varies Reflects only major variations
Osmolality, urine	Elevated (prerenal) Decreased (ATN)	More accurate than specific gravity Varies with hydration and ADH

impaired and the last to recover (Table 14-4). Urine specific gravity is a simple test of renal concentrating power that can be done at the patient's bedside or in a special care unit by nursing personnel. However, specific gravity is not extremely accurate and reflects only major deviations from normal (Tilkian, Conover, and Tilkian, 1979). In prerenal oliguria, the specific gravity is usually greater than 1.020 to 1.030, and in ATN the specific gravity is less than 1.012.

Measurement of urine osmolality is a more accurate test of the kidney's ability to concentrate and dilute urine. Osmolality is an expression of the total number of particles in a solution. Urine osmolality is related to plasma osmolality and ADH secretion. The normal osmolality of a random urine specimen is 500 to 800 mOsm/L, with a range of 50 to 1400 mOsm/L depending on the patient's hydration status and ADH secretion. The urine osmolality will be high in prerenal oliguria as an indication of concentrated urine. In ATN urine osmolality may be low.

In addition to the impairment of renal excretory function, other clinical problems are associated with the development of acute renal failure. The uremia that develops in renal failure affects the gastrointestinal system, producing nausea, vomiting, anorexia, and ulcerations. Use of magnesium-based antacids should be avoided because the kidney would be unable to excrete the magnesium. Uremia also affects the central nervous system, causing signs ranging from muscle twitching to seizures.

There is decreased production of erythropoietin from the injured kidney, contributing to the development of anemia in acute renal failure. The anemia can also be aggravated by increased bleeding tendencies in the gastrointestinal tract as a result of uremia. The patient's hemoglobin and hematocrit will be decreased and fatigue will develop as a result of the anemia. DIC and secondary infections caused by impaired healing can also occur. The nurse should be alert for signs of increased bruising or any abnormal bleeding. The patient's body temperature should also be measured frequently.

Therapeutic objectives

In the patient with impending acute renal failure, the primary therapeutic objective is to restore depleted vascular volume and support ineffective cardiac output. Improving renal blood flow will relieve renal ischemia and reduce the chance that acute tubular necrosis will develop. According to Lucas (1976), when blood volume and cardiac output are restored following shock, renal vasoconstriction first subsides at the preglomerular capillary bed. This allows for early restoration of the glomerular filtration rate. Later vasoconstriction is reduced at the postglomerular capillary bed. Lucas et al., in another study (1978), found that the use of albumin to increase plasma volume in hypovolemic shock had little effect on increasing renal blood flow.

Use of diuretics

The use of osmotic and loop diuretics in acute renal failure is controversial. It has been suggested that the administration of diuretics such as mannitol and furosemide would reduce renal ischemia by increasing renal blood flow. In studies by Lucas and associates (1976, 1977) there were no significant changes in renal hemodynamics in patients with shock who received furosemide. It was concluded that even though water, salt, and osmolar excretion may increase, there was no increase in renal blood flow. In fact these diuretics may cause a further decrease in effective circulatory volume and increase the risk of renal ischemia and acute oliguric failure. There is a lack of sufficient evidence from controlled studies that indicates that furosemide may play a role in converting acute oliguric failure to nonoliguric failure (Popovtzer, 1979). Kashgarian et al. (1976) found that the effect of mannitol in reducing ischemia in acute renal failure was limited to those areas of the kidney that were better perfused. Brown et al. (1980) recommend volume replacement along with inotropic agents and loop diuretics in critically ill patients before the onset of oliguria.

The major patient care problems during the oliguric phase include the following:
1. Inability to excrete metabolic wastes
2. Inability to regulate electrolytes
3. Inability to excrete fluid loads
4. Difficulty in maintaining adequate nutrition
5. Increased potential for injury
6. Discomfort

The major problem during the diuretic phase is an inability to appropriately conserve fluids and electrolytes (Phipps, Long, and Woods, 1979).

The management of acute renal failure during the oliguric phase includes the following:
1. Restriction of fluid intake
2. Control of potassium excess
3. Nutritional support
4. Prevention of infection
5. Protection from injury

Monitoring fluid and electrolyte balance

Daily fluid allowance for a patient during the oliguric phase should be calculated to replace basic insensible losses (500 to 1000 ml/day), the amount of urine excreted, and other fluid losses from diarrhea, vomiting, or fever. Approximately 100 ml of fluid

---

Calculating fluid intake and replacement

Intake
Oral (liquids, ice chips, food)
IV (fluids, medications)

Output
Urine
Insensible (500 to 1000 ml, increases with fever)
Other (diarrhea, vomiting, drainage)

---

should be added to the patient's fluid allowance for each degree Celsius increase in body temperature in 24 hours (Metheny and Snively, 1979). The nurse assumes an important role in accurately measuring all fluid losses from the body. Whenever possible, the patient's cooperation should be gained in spacing fluid intake during the 24-hour period. Some patients respond more positively to ice chips than water to control thirst and dry mouth. Ice chips contain approximately one-half the water volume of a glass of water. Frequent mouth care will also help relieve some of the discomfort experienced by the patient on fluid restriction. Thirst may be less of a problem for the patient when sodium intake is also controlled.

When assessing the patient's hydration status, the nurse should give attention to more than just the record of intake and output and daily weights. Assessment of the patient's fluid and electrolyte balance should include notation of the level of consciousness and mental activity, frequent measurement of pulse and blood pressure, evaluation of skin turgor, thirst, and mucous membrane moisture.

Since secondary infections can be a problem for the patient in acute renal failure, all possible sources of infection should be eliminated. Ideally, indwelling urinary catheters should be removed. However, this may not be possible when accurate measurement of urinary output cannot be obtained in other ways. In this situation, it is especially important to maintain a closed drainage system and carefully follow aseptic procedures for the care of the patient with an indwelling catheter. Special attention should be given to the use of sterile technique when collecting urine specimens from the drainage system.

Both intravenous and intra-arterial lines used to monitor the circulatory status of the patient also present a potential source of infection. Sterile technique should be used when caring for insertion sites, instilling fluids or medications, or changing intravenous tubings.

When serum potassium levels begin to increase above normal and represent a threat to myocardial function, several treatments can be used to reduce the potassium levels and protect the myocardium. Intravenous calcium in the form of calcium chloride or calcium gluconate can be given to counteract the harmful effects of potassium on the

---

Managing potassium excess

Treatment measures	Implications
Antagonize effect of potassium on myocardium (IV calcium)	Monitor ECG, does not change serum potassium
Shift potassium into cell (sodium bicarbonate, dextrose / insulin)	Short-term effect, may increase sodium and fluid load
Reduce intake (dietary, drugs)	
Increase excretion (exchange resins, dialysis)	May increase sodium load, causes diarrhea, careful monitoring of fluid and electrolyte balance

---

myocardium. The administration of sodium bicarbonate intravenously causes a rapid shift of potassium back into the cell. Hypertonic dextrose and regular insulin can be given intravenously to force potassium into the cell as glucose enters the cell. All of these measures are temporary, short-acting therapies. They may increase sodium levels and create a fluid overload.

There are several preventive measures that can be used to slow the increase in potassium levels or provide an alternate means of excretion from the body. Restricting the patient's intake of potassium can be done in several ways. The administration of drugs that either contain potassium or act to conserve body potassium should be avoided when possible. According to Metheny and Snively (1979), the use of blood that has been stored should be avoided since the blood can contain up to 30 mEq/L of potassium. If the patient can consume food or fluids orally, those high in potassium should be limited.

The excretion of potassium through the gastrointestinal tract can be accomplished through the use of cation-exchange resins. The resins, which can be given either orally or rectally in an enema, exchange sodium for potassium across the bowel wall. The bound potassium is excreted in the feces. A commonly used resin is sodium polystyrene sulfonate (Kayexalate). Sorbitol is added to the resin to promote an osmotic diarrhea. Because these resins exchange sodium for potassium at a rate of 2 mEq sodium for 1 mEq potassium, the patient should be observed for signs of sodium excess.

Dialysis

Hemodialysis is the quickest way to remove metabolic wastes from the blood and correct fluid and electrolyte abnormalities in acute renal failure. However, not all hospitals are equipped to perform hemodialysis, and the patient may not be stabilized sufficiently to allow transfer to a center where hemodialysis could be done. Peritoneal dialysis, on the other hand, can be used in any hospital setting. It does have the disadvantage, though, of being a slow, time-consuming process that may not achieve a rapid correction of symptoms. Gerhardt, Abdulla, Mach, and Hudson (1979) report the use of an isolated ultrafiltration device in patients with cardiogenic shock. The procedure reduced cardiac preload and produced an improvement in urine output. The device has the advantage of being quicker than peritoneal dialysis and safer than hemodialysis, which can cause low cardiac output and low systemic pressure.

Nutritional support

Nutritional support is an important aspect of care for the patient in acute renal failure. Sufficient nutrients must be provided to supply calories for energy needs and protein for tissue repair. The patient's oral intake may be limited by gastrointestinal distress and by the psychological barriers of a diet that is highly restrictive. Carbohydrates and fats are included to supply calories for energy and to spare the use of tissue protein. Thiele (1980) recommends a carbohydrate intake of 100 to 200 gm per day. This amount will help prevent protein catabolism and metabolic ketosis. There is controversy concerning the amount of protein to include in the diet for these patients. The goal is to provide enough protein to prevent tissue-protein catabolism without elevating the BUN level. Use of parenteral infusions of amino acids, as essential amino acids alone or in combination with nonessential amino acids, has been successful in nutritional support when oral feeding is not possible. When the diuretic phase begins and serum levels of urea nitrogen and creatinine begin to decrease, the patient's diet can be liberalized.

Prevention of complications

Monitoring the patient's response to drug therapy to prevent complications is another part of nursing care for the patient with renal impairment. Gastrointestinal problems in renal failure can limit the absorption of many drugs. The serum concentration of drugs in the body can be lowered by decreases in plasma proteins and increased fluid retention. Some of the pathways used for the normal metabolism of drugs may be slow and therefore increase the half-life of the drug. Also the byproducts of drug metabolism can accumulate in the patient, producing toxic side effects or prolonged therapeutic effects. Since most drugs are excreted by the kidney, their effects in the body will be prolonged. It is important to remember that alterations in electrolytes can also influence the patient's drug response. For example, changes in serum potassium levels in renal failure will affect the patient's response to digitalis preparations.

Orr (1981) recommends that either decreasing dosages or increasing the time interval between doses can help solve some of the problems associated with drug administration in the uremic patient. Careful nursing assessment of the patient is necessary. This requires the nurse to have knowledge of a drug's therapeutic action and its side effects. The nurse should give special attention to the patient on dialysis. Many drugs are dialyzable, and the patient may need an additional dose after dialysis.

The diuretic phase of acute renal failure signals the beginning of recovery for the injured kidneys. Serum levels of urea and creatinine may stay elevated for several days after increases in urine output. Major problems for the patient during this period include excessive fluid losses, hyponatremia, and hypokalemia. The ability of the kidney to conserve water and electrolytes is still impaired. The patient requires careful nursing assessment of fluid balance and special attention to sodium and potassium losses. Thirst will be an important indicator of water and sodium balance. Fluids and electrolytes will require liberal replacement.

Preparation of the patient for discharge should include diet instructions as needed and instruction concerning the importance of adequate fluid intake and self-monitoring of urine output. Complete recovery from an episode of acute renal failure may take 4 to 5 months. Preventing urinary tract infections and avoiding nephrotoxic substances should also be part of discharge education.

PATIENT VIGNETTE

Acute renal failure following traumatic shock

A 26-year-old woman was admitted to the emergency department in shock with a gunshot wound of the abdomen. Her blood pressure was 60 mm Hg by palpation. During surgery she required multiple transfusions and intravenous vasopressors to maintain a blood pressure of 80/60 mm Hg. Following surgery the patient's blood pressure stabilized at 110/70 and urine output was 30 to 60 ml/hr. Twenty-four hours postoperatively, her urine output dropped to less than 15 ml/hr. Her other vital signs remained normal. Over the next several days the BUN, serum creatinine, and serum potassium levels increased above normal. A 24-hour creatinine clearance showed a significant decrease in GFR. Hemodialysis was started using a shunt and the patient's fluid and electrolyte intake was restricted. Ten days postoperatively, the patient's urine output increased. Within 48 hours, the patient was voiding 5 L of urine in 24 hours. The BUN and creatinine levels began returning to normal. Three weeks postoperatively, a 24-hour creatinine clearance was within normal limits. The patient was discharged.

Questions

1. What would this patient's renal failure probably be classified as?
   a. Nonoliguric
   b. Postrenal
   c. Prerenal
   d. Renal, or intrinsic

2. Which of the following alterations would the nurse expect to find in assessing this patient's fluid balance during the oliguric phase?
   a. Increased blood pressure
   b. Flat neck veins
   c. Dependent edema
   d. All of the above

3. Why is creatinine clearance used as a measure of GFR?
   a. It has less variability than the BUN
   b. It can be done at the bedside
   c. Creatinine levels remain stable in acute renal failure
   d. Creatinine is excreted during filtration without secretion or reabsorption

4. Until dialysis can be initiated, how can serum potassium excess be managed?
   a. The use of ion-exchange resins
   b. Infusions of normal saline
   c. Administration of aluminum hydroxide antacids
   d. Administration of hypertonic dextrose and insulin

5. The patient is still experiencing postoperative incisional pain. What should the nurse understand when administering analgesics?
   a. The patient may require a smaller dosage than before renal failure began
   b. The patient is more prone to experience side effects
   c. The dosage may need to be repeated after dialysis
   d. All of the above

Answers

1. a. Prerenal oliguria as a form of acute renal failure occurs as a result of changes in circulation, such as shock. These changes cause a decrease in renal blood flow and eventually a decrease in glomerular filtration.
   Intrinsic renal failure is associated with situations that produce damage to the renal parenchyma. Postrenal oliguria results from damage to renal structures from the tubules to the urinary meatus.
2. a and c. During the oliguric phase, the kidney is unable to excrete body fluids. The fluid excess produces an increase in circulating blood volume that results in a rise in blood pressure. Dependent edema is also characteristic of fluid overload. The patient would also have distended rather than flat neck veins.
3. a and d. Many situations other than renal impairment can produce a rise in the BUN level. Creatinine is excreted during filtration and is not reabsorbed or secreted in the tubules. A creatinine clearance test will give a more accurate measure of GFR than the BUN. As GFR decreases in acute renal failure, the creatinine clearance drops and serum creatinine levels increase.
4. a and d. Hypertonic dextrose and insulin can be given intravenously to force potassium into the cell along with the glucose. This is a short-acting, temporary therapy. The use of resins that exchange sodium for potassium increase the intestinal elimination of potassium. Aluminum hydroxide antacids may be used to bind phosphates in the gut and increase its intestinal excretion.
5. d. Renal failure can alter the normal metabolism and excretion of drugs. This situation can result in increased drug half-life or accumulation of toxic byproducts.

Some analgesics are also dialyzable. The patient may require smaller doses or a longer time interval between dosages. Dosages given before dialysis may need to be repeated afterward.

REFERENCES

Brown, R., et al.: Renal function in critically ill postoperative patients: sequential assessment of creatinine, osmolar and free water clearance, Critical Care Medicine **8**:68-72, 1980.

Brundage, D.J.: Nursing management of renal problems, ed. 2, St. Louis, 1980, The C.V. Mosby Co.

Cronin, R.E., and Schrier, R.W.: Acute renal failure: diagnosis, pathogenesis and management, Hospital Medicine **12**(8):26-42, 1976.

Danovitch, G., Carvounis, C., Weinstein, E., and Levenson, S.: Nonoliguric acute renal failure, Israel Journal of Medical Sciences, **15**:5-8, 1979.

Ferguson, J.C., and Schenk, W.G., Jr.: Prostaglandin inhibition by indomethacin: effect on the renal vascular response to hemorrhage in anesthetized dogs, Surgical Forum **28**:10-11, 1977.

Freedman, P., and Smith, E.C.: Acute renal failure, Heart & Lung **4**:873-878, 1975.

Frega, N.S., DeBona, D.R., Guertler, B., and Leaf, A.: Ischemic renal injury, Kidney International, **10**(suppl. 6):17-25, 1976.

Gerhardt, R.E., Abdulla, A.M., Mach, S.J., and Hudson, J.B.: Isolated ultrafiltration in the treatment of fluid overload in cardiogenic shock, Archives of Internal Medicine **139**:358-359, 1979.

Johnson, H.K., Kowalski, LD., Brungardt, C.J., and Cotton, K.E.: Nursing care of the patient with acute renal failure, Nursing Clinics of North America **10**:421-430, 1975.

Jones, D.A., Dunbar, D.F., and Jivorec, M.M.: Medical-surgical nursing: a conceptual approach, New York, 1978, McGraw-Hill Book Co.

Kashgarian, M., et al.: Hemodynamic aspects in development and recovery phases of experimental postischemic acute renal failure, Kidney International **10**(suppl. 6):5160-5168, 1976.

Leaf, A., and Cotran, R.S.: Renal pathophysiology, ed. 2, New York, 1980, Oxford University Press, Inc.

Lucas, C.E.: The renal response to acute injury and sepsis, Surgical Clinics of North America **56**:953-975, 1976.

Lucas, C.E., et al.: Questionable value of furosemide in preventing renal failure, Surgery **82**:314-320, 1977.

Lucas, C.E., et al.: Effects of albumin versus non-albumin resuscitation on plasma volume and renal excretory function, Journal of Trauma **18**:564-570, 1978.

Metheny, N.M., and Snively, W.D., Jr.: Nurses' handbook of fluid balance, ed. 3, Philadelphia, 1979, J.B. Lippincott Co.

Meyers, C., Roxe, D.M., and Hano, J.E.: The clinical course of nonoliguric acute renal failure, Cardiovascular Medicine **2**:669-672, 1977.

Orr, M.L.: Drugs and renal disease, American Journal of Nursing **81**:969-971, 1981.

Phipps, W.J., Long, B.C., and Woods, N.F.: Medical-surgical nursing: concepts and clinical practice, St. Louis, 1979, The C.V. Mosby Co.

Pickering, L., and Robbins, D.: Fluid, electrolyte and acid-base balance in the renal patient, Nursing Clinics of North America **15**:577-592, 1980.

Popovtzer, M.M.: Acute renal failure, (editorial), Israel Journal of Medical Sciences **15**:1-4, 1979.

Rao, M.S., et al.: Infusion pyelography in anuric patients, Journal of Urology **116**:297-299, 1976.

Reubi, F.C., and Vorburger, C.: Renal hemodynamics in acute renal failure after shock in man, Kidney International **10**(suppl. 6):5137-5143, 1976.

Sorensen, K.C., and Luckmann, J.: Basic nursing: a psychophysiologic approach, Philadelphia, 1979, W.B. Saunders Co.

Thiele, V.F.: Clinical nutrition, ed. 2, St. Louis, 1980, The C.V. Mosby Co.

Tilkian, S.M., Conover, M.B., and Tilkian, A.G.: Clinical implications of laboratory tests, ed. 2, St. Louis, 1979, The C.V. Mosby Co.

Weinsier, R.L., and Butterworth, C.E., Jr.: Handbook of clinical nutrition, St. Louis, 1981, The C.V. Mosby Co.

Williams, S.R.: Nutrition and diet therapy, ed. 4, St. Louis, 1981, The C.V. Mosby Co.

Wilson, R.F., and Soullier, G.: The validity of two-hour creatinine clearance studies in critically ill patients, Critical Care Medicine **8**:281-284, 1980.

Index

A

Ao₂; *see* Oxygen saturation

Abbott/Shaw LifeCare Pump, 138

Abdominal injury, 129-130, 132, 262-264; *see also* Traumatic shock

Abortion, septic, 182

Abscesses, 182

Acetylcholine, 14, 28, 56, 202

Acid-base balance; *see also* Acidosis
- cardiogenic shock and, 157-158
- hypovolemia and, 142-143, 216
- nursing care and, 258-259
- renal failure and, 273, 274

Acidosis; *see also* Acid-base balance
- lactic, 96, 126, 128, 154
- metabolic
  - anaerobic metabolism and, 216
  - cardiogenic shock and, 154, 158
  - hypovolemic shock and, 126, 128
  - renal failure and, 269, 273
- microcirculation and, 52
- respiratory, 157-158

Acinetobacter, 188

Acral cyanosis, 253

ACTH; *see* Adrenocorticotropic hormone

Actin, 29, 35

Action potentials, 31, 32-33

Activity, 54, 216, 237

Acute renal failure; *see* Renal failure, acute

Acute tubular necrosis, 189, 190, 269, 274-275

Adenosine diphosphate, 246, 249, 251, 253

Adenosine triphosphate, 29, 98, 216

ADH; *see* Antidiuretic hormone

ADP; *see* Adenosine diphosphate

Adrenergic fibers, 13

Adrenergics, 30, 31

Adrenocortical steroids; *see also* Steroids
- adult respiratory distress syndrome and, 228
- anaphylaxis and, 206, 208

Adrenocorticotropic hormone, 128, 227, 228

Adult respiratory distress syndrome, 225-244
- albumin and, 138
- cardiac output and, 238
- causal factors in, 226
- conditions resembling, 225

Adult respiratory distress syndrome—cont'd
- endotoxin and, 179
- fluid balance and, 238-240
- humoral vasoactive substances and, 227, 228
- infection and, 240-241
- management of, 232-241
  - goals for, 232
- nursing assessment and, 229-232
- oxygenation and, 233-238
- pathophysiology of, 227-229
- patient vignette in, 242-244
- prognosis in, 241-242
- terms for, 226

Aerobacter, 188

Afterload, 12, 40
- cardiogenic shock and, 152
- intra-aortic balloon and, 164
- monitoring of, 123
- vasodilators and, 160

Airway
- artificial, 79; *see also* Mechanical ventilation
  - adult respiratory distress syndrome and, 233-236, 241
  - complications of, 85
- shock and
  - anaphylactic, 205, 206, 211
  - hypovolemic, 135-136
- supporting structures of, 65

Airway resistance, 70

Alanine, 218

Albumin
- infusions of, 239
  - fluid overload and, 143
  - hypovolemic shock and, 137, 138-139
  - septic shock and, 183
- serum, 223

Alcohol, 208

Aldosterone, 128

Alkalemia, 157, 158, 216

Alkaline phosphatase, 222-223

Alkalosis, 157, 158, 216

All or none principle, 33

Allen test, 105

Allergy, 195, 196-197, 198-199
- medical identification and, 208